AF365185

Pharmaceutics

Basic Principles and Formulations

Pharmaceutics
Basic Principles and Formulations

D. K. Tripathi

M. Pharm, Ph.D

Professor and Principal

Rungta College of Pharmaceutical Sciences and Research,

Bhilai, Chhattisgarh.

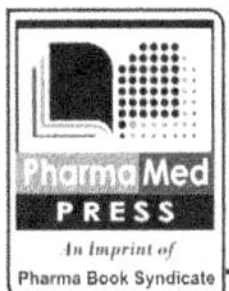

PharmaMed Press

An imprint of Pharma Book Syndicate

A unit of BSP Books Pvt. Ltd.

4-309/316, Giriraj Lane,

Sultan Bazar, Hyderabad - 500 095.

Pharmaceutics : Basic Principles and Formulations *by D. K. Tripathi*

Published by

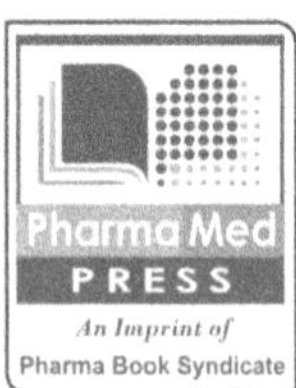

PharmaMed Press

An imprint of Pharma Book Syndicate
A unit of BSP Books Pvt. Ltd.
4-4-309/316, Giriraj Lane, Sultan Bazar, Hyderabad - 500 095.
Phone: 040-23445605, 23445688; Fax: 91+40-23445611
E-mail: info@pharmamedpress.com
www.pharmamedpress.com/pharmamedpress.net

ISBN: 978-93-5230-163-8 (Hardback)

Contents

Chapter 1   Introdution

Chapter 2 Solid Dosage Forms

Chapter 3   Semi Solid Dosage Forms

Chapter 4   Liquid Dosage Forms

Chapter 5   Sterile Preparations

Chapter 6   Gaseous Dosage Form

Chapter 7   Systems of Weights and Measures

Chapter 8   Pharmaceutical Calculations

Preface

This book has been written with an idea of introducing pharmacy students of undergraduate level, particularly of first years to the fundamentals of the subject, pharmaceutics. Although the contents have been designed in accordance with the syllabus of Chhattisgarh Swami Vivekanand Technical University, it will mostly cover the syllabus for first year B.Pharm course of other universities. The book contains nine chapters. The first chapter provides information about history of pharmacy, career opportunity in pharmacy, and development of pharmacopoeias, etc. Each of the other five chapters contains preliminary information about each type of the pharmaceutical dosage forms and their manufacture. Chapter 7 contains information about the systems of weights and measure and the chapter 9 deals with the pharmaceutical incompatibiliess. At the end, few annexure have been incorporated to furnish allied information.

Besides theoretical information about each dosage form, some classical examples of each type have been incorporated along with methods of manufacture to practice in the laboratory, so that, the students of higher semesters or years can use the book as the handbook for practical pharmaceutics.

The entire effort has been made to make this book a textbook for first year B.Pharm and practical handbook for all other students. The examples which can be conveniently performed in the laboratory have been provided.

However, the author shall be thankful to those who will communicate their views for further improvement or revision and their valuable suggestions shall be duly acknowledged in the revised edition also.

D. K. Tripathi

Acknowledgements

The journey of this project was initiated few years back. At different times, different types of obstruction came and the work got detained. Although one of my Student-cum-Colleague, Minaketan Tripathy had been constantly inspiring me to complete the book.

Ultimately, it has been completed. For completion, I must thank the people who helped me for this work. I express my thank to Azajuddin, M. D. Junaid Khan, Mr. Amit Alexander, Mr. Hemant Badwaik and Miss. Rashmi Chaurasia, my colleagues in this institute who helped me at various steps. I am also thankful to Sri Chinta Dilip, my office staff and to my elder son, Nirmalya for his assistance and at last I must name the person without whose cooperation nothing could have been done. She is my wife Bimala.

At last, I express my gratefulness to the management of this Institute under Santosh Rungta Group of Institutions for providing me the facility to complete the pending project.

D. K. Tripathi

Abbreviations

mol/l	Concentration, gram molecule of a substance per 1000 ml of solution.
n	Refractive index for electromagnetic radiation in a given medium, dimensionless, ratio of the sine of the angle of incidence of electromagnetic radiation on a medium to the sine of its angle of refraction in the medium.
20 n D	Refractive index, value measured at the wavelength of the sodium D-line (589.3 nm) and at a temperature of $20 \pm 0.5°C$.
NCIMB	National Collection of Industrial, Food and Marine Bacteria Ltd, 23 St Machar Drive, Aberdeen AB24 3RY, Scotland.
NCTC	National Collection of Type Cultures, Central Public Health laboratory, Colindale Avenue, London NW9 5HT, England.
NCYC	National Collection of Yeast Cultures, AFRC Food Research, Colney Lane, Norwich NR4 7UA, England. Probability of an event in statistical estimations.
pH	Dimensionless, physical quantity expressing the acidity or alkalinity of a solution, measured as the negative logarithm of the hydrogen ion concentration or hydrogen-ion activity expressed in moles per liter. The scale 0 to 7, represents the acidity and 7 to 14, represents the alkalinity. 7 indicates the neutral state. Increase of number indicates the increase of alkalinity.
ρ	Density of a substance at a particular temperature, mass per unit volume.
$ñ_{20}$	Density of a substance at a particular temperature of 20°C. ñ According to the International Pharmacopoeia, grams per millilitre (g/ml).
	Reagent.
R_f	Ratio of fronts, related to fronts. In paper or thin-layer chromatography, ratio of the distance travelled by the substance R to that travelled by the mobile phase.
R_r	In chromatography, ratio of the distances travelled by the substance to that of the reference substance.
RS	Reference substance.
SI	International System.
TS	Test solution.
VS	Volumetric solution.

Tables

Table 1 Aperture of Sieves

BSS (410/1969)	ASTM (11 – 70)	IS (469/1972)	MICRONS
4	5	4.00 mm	4000
5	6	3.35 mm	3353
6	7	2.80 mm	2812
7	8	2.36 mm	2411
8	10	2.00 mm	2057
10	12	1.70 mm	1680
12	14	1.40 mm	1405
14	16	1.18 mm	1204
16	18	1.00 mm	1003
18	20	0.850 mm	850
22	25	0.710 mm	710
25	30	0.600 mm	600
30	35	0.500 mm	500
36	40	0.425 mm	420
52	50	0.300 mm	300
60	60	0.250 mm	250
72	70	0.212 mm	210
85	80	0.180 mm	180
100	100	0.150 mm	150
120	120	0.125 mm	120
150	140	0.106 mm	105
170	170	0.090 mm	90
200	200	0.075 mm	75
240	230	0.063 mm	63
300	270	0.053 mm	53
350	325	0.045 mm	45
400	400	0.037 mm	37
500	-	0.025 mm	35

BSS	British Standard Specification.
ASTM	American Society for Testing and Materials.
IS	Indian Standards.

Table 2 Aperture size of Perforated Sieves

mm	Inch
4.75	3/16
6.3	1/4
8.0	5/16
10.0	3/8
12.5	1/2
16.0	5/8
20.0	3/4
25.0	1
31.5	5/4
40.0	3/2
50.0	2
63.0	5/2
80.0	3
100.0	4

Table 3 Atomic Weight, Atomic Number and Valence of Common Elements

Element	Atomic wt	Atomic No	Valence
H	1	1	+1
He	4.00	2	0
Li	6.9	3	+1
Be	9.0	4	+2
B	10.8	5	+3
C	12.01	6	+2, ±4
N	14.00	7	± 1,±2, ±3, +4, +5
O	15.99	8	-2
F	18.99	9	-1
Ne	20.17	10	0
Na	22.98	11	+1
Mg	24.30	12	+2
Al	26.98	13	+3
Si	28.08	14	+2, ±4
P	30.97	15	±3, +5
S	32.06	16	+4, +6, −2

Table 3 *contd…*

Element	Atomic wt	Atomic No	Valence
Cl	35.45	17	±1, +5, +7
Ar	39.95	18	0
K	39.09	19	+1
Ca	40.07	20	+2
Sc	44.95	21	+3
Ti	47.86	22	+2, +3, +4
V	50.94	23	+2, +3, +4, +5
Cr	51.99	24	+2, +3, +6
Mn	54.94	25	+2, +3, +4, +7
Fe	55.84	26	+2, +3
Co	58.93	27	+2, +3
Ni	58.69	28	+2, +3
Cu	63.54	29	+1, +2
Zn	65.4	30	+2
Ga	69.72	31	+3
Ge	72.64	32	+2, +4
As	74.92	33	±3, +5
Se	78.96	34	+4, +6,
Br	79.90	35	±1, +5 −2
Kr	83.79	36	0
Rb	85.47	37	+1
Sr	87.62	38	+2
Y	88.90	39	+3
Zr	91.22	40	+4
Nb	92.91	41	+3, +5
Mo	95.94	42	+6
Tc	97.91	43	+4, +6, +7
Ru	101.07	44	+3
Rh	102.90	45	+3
Pd	106.4	46	+2, +4
Ag	107.87	47	+1
Cd	112.41	48	+2
In	114.8	49	+3
Sn	118.7	50	+2, +6
Sb	121.76	51	±3, +5
Te	127.6	52	+4, +6, −2
I	126.90	53	±1, +5, +7

Table 3 *contd…*

Element	Atomic wt	Atomic No	Valence
Xe	131.29	54	0
Cs	132.9	55	+1
Ba	137.33	56	+2
La	138.90	57	+3
Ce	140.11	58	+3, +4
Pr	140.90	59	+3
Nd	144.24	60	+3
Pm	144.91	61	+3
Sm	150.36	62	+2, +3
Eu	151.96	63	+2, +3
Gd	157.25	64	+3
Tb	158.92	65	+3
Dy	162.50	66	+3
Ho	164.93	67	+3
Er	167.26	68	+3
Tm	168.93	69	+3
Yb	173.04	70	+2, +3
Lu	174.97	71	+3
Hf	178.49	71	+3
Ta	180.95	73	+5
W	183.84	74	+6
Re	186.21	75	+4, +6, +7
Os	190.23	76	+3, +4
Ir	192.22	77	+3, +4
Pt	195.08	78	+2, +4
Au	196.96	79	+1, +3
Hg	200.59	80	+1, +2
TI	204.38	81	+1, +3
Pb	207.2	82	+2, +4
Bi	208.98	83	+3, +5
Po	208.98	83	+3, +5
At	209.98	85	±1, +5, +7
Rn	222.01	86	0
Fr	223.02	87	+1
Ra	226.02	88	+2
Ac	223.02	87	+1
Th	232.04	90	+4

Table 3 *contd…*

Element	Atomic wt	Atomic No	Valence
Pa	231.03	91	+4, +5
U	238.03	92	+3, +4,+5, +6
Np	237.05	93	+3, +4, +5, +6
Pu	244.06	94	+3, +4, +5, +6
Am	243.06	95	+3, +4, +5, +6
Cm	247.07	96	+3
Bk	247.07	97	+3, +4
Cf	251.07	98	+3
Es	252.08	99	+3
Fm	257.09	100	+3
Md	258.09	101	+2, +3
No	259.10	102	+2, +3
Lr	262.11	103	+3
Rf	261.11	104	+4
Db	262.11	105	
Sg	266.12	106	
Bh	264.12	107	
Hs		108	
Mt	268.14	109	
Ds		110	
Rg	272.15	111	
*Uub		112	
*Uuq		114	
*Uuh		116	

Note: 1. * Symbols given in the Table is based on IUPAC systematic names.

2. Elements with atomic numbers 112 and above have been reported but not fully authenticated.

Table 4 Relative terms of Solubility

Solubility Term	Meaning
Very soluble	1 g of solute dissolves in less than 1 ml of solvent
Freely soluble	1 g of solute dissolves in 1-10 ml of solvent 1g
Soluble	Solute dissolves in 30-100 ml of solvent 1 g
Sparingly soluble	Solute dissolves in 30-100 ml of solvent 1 g
Slightly soluble	Solute dissolves in 100-1000 ml of solvent 1 g
Very slightly soluble	Solute dissolves in 1000-10,000 ml of solvent
Practically insoluble or insoluble	1 g of solute dissolves in more than 10,000 ml of solvent

Table 5 Sodium chloride Equivalents (E), Freezing point Depression (D) values of 1% solution of some common substances

Name of the substance	E	D
Apomorphine HCl Ascorbic acid	0.14	0.080
Atropine sulfate Bacitracin		0.105
Benzyl alcohol	0.13	0.075
	0.05	0.03
	0.17	0.09
Calcium chloride (2H$_2$O)	0.51	0.298
Calcium chloride (6H$_2$O)	0.35	0.2
Calcium chloride, anhydrous	0.68	0.39
Calcium gluconate	0.16	0.091
Calcium lactate	0.23	0.13
Carboxymethylcellulose sodium	0.03	0.017
Chloramphenicol sodium	0.14	0.07
Chlordiazepoxide HCl	0.22	0.125
Chlorobutanol (hydrated)	0.24	0.14
Chloroquine phosphate	0.14	0.082
Chloroquine sulfate	0.09	0.05
Chlorpheniramine maleate	0.15	0.085
Chlortetracycline HCl Citric acid	0.10	0.061
	0.18	0.10
Cocaine HCl	0.16	0.09
Codeine phosphate	0.14	0.08
Cupric sulfate	0.18	0.100
Chloroquine sulfate	0.09	0.05
Citric acid	0.18	0.10
Cocaine HCl	0.16	0.09
Dextrose	0.16	0.091
Dexamethasone sodium phosphate	0.17	0.095
Ephedrine HCl	0.30	0.165
Ephenephrine bitartrate	0.18	0.104
Dimethyl sulfoxide	0.42	0.245
Diperidon HCl	0.14	0.079
Ephedrine sulfate	0.23	0.13
Epinephrine HCl	0.29	0.16
Erythromycin lactobionate	0.07	0.04
Fluorescein sodium	0.31	0.181
Gentamicin sulfate	0.05	0.03
Homatropine HCl	0.17	0.097

Table 5 *contd…*

Name of the substance	E	D
Imipramine HCl	0.20	0.11
Kanamycin sulfate	0.32	0.184
Magnesium sulfate anhydrous	0.09	0.05 1
Methylprednisolone sodium succinate	0.15	0.086
Morphine HCl	0.14	0.079
Morphine sulfate		
Neomycin sulfate	0.11	0.063
Neostigmine bromide	0.22	0.127
Nicotinamide	0.26	0.148
Nicotinic acid	0.25	0.144
Novobiocin sodium	0.10	0.057
Papaverine HCl	0.10	0.061
Penicillin G potassium	0.18	0.102
Phenylephrine HCl	0.32	0.184
Pilocarpine HCl	0.24	0.138
Polysorbate 80	0.02	0.010
Polyvinylpyrrolidone	0.01	0.006
Potassium acetate	0.59	0.342
Potassium chloride	0.76	0.439
Potassium phosphate monobasic	0.44	0.25
Procainamide HCl	0.22	0.13
Kanamycin sulfate	0.07	0.04 1
Quinine bisulfate	0.09	0.05
Quinine HCl	0.14	0.077
Silver nitrate	0.33	0.190
Sodium ampicillin	0.16	0.090
Sodium benzoate	0.40	0.23 0
Sodium bicarbonate	0.65	0.375
Sodium borate	0.42	0.24 1
Sodium chloride	1.00	0.576
Sodium citrate	0.31	0.178
Sodium metabisulfite	0.67	0.3 86
Streptomycin sulfate	0.07	0.036
Sucrose	0.08	0.047
Sulphacetamide sodium	0.23	0.132
Tetracycline HCl	0.14	0.08 1
Urea	0.59	0.34
Vancomycin sulfate	0.05	0.028

1 Introduction

History of Pharmaceutical Practice through Ages

Prehistoric Pharmacy

Pharmacy has been a part of everyday life since ancient times. Excavations, such as Shanidar (30000 B.C.E) supports this fact. The ancient tribal healers, also called as Shamans often guarded this knowledge of healing properties of certain natural substances. But, the recognition of the medicinal plants, was so widespread that it obstructed any necessity for a special class of drug gatherers. Earlier people used to describe diseases in supernatural terms. They believed the beneficial medicines worked in supernatural ways. The magical medicines for curing were part of the duty of Shamans. Usually they were in charge of all supernatural things in a tribe, and hence, they diagnosed and treated most serious and chronic diseases. These remedial medicines, connected with supernatural world for thousands of years continues to fascinate us all even today. Thus we can consider that drugs have a dual heritage, a simple curing tool and special substance with supernatural powers.

Though ancient people have discovered a small number of drugs that heal human diseases, still this discovery can be considered as one of the humanity's greatest advances.

Afterwards, settled cultures provided tools (such as writings, weights, measures) to mushroom this rationale method of medical treatment, without which pharmaceutical sciences may have failed to progress.

Antiquity

The advancement of societies also started influencing the fundamentals of disease and healing. The changes can be verified from the remains of the civilizations of Mesopotamia and Egypt. From ancient records of Egyptian civilization, it can be concluded that pharmaceutical sciences rose greater heights in these times, with more dosage forms compounded from more detailed formula. The Egyptian medical texts shows a close connection between supernatural and natural healing. Recipes usually began with a prayer or hymn and ended with plant drugs.

In ancient Greece, there was a similar connection of drugs or *pharmakon*, means magic spell, remedy, poison. Most Greek medicines were prepared from plants and the first great study of plants was done by Theophrastus (370 – 285 BC), a student of Aristotle.

Middle Age

Traditionally, Middle Ages refers to the period from the first fall of Rome (400 AD) to the fall of Constantinople (1453). In the middle age the use of drugs went into another shift. Rational drug treatment was replaced by Church's teaching that sin and disease were related intimately. Monasteries became centres for healing, both spiritual and physical. At this age monks planted gardens to grow medicinal herbs, and inclined to credit their cures to the God, rather to their medical resources.

There were many cultures that dealt with medicines but there was no significant change that occurred in this period.

In western Europe, teachings of Mohammed was followed. Greek writings in medicines were translated into Arabic. As Arabs conquered this region, they brought new medicines with them. They rejected the idea that foul tasting medicines worked best. Arabic culture returned the classical knowledge of medicine to Europe. The debate on medicine among European academics were based on speculation but not on observation.

Hence, observation methodology was to be followed to bring down a significant change in the medical practice. This new experimental period was called *Renaissance*.

Indian Systems of Medicines

Indian Systems of Medicines includes the systems originated in India and the systems originated outside but adapted in India. These are Ayurveda, Unani, Siddha, Yoga, Naturopathy and Homeopathy.

Ayurveda

Ayurveda, the science of life, has arrived from the Vedas. Around 1000 BC, the knowledge of Ayurveda was comprehensively documented by Charak and Sushruta. Ayurveda considers both physical and spiritual aspects of man. According to the philosophy of Ayurveda, human being is a combination of the following structural and functional entities, three doshas, panchamahabhutas, sapta dhatu, panchaindriyas, manas, budhi and atman. Three doshas are vata (air), pitta (fire) and kapha (water and earth).

The principle of Ayurveda is to keep these structural and functional entities in a state of equilibrium to maintain a good health. The cause of illness is imbalance of these entities due to internal and external factors.

The diagnosis of any disease is done by questioning the patients and eight examinations, e.g. pulse, urine, faeces, tongue, eyes, visual examination and inference.

The factors, such as state of body, mind, temperament, sex, age, metabolic condition, etc,. are considered at the time of prescribing medicines. The system provides both preventive treatment and curative treatment.

Unani

This system was brought from Arab and Greece during 460-376 BC. According to this system the body has four humours-blood, phlem, yellow bile and black bile. Disease is a normal process of life and reactions of the body is symptom. The diagnosis and treatment are based on the principle of temperament, hot, cold, moist and dry. Any change in temperament is due to imbalance of humours. Medicines are made of herbal, animal and mineral origin. According to this system there is some natural self-preservation mechanism in human body. The function of the drugs is to stimulate and strengthen the defence mechanism and to normalise the imbalance in humours.

Siddha

Siddha means achievement or perfection. This system was originally practised in Tamilnadu. The manuscripts are written in Tamil. It is believed that eighteen Sidhars (saints or saintly persons), through the practice of yoga, developed this system of medicines which is mainly therapeutic in nature.

The principles of this system and of Ayurveda are similar. According to this system, the human body, the food and medicines are all replica of the universe. The concept of this system is based on tridosha and panchamahabhutas of Ayurveda. The method of diagnosis and treatment are similar to Ayurveda.

Homeopathy

The German physician Dr. Christian Frederic Sammuel Hahnemann introduced the basic principles of Homeopathy and translated Cullen's Materia Medica into German from English. Dr. Hahnemann discovered that any substance which produces artificial symptoms on healthy persons, can cure the symptoms in natural disease also. Thus, the concept of treatment is *Similia Similibus Curentur*. The symptoms disappear in the reverse order of their appearance. The doses sufficient to cure is administered. The treatment is done on individual symptoms basis, but not disease basis. Hence, detail study of symptoms in the patient and of the drug is of prime importance.

Yoga

Sage Patanjali proposed yoga. It contains eight components-restraint, observance of austerity, physical postures, breathing exercises, restraining of sense organs, contemplation, meditation and samidhi. Yoga is a way of life. Practice of yoga improves behaviour, keeps through better circulation of oxygenated blood in the body, restrain the sense organs and mind, and induce tranquillity. It prevents psychosomatic disorders and improves the ability to overcome stress. It also improves the intelligence and memory.

Naturopathy

Treatment of disease without drug and application of simple laws of nature are the basic concepts of this system. The fundamental principle of this system is similar to that of Ayurveda. There are two groups-one believes in practising ancient Indian methods and the other believes in practising western methods similar to physiotherapy. The practitioner regulates the eating and living habits, methods of purification, hydrotherapy, fasting, cold packs, mud packs, baths, massages etc., and treat the patients.

Pharmacy in Relation to Allied Health Profession

The goal of medical therapy is to improve the patients' health and quality of life. Optimal medical therapy should be safe, effective and appropriate. An accurate and up to date information are necessary to provide best medical care for the patients as well as for the providers.

The responsibilities of physicians and pharmacists are complementary and supportive to meet the goal of providing optimal medical therapy. This requires communication, respect, trust and mutual recognition of each other's professional competence. During counselling the patients, the physician may focus on the goal of therapy, the risks and benefits and side effects. The pharmacists on the other hand may focus on correct usage, treatment adherence, dosage, precautions and storage information.

Responsibilities of a pharmacist during a medical therapy:

1. To ensure safe procurement, storage, adequate dosage and dispensing of medicines as per the prescription,

2. To furnish information to the patients, which may include the name of the medicine, its purpose, potential interactions and side effects, correct usage and storage,

3. To review prescription orders to identify interactions, allergic reactions, contraindications and therapeutic duplications. Significant matters should be discussed with the prescriber (physician),

4. To consult with the physician for the preparation and revision of therapeutic plans of the treatment with the medicines,

5. To discuss medicine related problems or concerns with regard to the prescribed medicines, if requested by the patient,

6. To advise patients on the selection and use of non-prescription medicines and how to manage the minor symptoms or ailments,

7. To advise the patient where self-medication is not appropriate and the respective physician to be consulted for diagnosis and treatment,

8. To report adverse reactions of medicines to health authorities, when necessary,

9. To provide and share general as well as specific medicine related information and to advise the public and health care providers,

10. To update the knowledge on medical therapy regularly through continuous professional development.

When the pharmacist and physician start exchanging information, each provider can understand other's performance. Such understanding ultimately helps to recognize each other's value, to build mutual trust and to develop satisfaction with the relationship. The net benefit of each exchange among service partners adds value to professional collaboration. Similarly, when expectations are met, the satisfaction with exchange partners may result. The continued meeting of expectations also can contribute to the development of trust.

Apart from the above discussed responsibilities, a pharmacist also co-ordinates with and assists the nursing staff at different levels or stages of therapy.

1. Proper administration of drugs i.e., to take right drug at right time. Whether the drug has to be administered before or after meals, frequency of administration, and dose of drugs to be administered in emergencies. All these are monitored by the pharmacist along with nurses,

2. A pharmacist also provides information to the nurse about the diet plan which should be followed by the patient during the drug therapy. A pharmacist is the best person who knows about the drug-food interactions and thus, he decides the diet plan which should be advised and monitored by the nurses.

3. The pharmacist also guides the nurses about the safe handling of drugs. He provides information regarding proper dispensing, storage of drugs and disposal of waste containers.

4. The pharmacist assists the nurses in documentation which includes recording of day to day and patient to patient plan of drug administration, recording of drug administered and to be administered. He can also assist in documentation of various clinical parameters at regular interval of time.

5. The pharmacist can also train the nurses about the use and sterilisation techniques of surgical instruments.

6. A pharmacist also acts as an active member of the health care team which includes physician and nurse, which can ultimately provide maximum benefits to the patients.

In the health care service the position of a pharmacist can be depicted as shown below.

Pharmacy as a Career

Pharmacy is a word derived from the Greek word *pharmakon* meaning drug. Pharmacy is a branch of science related to healthcare services and Pharmacist is a core healthcare professional. Today, the discipline of pharmacy has made enormous progress and is a distinctly independent discipline, known as pharmaceutical sciences & technology with the wealth of knowledge, research and art of technology. Unlike other curricula, pharmacy is a product as well as service related discipline. Pharmacist works in all stages related to drug, starting from drug discovery, development, safety, quality control, packaging, storage, use, marketing, sale and also in governing the manufacture, sale, export and import of drugs in the country, i.e. in drug control administration. Precisely, in the real sense, pharmacist is a drug expert.

In the changing global scenario and in post implementation of GATT (General Agreement on Tariff and Trade) and TRIPS (Trade Related aspects of Intellectual Property Rights) in India, Indian pharmaceutical sector is witnessing tremendous growth with contract research and clinical trial business. The new patent regime is also opening avenues for Indian players. The Indian pharmaceutical industry presently has become the front line player in the global pharmaceutical business. The sector is estimated to be worth of about 8 billion US$ with an annual growth of about 13%.

Indian pharmaceutical industry globally ranks 4th in terms of volume with about 8% share in global business, ranks 13th in terms of value. Indian pharmaceutical industry is now producing about 24% of the global generic drugs in terms of value. India is one of the 5 top producers of active pharmaceutical ingredients (API) with a share of about 6.5% globally. We are now supplying formulations to many countries of the world and catering about 70% of the demand for bulk drugs.

India ranks 17th with respect to exports value of bulk drugs and dosage forms. The factors that help Indian pharmaceutical industry to grow are, low cost of R&D, low cost of production, innovative scientific manpower and the strength of national laboratories.

With these advantages, India can now be able to export nearly 40% of the production which constitutes 55% of formulations and 45% of the bulk drugs.

According to Mckinsey report 'Indian pharmaceutical market will grow to USD 55 billion by 2020 driven by a steady increase in affordability and a step jump in market access. At the projected scale, this market will be comparable to all developed markets other than the US, Japan and China. In terms of volumes, India will be at the top, a close second only to the US market

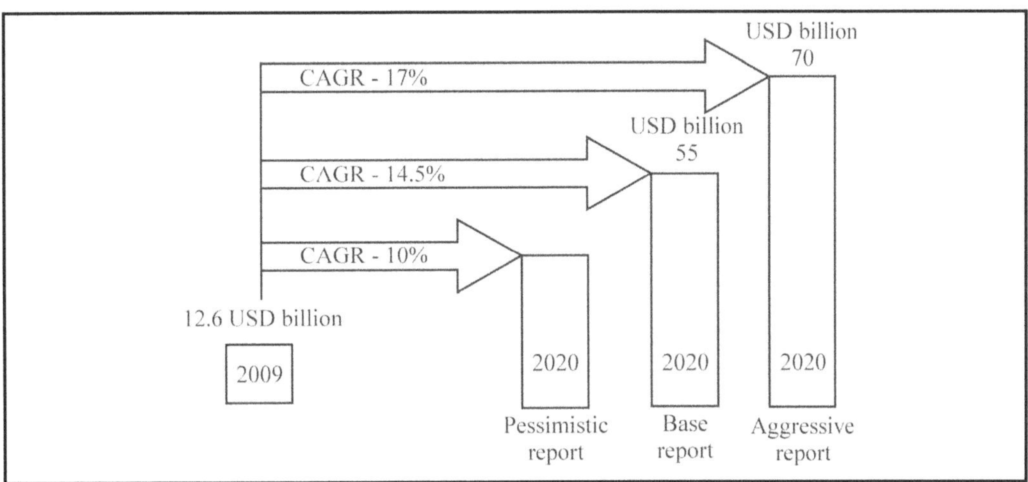

Figure 1.1 Projected size of Indian Pharma Market.

Source: Mckinsey analysis: secondary research

On account of inventory rationalization and reduction in Research and Development (R&D) budget by multinational pharmaceutical companies in the face of global slowdown the growth rate for Indian CRAMS (Contract Research and Manufacturing Services) players slowed down to 5-8% CAGR (Cumulative Annualised Growth Rate) during 2009-2011. The industry has undergone tough times. However, in subsequent years the growth rate gradually picked up to low double digits. CARE Ratings expects gradual improvement (expected CAGR 18-20%) on the back of recovery signs witnessed in US markets. Some of the major drugs are going off patent during 2014-2020.

As per the report of a global pharmaceutical market intelligence company, IMS Health, the Indian Generic Manufacturers will grow to more than 70 billion US$ within couple of years as the patent of some drugs worth of 20 billion US$ annual sales value had expired in 2008 and the patent of some best selling drugs worth of about 80 billion US$ will expire by 2012.

Thus, it is clearly evident that the employment potential in pharmaceutical sector is growing faster in this country.

Career Opportunities

There are various options a pharmacy professional do have for their career growth.

1. Pharmaceutical Industries
   Production – Manufacturing, Packaging, Store & Purchase
   Quality Control & Quality Assurance
   Research & Development
2. Pharmaceutical Marketing
3. Hospital & Clinical Pharmacy
4. Community Pharmacy
5. Regulatory Affairs
6. Academics
7. Consultancy
8. Library Information Service and Pharmaceutical Journalism
9. Opportunities Abroad

1. Pharmaceutical Manufacturing

Whether it is allopathic, ayurvedic or homoeopathic drug manufacturing unit. Each manufacturing unit comprises various major sections like production, packaging, inventory and purchase. Based on type of dosage forms being manufactured the number of sections vary. A pharmacy professional is most desired technical person for production of bulk drugs, intermediates and formulations. The job is supervisory in nature and the initial designation, chemist, supervisor, executive, etc varies from company to company. Based on efficiency and experience the candidate can become Manager, General Manager, Vice-President and President, the top most position.

In cosmetic, soaps and toiletries industry the pharmacy professionals are also preferred as suitable technical persons. For production of Blood and Plasma products pharmacy professionals are appointed as supervisors.

Packaging of pharmaceutical products is of great importance and requires technical supervision. Similarly store & purchase are two major operations associated with production on which the quality of a product depends. Hence, many pharmaceutical companies appoint pharmacy professional for supervising these activities.

Quality control and Quality assurance are two major departments of any manufacturing industry. Of course there are official standards for drugs and drug products with permissible limits of impurities and purities for every raw material and finished product, but most of the pharmaceutical industries have their own internal standards for input materials and products, which are more specific and process based. Hence, it is very essential to adhere to established methods and standards, so that the final quality of the manufactured products is achieved consistently. Highly specialised and trained staff is required to operate most sensitive and sophisticated analytical instruments. In general professionals with M.Pharm or M.Pharm, Ph.D are most preferred.

Research and Development is heart of an industry. For sustenance and growth every industry should have its own R&D department. In pharmaceutical industry it is very much essential, because the discovery of a drug molecule and development of a suitable dosage form are continuous processes as the type of disease and its treatment are changing. Even for better treatment of the existing diseases the development of the drug delivery systems are necessary. Hence, a lot of job opportunity exist in this area and persons having M. Pharm or M. Pharm, Ph. D qualication are most suitable.

2. Pharmaceutical Marketing

Without marketing and sales of its products no business can be viable. The pharmaceutical marketing and sales are highly technical in nature, the prescribing physician needs to be aware of the dose, use and contraindication of every drug product. And this is done by the representative of the manufacturer visiting the doctor. Hence, this is a specialised job and needs a person who is fully aware of the subject. Pharmacy professional can do this successfully. Even the retailer needs to be trained on proper storage of a particular drug product and how the patient should take the preparation. This is field job. Scope of promotion is maximum and within short period one can reach to top position with basic qualification only.

Product management is another area of marketing where the person having some field experience can do excellently. This is not field job. Great scope of earning exists if the person has innovative ideas.

3. Hospital and Clinical Pharmacy

For pharmacy professionals this is one more opportunity to work as *Registered Pharmacist* in the hospitals or drug store. In fact, in most of the countries abroad this is a prestigious job and the pharmacist is the only authorized person to prescribe a medicine. The physician only diagnoses the disease but cannot prescribe a medicine. This requires the knowledge of drug-drug interaction, drug-food interaction, pharmacokinetics of the drug. After careful consideration of the patient's medical history, disease state, health condition, incompatibility with other medicines, if being taken, etc., the pharmacist selects the suitable drug, decides the proper dose and its administration schedule.

4. Community Pharmacy

As such this concept is existing in developed countries. Through the community pharmacy a pharmacist plays a vital role during treatment of a patient. The pharmacist through his service becomes a link between the patient and treating physician, i.e., as a link between the patient and drug. The duties of the pharmacist in a clinical pharmacy are,

- Counselling the patients regarding the use of the drugs and dosage forms,
- Providing up-to-date information about the drug/dosage form to the patient, as well as to the medical staff,
- Maintaining the patient record and disease-treatment history,
- Training of the patient regarding use of self-diagnostic kits for certain disease like diabetes, hypertension, etc,.
- Providing supply of home care dosage forms.

5. Regulatory Affairs

In India Drugs Control Administration is the main regulatory body that governs the manufacture, sale, import and export of drug and drug products. Every state has its own Directorate of Drug Control Administration, over and above there is Central Drug Control Administration. In each set up there are Inspectors of Drugs who visit the retail counters, manufacturing units, etc and draw samples for quality check. The state directorate is headed by State Drugs Controller and the central administration is headed by the Drugs Controller of India. In between the Director and Drug Inspector, the Deputy Director and Assistant Directors are there. The minimum eligible qualification for such job is B. Pharm.

6. Academics

Excellent opportunities in teaching profession are available throughout the country. There are many Institutions in the country managed by government and private institutions where vacancies at different levels are still in existence. The minimum eligible qualification at lecturer level is M.Pharm and with Ph.D one reach up to Professor level.

7. Consultancy

For highly technical and experienced pharmacy professional this is an ideal opportunity to earn handsomely as a self-employed entrepreneur. There is no age limit for this profession. The consultancy fees depends on the type of service and field, like regulatory affairs, documentation, approval, manufacturing process know-how, analytical technique, research, market survey and sales promotion, information retrieval, data management, turn key project, etc.

8. Library Information Service and Pharmaceutical Journalism

In the recent times the regulatory affairs and patenting processes involve a lot of documentation work to be done and submitted to the concerned Regulatory Authorities within a definite time schedule, for which a special work force is necessary. Hence, most of the large scale companies have separate department for this purpose and pharmacy professional are best suited for such activities.

Similarly, the Research & Development and Q.C departments need to collect technical information across the world. This needs to be regularly updated to match the pace of global competition. So, library information service is another area of growing demand in pharmaceutical industries. Moreover, Bio-informatics and Electronic Data Retrieval systems are also promising area where a pharmacy professional can find growth.

9. Opportunities Abroad

There are golden opportunities for pharmacy professional to work abroad. Countries like USA, Canada, UK, France, Germany, Australia, African countries, Saudi Arabia, Japan, etc., still importing pharmacy professionals for different types of jobs like industrial, academics and clinical pharmacy.

One with B. Pharm degree can pursue higher education in developed western countries and can find highest career growth.

Pharmacy Education and Regulatory Bodies in India

Pharmacy education in India is a two-tier system. After 12th, science students of state or central board one can opt for any of the three courses, D.Pharm, B.Pharm and M.Pharm. The duration of these courses are 2, 4 and 2 years respectively. After D.Pharm one can persue B. Pharm course being admitted to 2nd year. After completion of M.Pharm course, one can persue Ph.D. Presently, the Pharm. D, a 6 years' course has been started which is a Doctorate course in pharmacy.

The pharmacy education in India is regulated by the All India Council for Technical Education (AICTE) and the Pharmacy Council of India (PCI). The Universities are affiliating bodies.

Dosage Forms

Drug is a substance which is used for diagnosis, mitigation, treatment, cure or prevention of a disease in human beings or in the animals.

Drug(s) are as such rarely administered but are administered as a particular form - known as *dosage form*, wherein certain substances which are non-toxic, therapeutically inactive and compatible with the drug(s) substances are mixed with the drugs to prepare the dosage forms. These substances are termed as *excipients or adjuvants or additives*. Each of these has a specific role or function for being used in a particular dosage form.

Hence, the term **Dosage form** may be defined as a pharmaceutical preparation designed for administration of a drug into the body through a suitable route.

Each dosage form must have the following characteristics:

- Therapeutic effectiveness,
- Physiochemical stability, ability to deliver the correct dose of the drug at the correct site and at the desired time,
- Acceptability to the patient and
- Reasonable cost.

The formulation or dosage form of a drug may be generic or branded. A drug which is

1. No longer under patent protection, which may be produced by any manufacturer following GMP,
2. Is sold under the generic name, is called as **generic product** and the label of the product shall mention only the official name of the drug and its formulation.

For example, if on the label the name of the product is given, *Paracetamol Tablets IP*, it is *generic*, but if any name other than this, is given to the formulation by the manufacturer for its promotional purpose, and the name of the drug (paracetamol, here) is only known through the composition, it is **branded**.

Advantages of Dosage Forms

- Through a dosage form accurate dose of the drug can be administered.
- It can protect the drug from its degradation.

- The unpleasant odour and taste can be masked.
- Depending on the requirement a drug can be formulated as solid, semisolid, liquid or gaseous   dosage form.
- The palatability of a liquid dosage form can be improved by addition of suitable excipient.
- The therapeutic action of a drug can be modified through a formulation, e.g. sustained, delayed, controlled release formulation.
- A properly designed formulation can be inserted into any part of the body for desired therapeutic action, e.g. suppositories, inserts and dental cones etc,.
- For dispensing to various category of patients, e.g. children, adult, elderly, bed ridden, a drug can be formulated differently.

Classification of Dosage Form

The dosage forms may be classified on the basis of their routes of administration, the physical state and method of manufacture.

Physical state	Dosage form
Solid	Tablet, Capsule, Granules and Powders.
Semi-solid	Ointment, Cream, Paste, gel.
Liquid	Solution, Suspension, Emulsion.
Gas	Inhalations.

Route of administration	Dosage form
Oral	Tablet, Capsule, Granules, Powders, Solution, Syrup, Elixir, Suspension, emulsion, Gel.
Parenteral	Injection (in the form of solution, suspension, emulsion), Implant.
Topical	Ointment, Cream, Paste, Lotion, Gel, Solution, Aerosol.
Eye	Solution, Ointment.
Ear	Solution, Suspension, Ointment.
Nasal	Solution, Inhalation.
Lung	Aerosol (in the form of solution, suspension, powder), sprays, Gases, Inhalation.
Rectal/Vaginal	Suppositories, Ointment, Cream, Powder, Lotion.

Method of Manufacture	Dosage form
Aseptic	Sterile (Parenterals, Opthalmics)
Non-aseptic	Non-sterile (Solutions, syrups and others)
Special	Novel Drug Delivery systems (Controlled drug delivery)

Routes of Drug Administration

The routes through which a drug may be administered are: oral, buccal or sublingual, inhalation, rectal, parenteral and topical. The route of administration is selected on the basis of necessity and convenience.

Oral Route

This is the most convenient route because a patient does not require anybody to take a dose of a drug. Only a child, very elderly or bed ridden cannot take the drug without the help of anybody. Most of the drugs are capable of reaching systemic circulation adequately within a reasonable time limit and can elicit expected therapeutic effect. Most of the drugs are absorbed from the gastrointestinal tract. However, there are certain exceptions.

Buccal or Sublingual Route

Although by swallowing a dosage form, adequate plasma concentration of a drug is achieved within a reasonable time, sometimes for faster response and to avoid degradation of the drug in the liver, a drug may be given through buccal or sublingual route. For example, in case of angina pectoris a patient can get relief by taking drug through this route and parenteral route may by avoided. Limited drugs are administered by this route.

Inhalation Route

This route is used to deliver either the gaseous or volatile drug substances or through a gaseous or volatile carrier into the systemic circulation. For example general anaesthetics. The drug is administered through lungs to the alveoli. As the alveolar and vascular membrane are penetrable to the drugs, flow of blood is abundant and the surface area is large, the absorption of drug is also high. Because of certain problems this route is not used largely. It is mostly useful when the drug is supposed to act on the respiratory tract.

Rectal Route and Vaginal Route

Usually the drugs which are administered orally can be administered rectally also. It has three distinct advantages:

1. The drug administered rectally can exert a direct action on the rectum,
2. It can evacuate the bowel, and
3. Can provide a systemic effect.

In earlier days, rectal suppositories and retention enemas were more popular, but due to improvement in parenteral preparations their popularity has been decreased. Still with certain limitation this route is in use and, sometimes, very important for administration of drugs, particularly in paediatrics and geriatrics. In some cases, the retention enemas become very useful substitute for oral route.

Parenteral Routes

There are various routes of administration of a drug parenterally. Depending on the need and the drug, the solution of a drug is injected through one of the following parenteral routes.

1. ***Intracutaneous or Intradermal Injection:*** The drug solution is injected into the skin, between the epidermis (outer layer of the skin) and dermis (inner layer). The volume of injection, usually small, 0.1 to 0.2 ml and normally the skin of left forearm is the site. Main purpose of such injection is diagnostic or investigation of immunity or allergy.

2. ***Subcutaneous or Hypodermic Injection:*** This is given under the skin. That is, into the subcutaneous tissue, and the maximum volume of injection is up to 1 ml. Oily solution or suspension in oil or water cannot be given through this route as these cause pain or irritation.

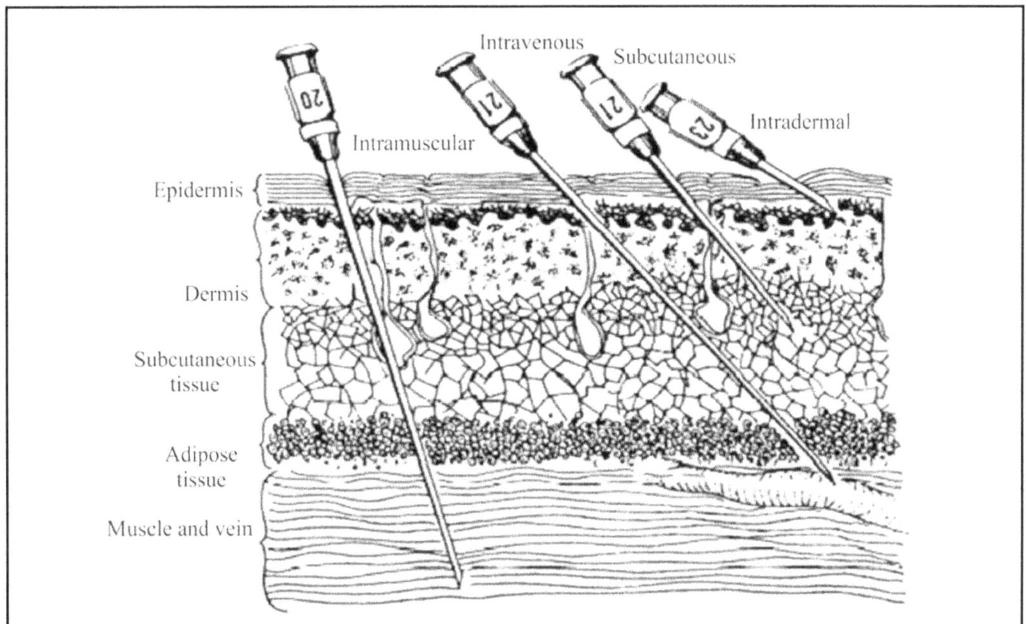

Figure 1.2 Routes of Parenterals Administration.

3. ***Intramuscular Injection:*** These injections are given inside a muscle penetrating the subcutaneous tissue and muscle membrane. The common sites are muscles of shoulder, thigh or of buttock. The maximum volume injected is 4-5 ml. As the muscle can tolerate pain, irritation and there is little fear of blockage, the oily solution or suspension in oil or water can be administered

through this route in small volumes. The rate of administration should be slow in such cases.

4. *Intravenous Injection:* These are given to the vein and hence, directly to the blood stream. This is the route of choice when immediate response is desired. Most common site of injection is the median basilic vein, near anterior surface of the elbow. The volume of injection may range from 1 ml to 500 ml or more. For immediate therapeutic action the small injections are given. Large volume is given usually for replacement of body fluids or eletrolytes.

5. *Intra-arterial Injection:* This is almost similar to intravenous injection. This is given when immediate effect is required in peripheral area. For example, in early gangrene when arterial flow is restricted, this injection is given to improve the flow.

6. *Intracardiac Injection:* In emergency only, this is given into the heart muscle or ventricle. For example, in cardiac arrest injection of adrenaline or isoprenaline sulphate is given through this route.

7. *Intrathecal Injection:* This is given into the subarachnoid space surrounding the spinal cord. That is the space, between arachnoid and pia matter, containing a fluid known as cerebrospinal fluid. Such injection requires special skill so that the injection is made without entering the spinal cord and causing serious damage. The volume injected normally within 20 ml and in extreme cases like in spinal anaesthesia, tubercular meningitis the drug is given in this route. In the same way the cerebrospinal fluid is taken for diagnostic purpose also.

8. *Peridural Injection:* The injection is made into the peridural space between the dura matter and the inner aspect of the vertebrae. The peridural space is narrow but extended throughout the spinal column length wise. Hence, a special skill is necessary for injection.

9. *Intracisternal Injection:* This is another special route and requires special skill, used either to withdraw the cerebrospinal fluid or to inject a dye for investigation purpose, or to administer an antibiotic for treatment. The needle is inserted between the first and second vertebrae, and into the cisterna magna. This is done when intrathecal route is failed.

10. *Intra-articular injection:* This injection is made into the synovial fluid that lubricates the articulating ends of bones in a joint. Usually anti-inflammatory drugs are administered through this route.

Topical Route

This route refers to the application of a drug over the skin either for its local effect or for systemic effect. For example, a dermatological preparation is meant for treating skin disorder, the skin is the target organ. A transdermal preparation is intended to deliver the drug to the systemic circulation through the skin, skin is not the target organ.

Pharmacopoeia

The term Pharmacopoeia came from two Greek words, *Pharmakon* (means drug) and *Poiein* (means make). In Bergamo, Italy in the year 1580 this term Pharmacopoea was first used for a book on the standards of drugs. Subsequently many countries started using this word for their books on drug standards. Now almost every country of the world has its own national Pharmacopoeia. This is the official book of standards for drugs and their formulations.

Indian Pharmacopoeia

The Indian Pharmacopoeia originated in the year 1844 in the name of Bengal Pharmacopoeia and General Conspectus of Medicinal Plants commonly known as Bengal pharmacopoeia. It was prepared by William Brooke O'Shaughnessy and published by the order of the Government. The principal focus of this was on indigenous drugs along with some products imported from Europe.

Later in the year 1865 the Indian Pharmacopoeia Committee was constituted, which in the year 1868 published the first Pharmacopoeia of India under the authority of the Secretary of State for India in Council. The Pharmacopoeia was edited by Edward John Waring. It contained the drugs, official in the British Pharmacopoeia 1867 along with some indigenous drugs. A Supplement to the Pharmacopoeia of India was prepared by Moodeen Sheriff which was published in 1869. Till 1885 the Pharmacopoeia of India had been in use. When British Pharmacopoeia 1885 was published, the Government made this Pharmacopoeia the sole authority on all matters relating to pharmacy in India. In 1900, the Indian and Colonial Addendum to the British Pharmacopoeia 1898 was published and in 1901, it was published as the Government of India Edition with certain minor modifications. The important articles of this Addendum were subsequently included into the general body of the British Pharmacopoeia 1914. The British Pharmacopoeia Commission also made provision for publication of Supplement or Addenda according to the local requirements and the Indian Pharmacopoeia List 1946 was accordingly prepared to serve as the Indian Supplement to the British Pharmacopoeia 1932. After independence, in the year 1948 an Indian Pharmacopoeia Committee was constituted for preparation of the Pharmacopoeia of India (The Indian Pharmacopoeia) 1955. In 1960, a Supplement to it was published. This Pharmacopoeia contained western as well as traditional drugs. The Indian Pharmacopoeia 1966 and its Addenda 1975 were prepared as per the same policy. Next edition of the Pharmacopoeia of India 1985 and its Addenda 1989 and 1991 also did not include the traditional drugs in general. The traditional drugs were considered separately and only those herbal drugs having definite quality control standards were included.

The Government of India Ministry of Health & Family Welfare, vide their Resolution No. X.19020/1/89-DMS & PFA dated 12th August, 1991 reconstituted the Indian

Pharmacopoeia Committee for a period of five years for preparation of the next edition of the Indian Pharmacopoeia under the Chairmanship of Dr. Nityanand, Ex-Director, Central Drug Research Institute, Lucknow.

To expedite the preparation of the new edition of the Indian Pharmacopoeia, the Committee constituted various Sub-Committees, Working Groups having expert representatives from the Pharmaceutical industries, Drug control laboratories, Research and Teaching Institutions of the country for preparation of draft monographs and appendices, for examination of the comments received on those and for suitable recommendation there on to the Committee.

It was also felt necessary to prepare a Veterinary Supplement to this new edition. Since the drugs for veterinary use needed specialised information, a group was formed for this purpose.

Accordingly, the committee finalised the monographs, appendices and general notices prepared by the Working Groups and in 1996, the Indian Pharmacopoeia was published. For the said purpose other Pharmacopoeias like the British Pharmacopoeia (BP), European Pharmacopoeia (EP), the United States Pharmacopoeia (USP), National Formulary, the Pharmacopoeia of Japan, the Pharmaceutical Codex, the International Pharmacopoeia, the Marck Index and the standards published by the Bureau of Indian Standards were also consulted.

The full name or title of the Pharmacopoeia including Addenda there to, has been changed to Indian Pharmacopoeia 1996 and abbreviated to IP 1996 because of convenience to all and the initial name, Pharmacopoeia of India has been dropped. Current edition of Indian Pharmacopoeia is its 7th edition which has been published in 2014.

United States Pharmacopoeia

In January 1817, Dr. Lyman Spalding of New York City of the United States submitted to the Medical society of the Country a proposal to develop a national Pharmacopoeia. He proposed:

1. To divide the country into four districts - northern, southern, western and middle,
2. To call for *Convention* in each district with delegates from all medical societies and medical schools of the respective district,
3. To prepare a draft for pharmacopoeia and,
4. To appoint delegates for *General Convention* to be held later in Washington, D.C.

Accordingly the drafts were submitted only by the northern and middle districts.

In the General Convention held in January, 1820, these drafts were thoroughly reviewed and consolidated. In December 1820, the first United States Pharmacopoeia was published in two languages, English and Latin. Latin was the then international language of medicine. It was of 272 pages and 217 drugs were included. The convention also resolved that the USP would be revised every 10 years. Because of the extensive efforts extended for preparing the USP, Dr. Spadling is called as the *Father of the USP*.

In 1900, the Pharmacopoeial Convention decided to issue Supplements to the USP as and when necessary to maintain satisfactory standards. In 1940, the Convention decided to revise the USP every 5 years with periodic issuance of Supplements.

The USP is a non-governmental, non-profit public health organisation which independently works to set scientific and recognized standards.

In more than 130 countries across the globe USP's standards are recognized and used. To ensure quality medicines, food ingredients and other health care products USP establishes documentary and reference standards. These documentary standards and references are used by regulatory agencies and manufacturers of pharmaceuticals, dietary supplements and food ingredients to ensure appropriate strength, quality and purity of the ingredients and the products.

USP develops information relating to various aspects of drug-use and circulates this information to physicians, pharmacists and others who are associated with health care profession.

USP also acts to improve health and promote optimal public health care delivery around the world by running operations at various places like Europe, middle East, Africa, India, China and at Brazil.

Since 2002, the USP-NF has been revised and published annually. The current edition USP 39-NF 34 was published on 1, May 2016.

National Formulary

Till 1852, the third revision of USP was the only recognized and authoritative book of drug standards in the United States. The drugs having established therapeutic value were included in the USP. Many drugs and formulas being used by the medical practitioners were not included in the USP due to strict selectivity.

Hence, in 1852, the American Pharmaceutical Association (APhA) organised and prepared a Formulary containing some drugs and formulas which were not included in the USP. In 1888 the first edition of the Formulary was published under the title, National Formulary of Unofficial Preparations. The term unofficial indicated a kind of protest and to distinguish it from the USP in which the term official was used. In 1906 the title was changed to National Formulary (NF) and both USP and NF were made legal books of standards as per the first federal Pure Food and Drug Act under the signature of the then president, Theodore Roosevelt. Hence, according to the law the formulations carried the name USP or NF in their labels were bound to conform to the physical and chemical standards mentioned in the respective monographs.

The initial editions of NF provided uniform names of the drugs, their preparations and working directions as a convenient means to the practicing pharmacists and to the small scale manufacturers of popular preparations prescribed by the physicians.

Till 1940, like USP, the NF had been revised every 10 years and thereafter every 5 years with periodical issuance of supplements as and when necessary.

In 1975 both USP and NF were unified and the first combined compendiam USPXX-NF XV was published in 1980. The USP section contained all monographs on the drug substances and the NF section contained the monographs on pharmaceutical agents. The USP25-NF20 became an annual publication in 2002. The next edition of USP26-NF21 with about 4000 drug monographs was published and made available in both hard and soft copy.

All the members related to health care including pharmacists, physicians, dentists, veterinarians, nurses, manufacturers and suppliers of bulk drugs, chemicals and pharmaceutical products, public health agencies, drug regulatory and enforcement agencies and others were made responsible to adhere to the norms and standards mentioned in the USP-NF.

Since 2002 the USP-NF has been revised and published annually. The current USP33-NF28 shall be published in the year 2010. Currently USP 39 NF 34 is available.

British Pharmacopoeia

Since 1491 – 1547 the regulation of medicinal products had been regulated by officials in the United Kingdom. Physicians of The Royal College, London were empowered to inspect the products of apothecaries in the London area and to destroy the defective stocks. The first list of approved drugs and their manufacturing guidelines were published in London in 1618 as London Pharmacopoeia. In Great Britain, there were three city-pharmacopoeias – the London, the Edinburgh and the Dublin. These were official till the first British Pharmacopoeia (BP) was published in 1864 and all those three pharmacopoeias were merged. In 1907, a Commission was appointed by the General Medical Council and the body was made responsible statutorily under the Medical Act, 1858 to produce a British Pharmacopoeia on national basis. In 1907, the British Pharmaceutical Codex was published with the information and standards for drugs and other pharmaceutical substances not included in the BP.

The 1968 Medicines Act established the legal status of the British Pharmacopoeia Commission and of the British Pharmacopoeia as the standards for medicinal products in the United Kingdom under the section 4 of the Act. Since then, the British Pharmacopoeia Commission continued the work of the earlier Commissions appointed by the General Medical Council and was responsible for preparing new editions of the British Pharmacopoeia and the British Pharmacopoeia (Veterinary) and for keeping those up-to-date. Since 1864, the distribution of BP has grown throughout the world and is now used in more than 100 countries. Australia and Canada have adopted the BP as their national standard and in other countries, e.g. Korea, BP is recognized as an internationally acceptable standard.

The British Pharmacopoeia is prepared by the Pharmacopoeial Secretariat in collaboration with the BP Laboratory, the British Pharmacopoeia Commission and its Expert Advisory Groups and Advisory Panels. The input information are collected from relevant industries, hospitals, academia, professional bodies and governmental sources, inside and outside the UK.

The current edition of the British Pharmacopoeia contains six volumes with about 3000 monographs for drug substances, excipients and formulations along with supporting General Notices, Appendices and Reference Spectra used in the practice of medicines. BP (Veterinary) contains all items used exclusively in veterinary medicines in the UK.

Volume I and II contain medicinal substances, Volume III contains formulations, blood related products, immulogical products, radiopharmaceutical preparations, surgical materials and homeopathic preparations. Volume IV comprises Appendices, Infrared Reference Spectra and Index. Volume V is British Pharmacopoeia (Veterinary), Volume VI contains CD-ROM version of British Pharmacopoeia, British Pharmacopoeia (Veterinary) and British Approved Names.

Till 1996, the British Pharmacopoeia has been revised and published every 5 years. Since 1998 it has been revised and published annually.

International Pharmacopoeia

The history of the International Pharmacopoeia dates back to 1874. The first conference was called by the Belgian Government in Brussels in 1902 and an Agreement for the Unification of the Formula of Potent drugs which was ratified by 19 countries in 1906.

A second agreement, the Brussels Agreement, was drawn up in 1925 and ratified in 1929. It was resolved that the League of Nations would be responsible for the administrative work to produce a unified Pharmacopoeia, and a permanent secretariat of an international organisation would coordinate the work of National Pharmacopoeial Commissions. General principles for the preparation of galenicals, maximal doses, nomenclatures and biological testing of arsenobenzones were included in the articles of this agreement along with a table of dosage strengths and descriptions for 77 drug substances and preparations.

In response to the repeated calls from pharmaceutical experts in various countries, the health organisation of the League of Nations set up a Technical Commission of Pharmacopoeial Experts in 1937. In 1947, the Interim commission of WHO (World Health Organisation) took over the work of pharmacopoeias and in 1948, the first World Health Assembly approved the establishment of the Expert Committee on the International Pharmacopoeia.

The third World Health Assembly held in May, 1950, formally approved the publication of the *Pharmacopoea Internationalis*. This was not intended to be legal pharmacopoeia in any country unless adopted by the pharmacopoeial authority of that country. From that time WHO constituted a permanent International Pharmacopoeial Secretariat. Accordingly, the first edition of International Pharmacopoeia was published in 2 volumes, one in 1951 and the other in 1955. In 1959, a supplement was published. These were published in English, French and Spanish, subsequently translated into German and Japanese languages. Altogether, it included 344 monographs on drug substances, 183 monographs on dosage forms and 84 tests, methods and general requirements. A large number of national pharmacopoeias and official lists were examined and assistance from International Pharmaceutical Federation (FIP) was also obtained to select substances and products for their inclusion in the pharmacopoeia.

The second edition was published in 1967, the third edition in 1975, and in 2006 the forth edition was published. The current edition is published in 2015 and this is the fifth edition. This serves as the source material for reference or adaptation by any WHO Member State wishing to establish pharmaceutical requirements.

European Pharmacopoeia

In the year 1964, a Convention was organised by the European countries- Belgium, France, Germany, Italy, Netherlands, Switzerland, Luxembouurg and United Kingdom under the banner of Council of Europe and decided to prepare an European Pharmacopoeia. The objectives were to make uniform specifications for medicinal substances of general interest to the people of Europe and to prepare the specifications for the growing number of new medicinal substances coming to the market.

Based on these objectives the European Pharmacopoeia was created and published in the year 1967 comprising monographs and became official standards applicable to the territories of the countries which were contracting parties to the convention. The second edition was published in 1980.

On 16th November, 1989, a protocol to this convention was signed in order to enable the European community to accede to it and since 1st November 1992, it was entered into force.

In 1996 the European Directorate for the Quality of Medicines & Health Care (EDQM) came into force. It is an organ of the Council of Europe. It consists of the Technical Secretariat of the European Pharmacopoeial Commission, set up in 1964 by the European Pharmacopoeia Convention. The EDQM is in charge for

- Preparing and publishing adopted text (printed, CD-ROM, and Internet version) and distributing the European Pharmacopoeia and other publications.

- Checking the text experimentally in the laboratory, the laboratory also carries out analytical studies and organises collaborative studies to establish European Pharmacopoeia chemical or biological reference substances or preparations.

- Preparing, managing and dispatching European Pharmacopoeia reference substances.

- Organising regularly congresses on new scientific and technical subjects, as well as seminars and training sessions on subjects related to European Pharmacopoeia.

The European Pharmacopoeia currently has 37 European Members including the European Union (EU). There are 21 observer countries for European Pharmacopoeia including the WHO.

The 2005 edition, the 5th edition, includes 1800 specific and general monographs , including various chemical substances, antibiotics, biological substances; Vaccines for human or veterinary use; Immunosera; Radiopharmaceutical preparations; Herbal drugs; Homoeopathic preparations and Homoeopathic stocks. It also contains Dosage forms, General monographs, Materials and Containers, Sutures; 268 General methods with figures or chromatograms and 2210 reagents are described.

The current edition is the 8th edition, published in the year 2014 and consists of a two-volume main edition with supplements. But since 1st January 2017 the 9th edition shall be effective.

The texts and monographs of the European Pharmacopoeia form an integral part of the British Pharmacopoeia.

Extra Pharmacopoeia

It was published in 1883 under the title, Martindale: *The Extra Pharmacopoeia*. Presently it is being published as Martindale : *The Complete Drug Reference*. It is a reference book with information of about 6000 drugs and medicines, and 146000 proprietary preparations. It also includes 668 disease treatment reviews along with some selected investigational and veterinary drugs, herbal and complementary medicines, pharmaceutical excipients, vitamins and nutritional agents, vaccines, radio-pharmaceuticals, diagnostic agents, contrast media, medicinal gases, drugs of abuse, recreational drugs, toxic substances, disinfectants and pesticides.

The purpose of Martindale is to provide information on drugs and related substances reported to have clinical value anywhere in the world. It is also a source of useful information for patients arriving from different country to search their existing medication, available in different brand name. If not available, their substitutes.

The monographs include Chemical Abstract Services (CAS) and Anatomical Therapeutic Chemical Classification System (ATC) numbers, so that a reader can refer to other information system.

Martindale has two main parts, Monographs and Preparations plus two extensive indexes, Directory of manufacturers and General index.

Monographs on drugs and ancillary substances, - about 5827 monographs are arranged in 53 chapters based on clinical use with reference to disease treatment reviews. Monograph contains nomenclature, properties and actions of each substance. A chapter on supplementary drugs and other substances covers about 980 monographs on new drugs, not easily classified, herbals and drugs which are not even clinically used, but reported to be of clinical interest. Monographs of some toxic substances are also included.

Preparations about 1,46,000 preparations from various countries of the world are included in this portion.

Directory of Manufacturers contains about 13,000 names of manufacturers.

General index contains approved names, synonyms and chemical names.

In the digital version, additional 1000 drug monographs, 30,000 preparation names and 5000 manufacturers are provided.

Some Important Compendial Terms

Monographs: The format of the text given in a Pharmacopoeia containing the official title, the primary informations and the all the requirements given under the heading, **STANDARDS** for a pharmaceutical ingredient or for a formulation.

General Monographs are the monographs which describe official preparations, requirements of general application and requirements of tests applicable to all monographs for the relevant dosage forms, unless otherwise mentioned in the individual monograph.

Official Standards: It refers to the requirements mentioned in a monograph of the Pharmacopoeia applicable for a substance or its product intended for medicinal use, not for other purpose. A monograph shall be construed according to any general monograph, notice, note, any appendix, or any other explanatory material given in the Pharmacopoeia and those shall be applicable to that monograph.

Under the heading **STANDARDS** in a monograph all the statements shall refer to as standards, if there is no specific general notice indicating otherwise is given and no material can be considered as of *pharmacopoeial quality* unless it comply with all the requirements stated in the monograph. The monograph limits the presence of potential impurities only. Any material, if found to contain any impurity, contaminant or adulterant which cannot be detected by the prescribed tests, cannot be declared as *not of pharmacopoeial quality* unless the nature and amount of such substance is found objectionable under the conditions of use or is incompatible with good pharmaceutical practice.

Usual Strength: In any individual monograph of a preparation the strength is mentioned as a general information to the pharmacist or the medical practitioner and does not prevent any manufacturer from manufacture and market the formulation of different strength with the approval of appropriate authority.

Storage: The storage conditions mentioned in a monograph are not mandatory, only a advice type to maintain the appropriate conditions to protect a substance or a product from the effects of atmosphere, moisture, heat, light and to prevent deterioration and contamination. The terms mentioned as storage condition with respect to temperature are;

Cold: Any temperature within the range from $2^\circ - 8^\circ$C, a refrigerator is a cold place.

Cool: Any temperature within the range from $8^\circ - 25^\circ$C, unless otherwise mentioned, a refrigerator can be used as a cool place.

Room temperature: The temperature prevailing in a particular place of work.

Warm: Any temperature within $30^\circ - 40^\circ$C.

Excessive heat: Any temperature more than 40°C.

Protection from freezing: Where it is known that freezing may cause breakage of the container, alter the characteristics of the contents in terms of strength or potency or any other, the precautionary note is provided in the monographs.

Storage under non-specific conditions: Where there is no specific storage condition is mentioned in the monograph, the material is to be kept away from moisture, freezing and excessive heat.

Containers: Container is a device to hold a material. The closure is a part of container. The immediate container is that which always remains in direct contact with the material, e.g., an ampoule, bottle, etc. Since it has a role in protecting the material from contamination and deterioration, requirements and guiding information are provided in the Pharmacopoeia. Despite that in certain individual monographs requirements for containers are also provided. However, any other newly developed or designed container which satisfy the requirements and serve the purpose, but not included in the pharmacopoeia, can be used with the permission of the appropriate authority.

The primary functions of a container are;

- To provide the required degree of protection to the contents from the environment,
- To provide convenient transfer of the content from the container,
- To ensure that the safety and quality of the contents are not changed,
- There should be no interaction between the container and contents,
- To ensure that no extraneous material is introduced into or onto the contents.

Thus, the container should be properly cleaned.

Light-resistant Container means a container that protects the contents from the effects of actinic light by means of,

- Light resistant property of the container itself,
- By wrapping the container with an opaque cover,
- Storing the container in dark place.

In the later cases the label on the container should clearly mention the instructions for storage.

Well-closed Container should ensure - protection of the contents from extraneous solids and liquids, and – no loss of content under normal conditions of, handling, shipment and distribution, storage.

Tightly-closed Container should ensure - protection of the contents from extraneous solids, liquids, or vapours, – no loss or deterioration of content from effervescence, deliquescence or evaporation under normal conditions of, handling, shipment and distribution, storage.

A tightly-closed container should be capable of being closed tightly after opening the container.

Where a tightly-closed container is specified, a hermetically sealed container can be used for a single dose of a formulation.

Hermetically Sealed Container is a container impervious to air or any other gas under normal condition of handling, shipment, distribution and storage. It may be closed either by fusion of the material of the container, e.g. ampoule, or by any other means, e.g. sealed container used for powder for injection as mentioned in an individual monograph of the Pharmacopoeia.

Single Unit Container is designed to hold a single dose of a preparation and intended for use immediately after opening the container. The immediate container and/or outer container or protective packaging is also designed in such a way that any tampering with the contents can be seen.

Single Dose Container is intended for holding a single dose parenteral preparation or an amount of a drug sufficient for its single dose.

Unit Dose Container is a container to hold a single dose of a non-parenteral preparation which can be administered directly from the container.

Multiple Unit Container is a container which holds multiple doses of a preparation and allows withdrawal of contents repeatedly without affecting the strength, quality or purity of the remaining portions in the container.

Multiple Dose Container is a multiple unit container intended for holding multiple doses of a parenteral preparation.

Tamper-evident Container is a container fitted with a device or mechanism that reveals irreversibly whether the container has been opened.

Labelling: The labelling of drugs and pharmaceuticals, in general, is governed by the Rules made under the Drugs and Cosmetics Act, 1940 and a drug or its product must bear a label stating the information necessary for it. No deviation is permitted. In the pharmacopoeial monograph the statement given under the heading Labelling is mere a recommendation.

General Guidelines for Manufacturing

The experiment may be performed either on the basis of an established formula (composition and method of manufacture) or after designing a formula. The former will be a demonstration or practice case while the latter shall be considered as a project work.

In either case the following procedures must be followed to approach a *zero-error* result.

1. Fix up the *lot size* of the product to be manufactured.
2. Decide which method is to be followed.
3. Accordingly make a list of ingredients both *active ingredients* and *excipients,* necessary for the lot.
4. Write down the different *steps* of manufacturing.
5. Make a list of *machineries, equipments* and *apparatus* required for the experiment.
6. *Clean* each equipment and machine, *calibrate* each of these.
7. Clean the *work place.*
8. Examine all the materials required for the experiment with respect to their *appearance, assay* and *impurities.*
9. The materials to be used as *dried form*, dry them properly at a temperature quite below their melting point; if to be *sieved* or *filtered,* sieve or filter before *weighing*

the required quantity for the lot. While calculating the required quantity take the *purity (assay value)* of the *drug substance(s)* into consideration.

10. Make *list of tests* to be carried out during processing (*process control test*) and after completion (*final tests*). Ensure the availability of *testing facility* and *calibrate* the *instruments* accordingly.

11. Also, check the *working environment*, e.g. room temperature, humidity, sterility, etc., as appropriate to the product being manufactured, is maintained.

Record all the *information* properly and sequentially in the practical note book.

Contents or Parts of a Label

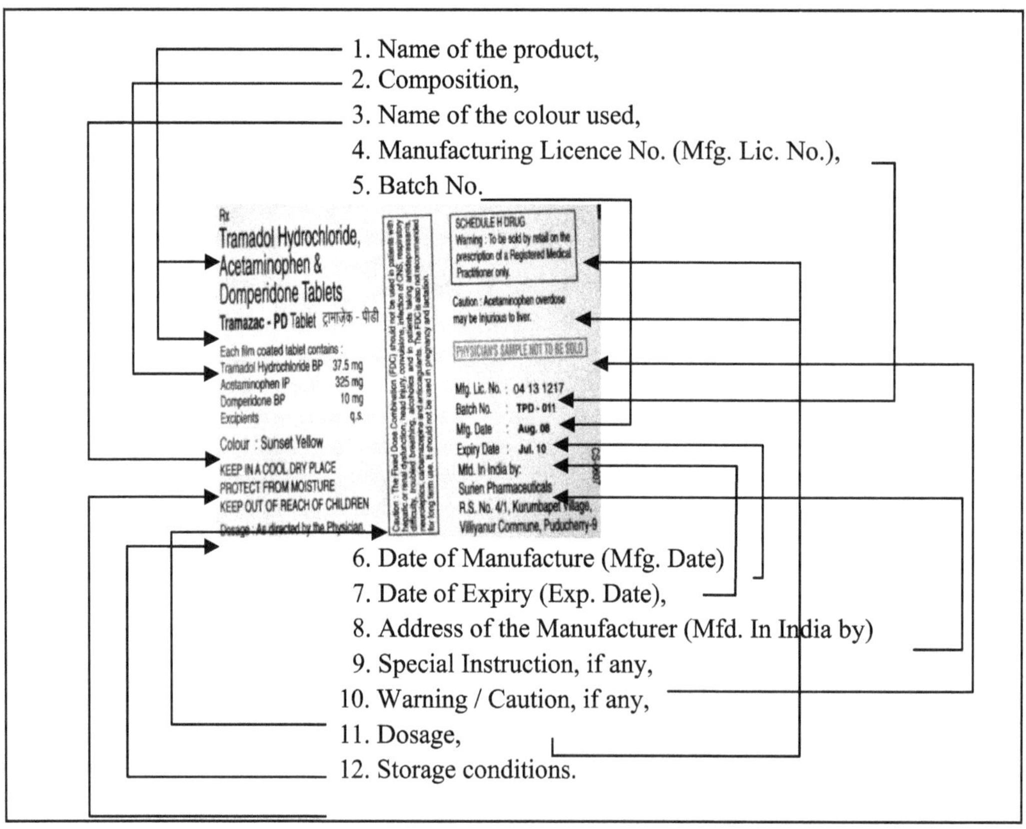

Exercises

Short Questions

1. (a) What do you mean by Shanidar and Mangical medicines?

   (b) How the pharmacy had been practiced during middle age?

   (c) Which period is called Renaissance and why?

   (d) What are other professionals related to health care system?

   (e) What are in-patient and out-patient counselling?

   (f) What is community pharmacy?

   (g) Name the bodies who regulate pharmacy education in India.

   (h) Define drug, dose, dosage form and excipient.

   (i) Write down the characteristics of a dosage form.

   (j) What are generic and branded dosage forms?

   (k) How can a generic product be identified from the label?

   (l) What is a Pharmacopoeia?

   (m) What are full form of IP, USP, BP, EP, NF, BPC?

   (n) Define the term Monograph.

   (o) What do you understand by Official Standard?

   (p) What are temperatures referred to as cold, cool and warm?

   (q) What are single dose container and unit dose container?

2. Discuss how the pharmacy has been developed.

3. Enumerate the role of pharmacist in health care system.

4. How can a pharmacist assist a nursing staff during various stages of therapy?

5. What are the career opportunities in pharmacy?

6. Classify the dosage forms according to their method of manufacturing, physical state and route of administration.

7. Discuss briefly the developmental history of IP/BP/USP/Extra Pharmacopoeia.

8. Explain briefly the importance of a Pharmacopoeia in a country. What does it contain? How it is related to pharmacy?

9. Present a label and mention the various parts.

10. Briefly write down the measures to be taken during manufacture of a dosage form.

11. Write short notes on:

    (a) Parenteral Route of Administration

    (b) Antiquity

    (c) Patient counselling

    (d) Dosage Forms

    (e) Community Pharmacy

    (f) International Pharmacopoeia

    (g) National Formulary

    (h) AICTE,

    (i) PCI

    (j) Importance of a label

2 Solid Dosage Forms

Among the pharmaceutical dosage forms the most popular one is the solid dosage form because it is convenient to use/administer. History reports the dispensing of medicament in the form of moulded tablets even before 3000 years. The solid dosage forms are considered to be more stable if they are properly formulated, packed and stored. There are various types of solid dosage forms. Each type has certain specific use.

These are tablets, troches and lozenges, capsules, powders, granules, cachets, suppositories and pessaries.

Tablets

In 1843 Brockend on first formulated the compressed tablets. Since, mid of 19th century the development in the field of tablet formulation has been continued and has gained the maximum popularity.

Tablets are usually single-dose, solid dosage form either compressed or moulded into suitable shapes containing a mixture of the active ingredient(s) (drug substances) and other suitable excipients. These are so formulated that the active ingredient(s) would be released within a desired time at the desired site of gastrointestinal tract from where the drug can be absorbed into the system.

Types of Tablets

Compressed, moulded, effervescent, chewable, sustained-release or modified release, buccal and sublingual, bolus, etc.

The tablets may be uncoated or coated. The coat may be enteric or non-enteric. The tablets are packed either in container of glass or plastic or individually in strips of aluminium, or plastic coated paper foil.

Compressed Tablets

Most of the tablets are of this type and manufactured by compressing the granules made with a mixture of drug substance(s) and other excipients using suitable die and punch.

The granules for compression may be prepared either by dry process or by wet process depending on the physico-chemical properties of the drug substance(s) or for convenience.

Necessary excipients are selected accordingly. Some tablets are prepared by direct compression of the drug substance.

Moulded Tablets

These are small discs usually containing medicament diluted with excipients, e.g., lactose, sucrose, dextrose, mannitol, etc. The mixture is then moistened with alcohol, hydroalcohol or any other suitable solvent. By pressing the moist mass into standardized mould of metal, plastic or rubber to make the tablets. The tablets so made are dried at room temperature.

Before making the moulded tablets the moulds should be calibrated experimentally for maintenance of the average weight of the tablets.

Chewable Tablets

These tablets are intended to be chewed in the mouth, not to be swallowed intact. The reason for making these tablets is to provide quick and better therapeutic action of the medicament. For example, chewable antacid tablet when chewed acid neutralization may be better as the antacid activity depends on the particle size. Such tablets do not have any disintegration time limit and contain sweetening agent, colour and flavour to enhance the palatability.

Effervescent Tablets

These tablets are prepared in such a way that when a tablet is put into water, rapid dissolution of the drug takes place with effervescence (evolution of carbon dioxide). These tablets contain an organic acid, e.g., citric acid, tartaric acid, etc. and a base, e.g. sodium bicarbonate, calcium carbonate, etc. in addition to other excipients. When such tablet comes in contact with water, a chemical reaction between acid and base takes place resulting faster dissolution there by faster release of the medicament from the tablet with evolution of carbon dioxide. The carbon dioxide generated has the ability to mask the taste of certain drugs. When all the ingredients, drug and excipients, present in the tablet are water soluble a clear solution is produced. Otherwise a suspension of fine particles is produced. Soluble aspirin tablet is the most common effervescent tablet. The main disadvantage of this tablet formulation is its stability. Because the moisture present in air may be enough to initiate the effervescent reaction and the reaction continues with water produced in course of the reaction.

However, using combination of malic acid, fumaric acid or acid anhydride and sodium glycine carbonate or sesquicarbonates stability of effervescent tablets can be improved.

Buccal and Sublingual Tablets

These tablets contain medicaments intended for absorption directly through the oral mucosa. These are held in buccal cavity (buccal tablet) or beneath the tongue (sublingual tablet). These are small, usually flat tablets designed mostly for slow dissolution and for systemic absorption of the drug. When administered by this route the drug is absorbed directly into blood stream through oral mucosa avoiding bypass metabolism or first pass metabolism. This is the advantage over other tablets administered orally. However, these tablets should not contain any ingredient which can increase salivation; because, with excess saliva a portion of the drug may be swallowed and net quantity of the drug for mucosal absorption will be reduced. Usually, these tablets take 15 to 20 minutes for complete dissolution and absorption.

Dispensing Tablets

As the name implies these are to be added to a desired volume of water of known quality to produce a solution of a given concentration of the drug. These tablets do not contain any excipient that may react with any other ingredient resulting deleterious effect in the intended application of the solution. Water soluble ingredients are to be used for making these tablets.

In some cases the tablets may contain buffer substances or any substances to make the solution isotonic. These tablets are less commonly used on a routine basis and the solution prepared with these tablets should never be administered orally. The labels should indicate this caution.

Hypodermic Tablets

These tablets are formerly used to prepare a solution to be used parenterally. Hence, the tablets contained all water soluble ingredients including the drug substance. Although to prepare the drug solution sterile water for injection is used but it is very difficult to maintain sterility of the final solution and since, stable parenteral preparations of most of the drugs are available today these tablets have become obsolete.

These tablets are soft, readily soluble in water and moulded ones.

Depot Tablets

These are alternatively called as **implantation tablets** and meant for subcutaneous implantation in animal or man to provide a prolonged drug action for period from one month to a year. These tablets are small cylindrical or rosette shape. The major problems with their administration are, a surgical technique is required for both administration and for discontinuation, and tissue toxicity in the area of implantation site. Due to this disadvantage the use of these tablets in human is restricted. These are used for administration of hormone in food-producing animals.

Coated Tablets

Tablets are coated to mask unpleasant taste, odour, to protect the drug from light (photodegradation) and air or from a substance of potentially sensitizing or irritant nature (protective coating); to control the rate of release of drug in the body(sustained release coating); or to control the site of drug release in the body(enteric coating).

Mainly there are three coating processes 1. Pan coating, 2. Air suspension coating and 3. Compression coating.

Pan coating is the traditional method. The coating solution or suspension is either sprayed or poured over the tablets or granules being rotated in a suitable bowl. The process is repeated till a layer of desired thickness is obtained.

In the **Air-suspension** method by an upward current of air the tablets cores are fluidized and cycled inside a cylindrical vessel and the coating solution or suspension in a volatile solvent is sprayed.

Compression coating involves compression of dry granules of coating substances around the tablet core using punches and dies.

Sustained-release Tablets

These tablets are formulated in such a way that after release of a initial therapeutic dose of the drug further amounts are released slowly to maintain the therapeutic effect of the drug over a period of several hours. The main advantage of this product is reduction in the frequency of administration but the drug substance is allowed to remain in the body for an unduly extended period after withdrawal of the drug.

The tablets may be prepared from coated granules, or from the hydrophobic matrix where in the fine particles of the drug are embedded. By using inert porous carriers or by coating the inner cores of the drug with a resistant film these products may also be prepared. In some tablets a resistant core is coated by an outer layer from which the initial dose of the drug is rapidly released.

Advantages of the Tablet Dosage Form

 (i) Satisfactory dose precision,

 (ii) Light in weight and compact, low cost, easy to pack and carry,

 (iii) Convenient to administer,

 (iv) Easy to identify the product,

 (v) Better stability,

 (vi) Commercial production is not difficult,

 (vii) Easy to mask the unpleasant taste and odour by coating,

 (viii) Better scope for altering the drug-release pattern, and

 (ix) Consumers' acceptability.

 (x) Tamperproof.

Formulation Considerations

The advantages of a particular dosage form can be made available only through proper formulation design and the good manufacturing practices. As there are number of formulation variables that affect the product characteristics and these are sometimes so competitive in nature that proper formulation design becomes a problem. A scientific optimum adjustment among these characteristics is very much necessary to formulate a dosage form of desired quality.

Hence, some methodical studies are carried out on the drug, the additives and the processed materials (*e.g.*, granules, solution, etc.). These studies are termed as *Preformulation studies.*

Although usually the term preformulation is used to refer the first information / learning phase for the development of dosage forms with new drug substance, while, on the marketed drugs the studies are referred to as *formulation development studies* which exclude the fundamental studies carried out on the drug molecule for its characterization. Whether preformulation or formulation development, the studies are carried out for formulation design as well as for evaluation (analytical studies).

No additive that may interfere in the evaluation method should be used in the formulation.

List of tests to be carried out during formulation / product development studies for development of different types of dosage forms / formulations are given in the Table 2.1 below.

TABLE 2.1

The list of tests to be carried out during formulation development

SI No.	Test	Dosage form	Information
1.	**Solubility** pH-solubility profile ionization constant-pKa common ion effect-k_{sp} thermal effect solubilisation salt formation partition coefficient dissolution	Liquid	Purity, solvent, co-solvent selection pH, stability biological Performance, pro-drug formation, solubility < 1 mg needs for salt formation
2.	**Stability** solid state stability solution state stability bulk stability compatibility	solid semisolid liquid	selection of dosage form selection of stabilizer selection of buffer storage condition additives

Table 2.1 Contd...

Sl No.	Test	Dosage form	Information
3	**Microscopy** basic crystallography particle size analysis	mostly solid	selection of additives powder structure-polymorphism and solvate, dose uniformity and dissolution rate
4	**Powder flow** Bulk density angle of repose	solid, semisolid	selection of method of manufacture, selection of excipients, selection of packing materials, angle of repose, Θ < 25 – excellent flow properties, >40–very poor flow properties
5	**Compression properties**	solid (mostly tablets)	selection of excipients, method of manufacture

Processes for Tablet Manufacture

The manufacturing processes as well as the type of dosage form are designed based on pre-formulation data and the therapeutic need. For example, Aspirin is formulated as aspirin tablet or granules only, not as a solution because of its stability.

In the above paragraph paracetamol or Ibuprofen can be formulated as both solid and liquid dosage forms.

Sometimes the conventional formulation process needs to be changed for other reasons, *e.g.* cost reduction, substitution of additive(s), etc. Even in such cases the studies are carried out to assess the formulation parameters including the stability of the formulation and to examine the compatibility among all the ingredients used in the formulation.

Hence, there should be a thorough knowledge of the additives used for various types of dosage forms and the process to be adopted for manufacturing the tablets.

Direct Compression

Some medicaments, usually inorganic salts e.g., potassium chloride, potassium chlorate, ammonium chloride, etc., aspirin, paracetamol which have adequate flow properties, cohesiveness and also disintegrating property can be directly compressed into tablets after mixing with certain directly compressible excipients, e.g., spray-dried lactose, dicalcium phosphate (dehydrate), microcrystalline cellulose, starch, etc.

Dry Granulation

The traditional dry granulation method involves the blending of active ingredients with suitable excipients and precompression in a heavy duty tablet machine in the form of slugs. The slugs or cakes, so formed, are milled to granules of desired size range which after lubrication are compressed finally into tablets of desired size and shape.

Wet Granulation

The moist or wet granulation method is the most common and traditional for manufacturing compressed tablets. In this method a suitable binder in the form of paste or solution is used to make the granules comprising active ingredients and diluents. The dried granules after reduction to appropriate size range are lubricated and compressed into the tablets. The solvents used for making the paste or solution of binder are water, alcohol, or hydroalcohol.

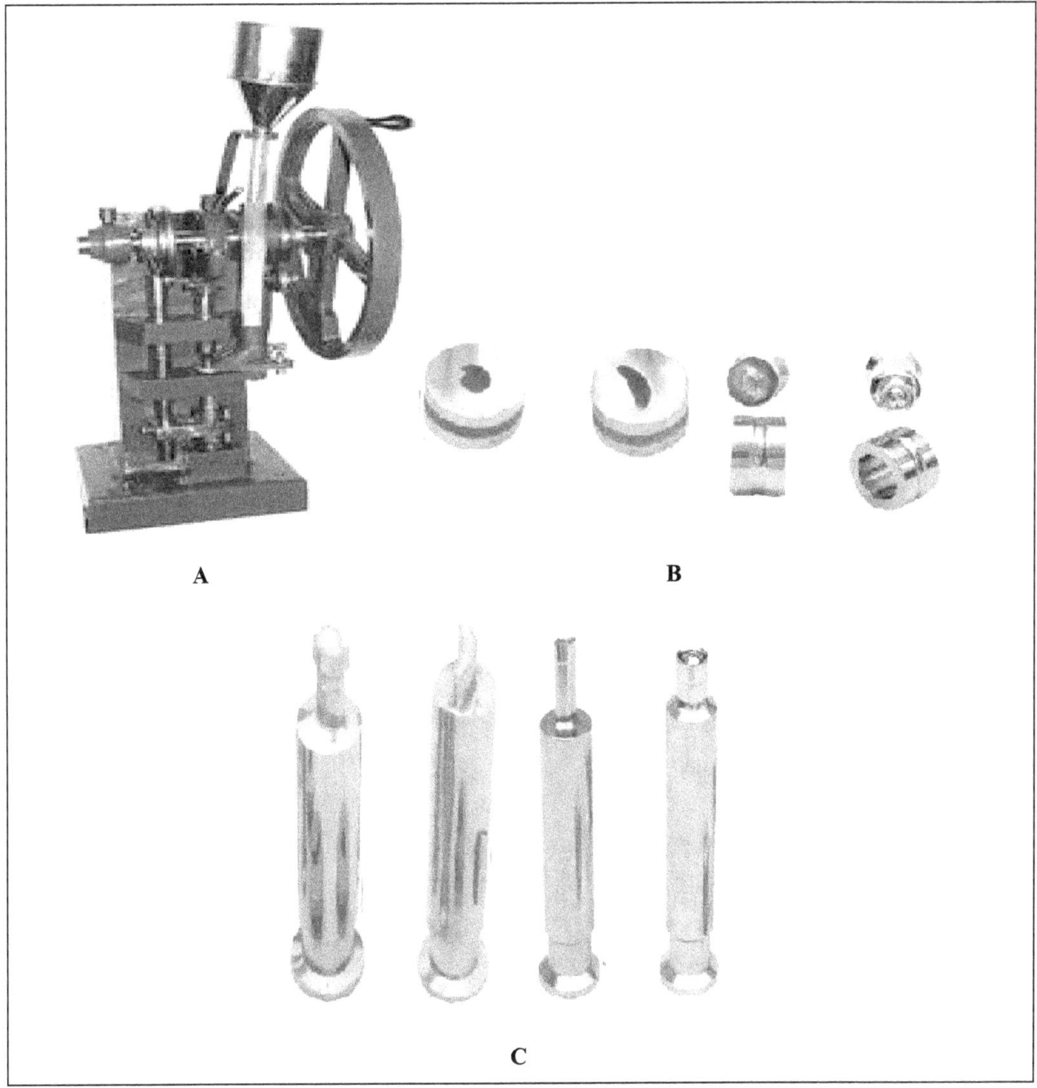

Figure 2.1 A-Tablet Compression Machine, B-Dies, C-Punches.

Types of Additives used in Tablet Dosage Form: The additives used in tablet formulations are presented below in the Table 2.2.

TABLE 2.2

The list of additives used in tablet formulations

Additives	Use or function
Diluent	Materials (additive) usually mixed with powder drug before granulation to increase the bulk.
Binder	Material which binds the powder mix to form the granules.
Disintegrant	Material which helps fragmentation/disintegration of the tablet in water.
Lubricant	Material that lubricates the granules so that the granules pour from the hopper into the die cavity freely.
Glidant	Material that enhances the flow ability of the granules.
Antiadherent	Material which helps ejection of tablets during compression.

Diluents used in direct compression: The diluents commonly used for direct compression of tablets are given in the Table 2.3.

TABLE 2.3

Dilutes used in direct compression

Name	Grade	Moisture content (%)
Lactose	Anhydrous	< 0.5
	Spray-dried	< 0.5
	Fast-flow	< 0.5
Sucrose	Di-Pac	< 0.8
	Nu-Tab	< 1.0
	Mannitab	< 2.0
	Sugartab	< 2.0
Dextrose	Emdex	< 9.0
Starch	Sta-Rx1500	< 12.0
Sorbitol	Crystalline	< 1.0
Mannitol	Granular	< 1.0
Microcrystalline Cellulose	Avicel PH 101	< 5.0
	Avicel PH 102	< 5.0

Diluents used in Wet Granulation: The diluents used commonly in wet granulation are shown in Table 2.4 below.

TABLE 2.4

The diluents used commonly in wet granulation

Diluents	
Lactose	Dextrose
Microcrystalline Cellulose	Sucrose
Calcium Sulphate	Starch and modified starch
DiCalcium Phosphate	Sorbitol
TriCalcium Pho	Mannitol
Polyethylene Glycol	Calcium Carbonate

Binders used in Wet Granulation: The list of binders with their approximate concentration used in wet granulation method for manufacturing tablets are shown in the Table 2.5 below.

TABLE 2.5

The list of binders used in wet granulation

Name	Concentration (%w/v) of solution/paste	Solvent
Gelatin	2 – 20	Water
Starch	5 – 10	Do
Sucrose	20 – 70	Do
Acacia	5 – 15	Do
Methylcelulose (MC)	1 – 5*	Do
Sodium carboxymethyl cellulose (sodiumCMC)	2 – 15*	Do
Polyvinylpyrrolidone (PVP)	2 – 10	water, alcohol or hydro alcohol
Ethyl cellulose (EC)	2 – 10*	alcohol or hydroalcohol
Hydroxypropylmethylcellulose (HPMC)	1 – 5*	Water alcohol, hydroalcohol
Tragacanth	1 – 4*	Water
Sodium Alginate	2 – 5*	Do
Polyacrylamides	2 – 10*	Do
Polyvinylalcohols	5 – 15*	Do
Veegum	2 – 5*	Do
Liquid Glucose	10 – 30	Do

Useful information about the Binders commonly used:

Gelatin: Use hot water to dissolve, use when warm; makes the tablets hard and results slow disintegration; most suitable for lozenges and chewable tablets.

Starch: Can use hot mucilage, on cooling better binding strength is available; proper mixing (wet) is necessary; it is better to use preservative in the mucilage.

Sucrose: Strong adhesive, on storage tablets may become hard.

Acacia: Use good quality, white acacia, particularly for white tablets, filter before use, low quality may darken the white tablets, never use excess, granules will be too hard.

Methylcellulose: Low viscosity grade is preferred.

Sodium CMC: Low viscosity grade is preferred, 2 – 10% mucilage is enough.

Sodium Alginate: May increase disintegration time.

Tragacanth: Most suitable for lozenges for its demulcent effect.

Liquid Glucose: Strong adhesive but tablets tend to soften under humid condition.

Dry Binders commonly used in Tablet formulations: The binders commonly used in dry form are given below in the Table 2.6.

TABLE 2.6

The list of dry binders

Dry binders	
Pregelatinized starch (Amijel)	Microcrystalline cellulose (MCC)
Direct compressible starch (Sta-Rx 1500)	Polyvinyl pyrrolidone (PVP)
Gum Acacia	

Adsorbents used commonly in Tablet formulations:

Silica gel, Silica aerogel, Aerosil.

Microcrystalline cellulose.

Aluminium Hydroxide.

Disintegrants used in Tablet Formulations: The list of disintegrants used in tablet formulations is given below in the Table 2.7.

TABLE 2.7

The list of disintegrants used in table formulations

Name	Concentration (%w/w)
Starch and modified starch	5 – 20
Microcrystalline cellulose (MCC)	5 – 20
Purified wood cellulose (solka-Floc BW40)	5 – 15
Guar Gum	5 – 10
Magnesium aluminium silicate (veegum)	5 – 15
Alginic acid	5 – 10
Sodium starch glycolate	5 – 15
Kaolin	5 – 15
Bentonite	5 – 15
Mixture of organic acids (citric, tartaric acid or fumaric a sodium carbonate or bicarbonate	2 – 15

Glidants and Antiadherents used in Tablet formulations: The glidants and antiadherents with their approximate concentrations commonly used in tablet formulations are given below in the Table 2.8.

TABLE 2.8

List of glidants and antiadherents

Glidants	Conc.(%w/w) used normally	Antiadherents	Conc.(%w/w) used normally
Aerosil (colloidal silica)	< 3	DL-Leucine	< 10
Talcum	about 5	Corn starch	< 10
Corn starch	5 – 10	Sodium Lauryl Sulphate	< 1
		Stearates, metallic	< 1

Lubricants used in Tablet Formulations: Commonly used lubricants and their usual concentrations are presented in the Table 2.9.

TABLE 2.9

The list of lubricants used in tablet formulations

Water soluble Lubricants	Usual conc. (%w/w)	Water insoluble lubricants	Usual conc. (%w/w)
Sodium Benzoate	1 – 5	Talcum	1 – 5
Sodium Acetate	1 – 5	Waxes of high melting point	1 – 5

Table 2.9 Contd...

Water soluble Lubricants	Usual conc. (%w/w)	Water insoluble lubricants	Usual conc. (%w/w)
Sodium Lauryl Sulphate	1 – 5	Hydrogenated vegetable oil (sterotex)	0.25
Boric Acid	1-2	Stearic Acid	0.25
Sodium Oleate	2-5	Sodium Stearate	Do
Magnesium Lauryl Sulphate	1 – 2	Magnesium Stearate	Do
DL-Leucine	1 – 5	Calcium Stearate	Do
Polyethylene glycol 4000	1 – 5	Zinc Stearate	Do
Polyethylene glycol 6000	1 – 5		

Problems in Tablet compression and some solutions:

1. Binding in the Die – Tablet ejection problem.

Observations	Solutions
Tablet sides/edges are rough, vertical scratches, score marks, edges of coloured tablets-light in colour;	Clean the die and punches properly, if worn change the die and punch. Lubricate the granules thoroughly with more efficient lubricant after screening through 80-100 mesh screen.
Cracking or crumbling apart	Moisten the granules, if necessary regranulate. Increase the die-punch clearance. Reduce granules size. Compress at lower temperature and/or humidity.

2. Capping and Lamination – Entrapment of air inside the tablets.

Observations	Solutions
Capping - cracking around the tablet edge, on shaking scale type portions come out of tablet's upper surface.	If capping or lamination is from a particular die-punch, the tooling is defective - check and rectify. Incorrect set up at the press. Development of wear ring – slow the tableting rate, use less concave punches, reduce the compression pressure.
Lamination – after ejection if the tablets splits or cracks on the sides and separates in layers.	Screen the granules and remove the fines. Change the lubricant or quantity of the lubricant. Check the moisture content of, if necessary, dry or moisten. Improve binding of granules. Add dry binders, if required.

3. **Chipping or Cracking** – Problem in binding/sticking/punch defect.

Observations	Solutions
Chipping – Tablets breaks or chips on the edge/faces.	Change the defective punches or polish the punch tips. Check tablet press take-off. Add dry binder to the granules. Moisten the granules. Remove fines from the granules. Reduce granules size.

4. **Sticking** – Sticking of granules to the punch faces.

Observations	Solutions
The loss of granules in the form of film from the tablet surface, usually from the lower face of the tablets; film is stuck to the punch face.	Dry the granules. If punch is Embossed/engraved, use punches with larger engraving/embossing. Either polish the punch surface with colloidal silica or change the punch sets. Clean and polish the punch face with a suitable cleaning liquid, e.g. mixture of light mineral oil and isopropyl alcohol (1:20). Increase binding of the granules. Add an adsorbent, e.g. aerosil, MCC

5. **Motling** – Unequal distribution of colour on the tablet surface.

Observation	Solution
Distribution of colour on the surface is not uniform. During drying dye migrate to surface.	Addition of dye to make uniform colour, Reduce the drying temperature, Reduce the particle size, if possible. Change the solvent or binder system, Add adhesive before granulating fluid and then dry colour additives

6. **Poor flow, Arching or Bridging** – Spasmodic movement of granules through the feed frame.

Observation	Solution
Incomplete fill of the dies, larger particles drift upwards and smaller particles sift downwards.	Make granules uniform in narrow size range, reduce fines as much as possible, lubricate the granules properly.

7. **Double impression** – Punches having a monogram or engraving.

Observation	Solution
Uncontrolled movement of lower and upper punches.	Avoid pre-compression, check set up of the press, use anti-turning device.

Manufacture of Tablets

Step-wise Processes involved in Tablet Manufacture

Direct Compression

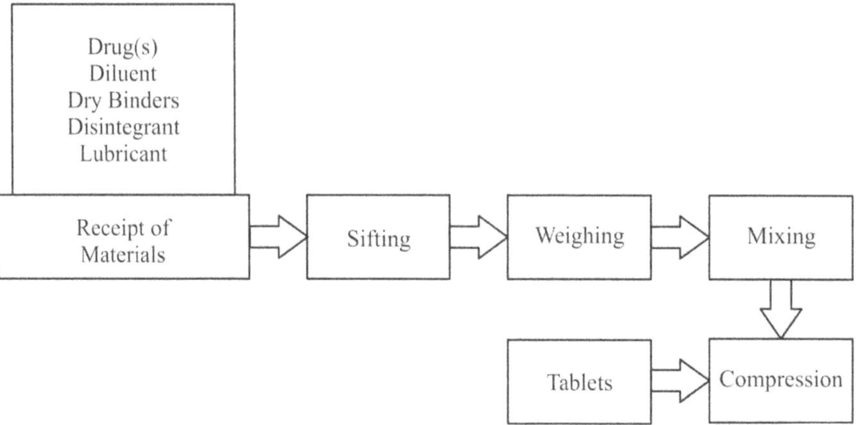

Dry Granulation

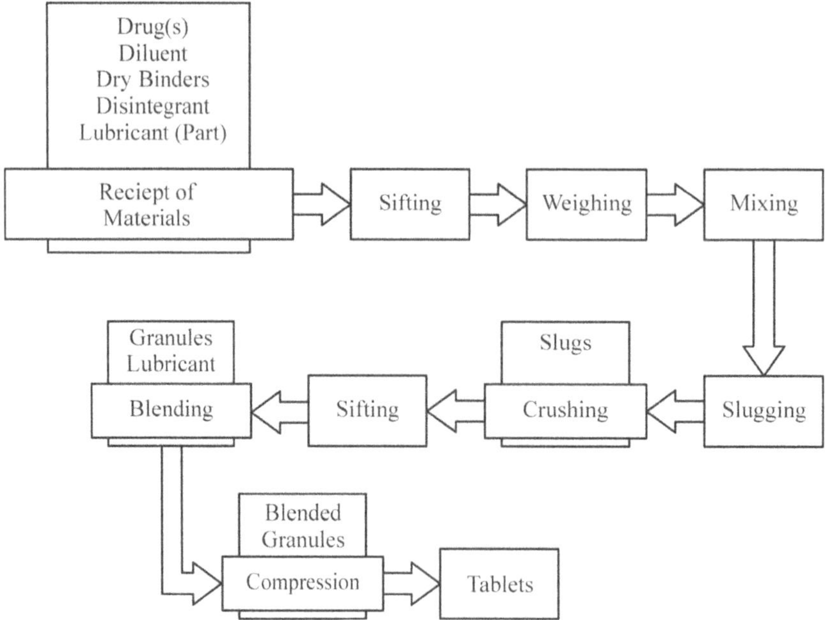

Wet Granulation

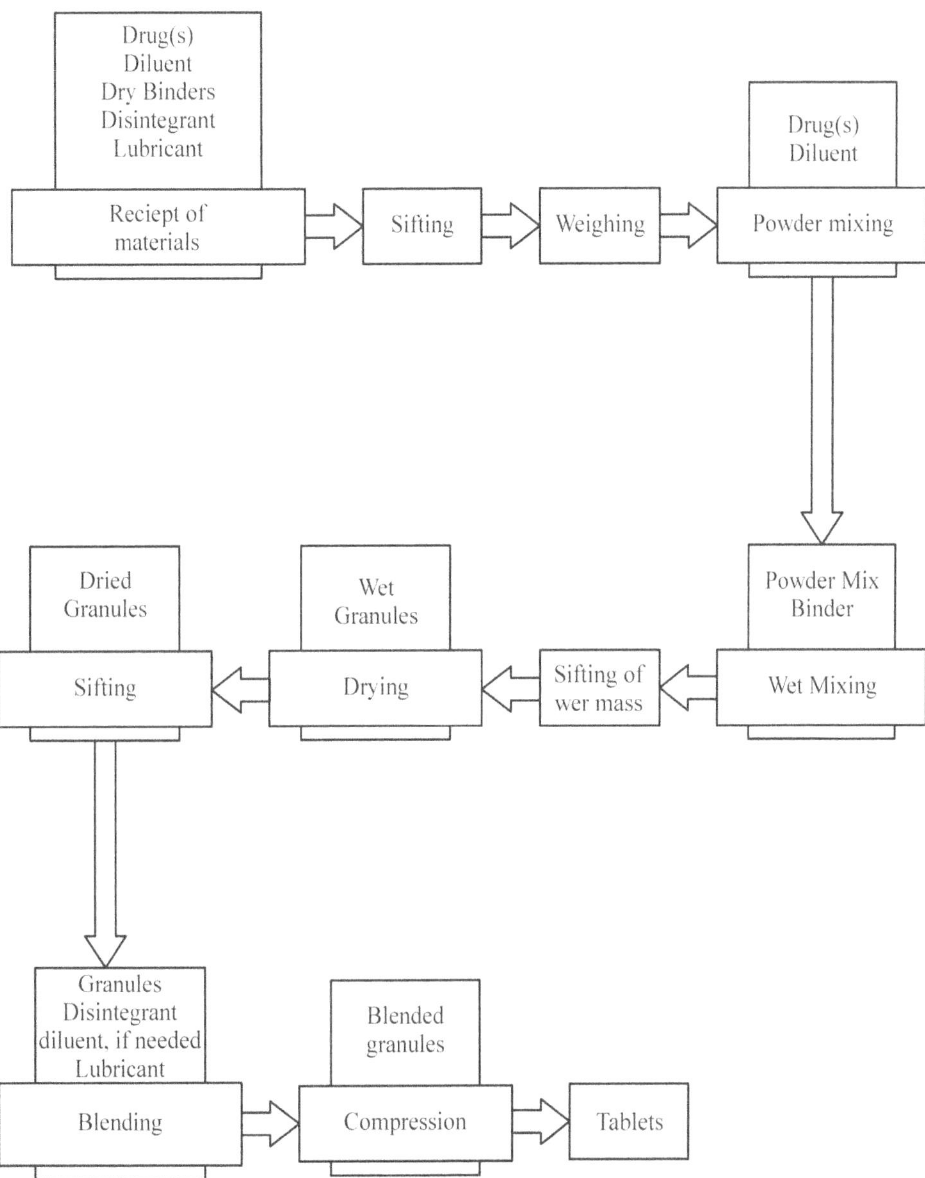

Process Control Tests for Tablets: The tests to be carried out during process control of tablet manufacturing are mentioned with respect to the step of manufacturing are given below in the Table 2.10.

TABLE 2.10

Process control tests with respect to the step of manufacturing

Manufacturing step	Test to be carried out
Granulation	(a) Assay of granules(content of active ingredient per gm of granules on dried basis. (b) Loss on drying.
Compression	Physical tests (a) Appearance, (b) Diameter and Thickness (c) Average weight (d) Individual weight variation (Uniformity of weight) of the tablets (e) Hardness and friability (f) Disintegration time (g) Dissolution test.
Strip packing	Chemical tests; (a) Content of active ingredient(assay of tablets) (b) Uniformity of content (c) Leak test

Method

Content of active ingredient in granules/tablets:

- Draw samples randomly and mix uniformly.
- Take 20 tablets or granules equivalent to weight of the 20 tablets.
- Finely powder in a clean, dried mortar pestle.
- Proceed as per the method described in the monograph or any established and
- approved method for assay.
- After taking required powder sample for assay, use the rest powder for loss on drying.
- Find out the content of active ingredient in the granules in terms of percent (%)w/w and in the tablets as mg per average weight of tablets.
- On the basis of drug content in the granules fix the average weight of the tablets during compression.

Fixing of average wt before tablet compression:

Example,

Manufacture of Nicotinamide Tablets USP. 100 mg

Say, as per the Manufacturing Formula the average weight of the tabs. (theoretical) is 125 mg.

Hence, 20 tabs. = 20 × 125 mg = 2.5 g of granules sampled and powdered.

According to the method of assay, sample equivalent to 25 mg of Nicotinamide is to be taken,

100 mg of Nicotinamide ≈ 125 mg of granules,

$$25 \text{ mg of Nicotinamide} \approx \frac{125 \times 25}{100} = 31.25 \text{ mg of granules.}$$

So, weigh accurately 31.25 mg of sample (powdered granules) and proceed as per USP monograph for the Assay (spectrophotometric method).

Say, actual weight of sample taken is 31.35 mg and actual weight of ref. standard(std.) taken is 24.95 mg.

Potency of ref. std. is 99.90%,

Absorbance (abs) of sample solution at 450 nm is 0.430 and

Absorbance of std. solution is 43

Then, the content of Nicotinamide in the sample

$$= \frac{\text{sample abs.} \times \text{std. potency} \times \text{std.wt(g)} \times 100}{\text{std.abs} \times 100 \times \text{sample wt(g)}}$$

$$= \frac{0.430 \times 99.90 \times 0.2430 \times 100}{0432 \times 100 \times 0.3135}$$

$$= 79.137\% \text{w/w} \approx 79.14\%$$

Fixing of av.wt. of the tablets; granules assay is 79.14%, that is,

79.14 mg of Nicotinamide is contained in 100 mg of granules,

So, 100 mg of Nicotinamide will be contained in $\dfrac{100}{79.14} \times 100$ = 126.36 mg of granules.

The general formula for fixing of average weight of tablets is given below,

$$\frac{\text{strength of the tablets (mg)} \times 100}{\text{content of active ingredient(s) in granules}\left(\%\dfrac{\text{w}}{\text{w}}\right)}$$

Loss on Drying

Loss on drying is the loss in weight in percent(%)w/w determined by any of the specific methods.

Method **I:**

- Transfer 1-2 g of the powdered sample, accurately weighed, into a clean, dried and tared weighing bottle. By shaking the bottle gently spread the powder evenly inside.
- The depth of the powder layer should not ordinarily exceed 5mm and for bulky material 10 mm.
- Place the bottle unstoppered in a drying chamber (Hot-Air Oven or Vacuum Dryer or Desiccator) as the case may be and maintain the required temperature $\pm2^{\circ}C$.
- Dry the sample till constant weight is attained or for the specified time period.
- Quickly stopper the bottle and put in a desiccator, allow to cool to room temperature.
- Weigh the bottle with its content.

Calculation:

Say, weight of the empty bottle = x gm

weight of the bottle + sample(before drying) = y gm

weight of the bottle + sample(after drying) = z gm

then, % Loss on drying = $\dfrac{(z-y)\times100}{(y-x)}$

Note: *Dry the empty bottle properly, cool it to room temperature in a desiccator, then weigh.*

If there is no drying-time mentioned, dry the sample at least for 1 − 2 hrs in hot air oven, or for 3 − 4 hrs. in vacuum dryer.

If there is no drying-temperature mentioned, dry the sample at a temperature 5-10 °C below the melting temperature.

Method II: Thermo-gravimetric method

This method is described in the Indian Pharmacopoeia. In brief the instrument consists of a thermobalance fitted to device for heating and cooling of the substance as per the temperature programme, a sample holder in a controlled atmosphere, an electrobalance and a recorder. The actual procedure and calculations to be followed depends on the particular instrument used. The loss of weight (loss on drying) of the substance being examined is calculated from the distance measured on the graph obtained and expressed in terms of percentage.

Method **III:**

For routine work IR Moisture Balance may be used. An infrared dryer causes water, readily volatile and non-volatile components to evaporate. The total moisture content of the sample is analyzed by determining the energy absorption caused by the intense heat. The results achieved are usually greater than with the drying oven reference method. Briefly the general procedure is (1) tare the sample pan, (2) place weighed sample on pan, (3) lower the hood, (4) shut off the test automatically, (5) the result is calculated automatically. However, the actual procedure depends on the particular instrument used.

Physical Tests for tablets

Appearance: Inspect the tablets for their colour, odour, shape, etc.

Check whether there is any sign of compression defects on the tablets.

Average weight of the tablets: Randomly collect 20 or 40 tablets depending on the drug content and weigh accurately.

$$\text{Average weight of the tablets} = \frac{\text{wt. of 20 tablets}}{20}\,\text{g}$$

Uniformity of weight (Individual weight variation)

Weigh each of 20 or 40 tablets depending on the drug content. As per I.P the individual weights of at least 18 tablets out of 20 should remain within the limits specified in the Table 2.11. None of the weights of the tablets can deviate by more than twice the limits.

Table 2.11 Limits of deviation of tablets

Average weight of the tabs.	Limits of deviation from Av.wt.
80 mg or less	± 10%
more than 80 mg and less than 250 mg	± 7.5%
250 mg or more	± 5%

Example:

Say, the wt. of 20 tabs is 3.4642 gm.

So, the average weight of the tablets $= \dfrac{3.464 \times 1000}{20} = 173.21$ mg

The limits of deviation as per Table is ± 7.5% of the av. wt.(173.21mg) i.e., ± 12.991 mg

Hence, the upper limit is 173.21 + 12.991= 186.20 mg

And the lower limit is 173.21-12.991 = 160.22 mg.

As per I.P the individual weights of atleast 18 tabs out of 20 should remain within 160.22 – 186.20 mg and no weight should remain within 147.23 – 199.19 mg (± 15% of 173.21 mg).

Diameter and Thickness

Measure the diameter and thickness of at least 20 tabs randomly collected using a standard slide calliper. The diameter of the tablet is the punch diameter which should not vary. While the thickness of the tablet will vary with the compression pressure. Thickness should be controlled so that lot to lot variation of a same product should remain within 5% or less of a standard value. Otherwise problem in packaging particularly in strip packing will be observed.

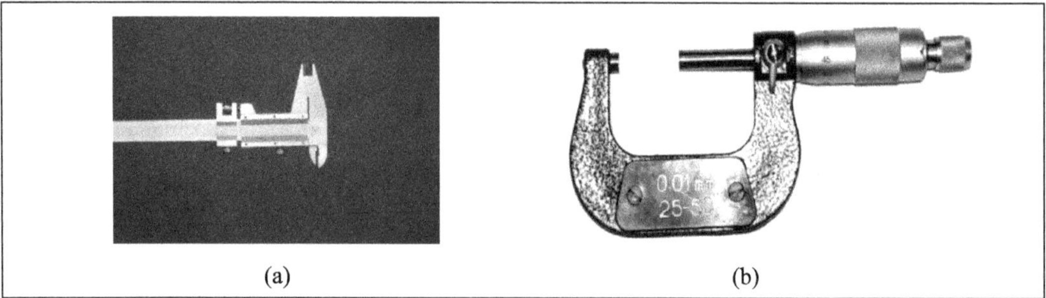
(a)   (b)

Figure 2.2 (a) Slide Calliper, (b) Screw Gauze.

Hardness and Friability

Hardness

To withstand mechanical shocks of handling, manufacture, packaging and shipping a tablet should have a minimum strength which is called as its hardness.

The hardness of a tablet may be defined as the force required to break or crush it a diametrical compression test. This is measured by using various instruments/devices called hardness tester, e.g. Monsanto tester, Strong-Cobb tester, Pfizer tester, Erweka tester, etc,.

Method for Monsanto tester: It consists of a barrel having a compressible spring held between two plunges. The tablet is placed diametrically in contact with the lower plunger and a zero reading is set on the gauge fixed with the barrel and by turning the upper plunger just to hold the tablet. Then the upper plunger is forced against the spring by turning a threaded bolt till the tablet is crushed. During turning of the bolt (i.e. compression of the spring) a pointer set at zero starts riding along the gauge to indicate pressure.

When the tablet breaks, the pointer stops riding and on the gauge where it stops indicates the hardness of the tablet in terms of kg/sq.cm.

For Strong-Cobb tester: In this device the movable plunger is moved by pumping a lever arm which forces an anvil against a stationary platform by hydraulic pressure. The force required to crush the tablet is read from a hydraulic gauge.

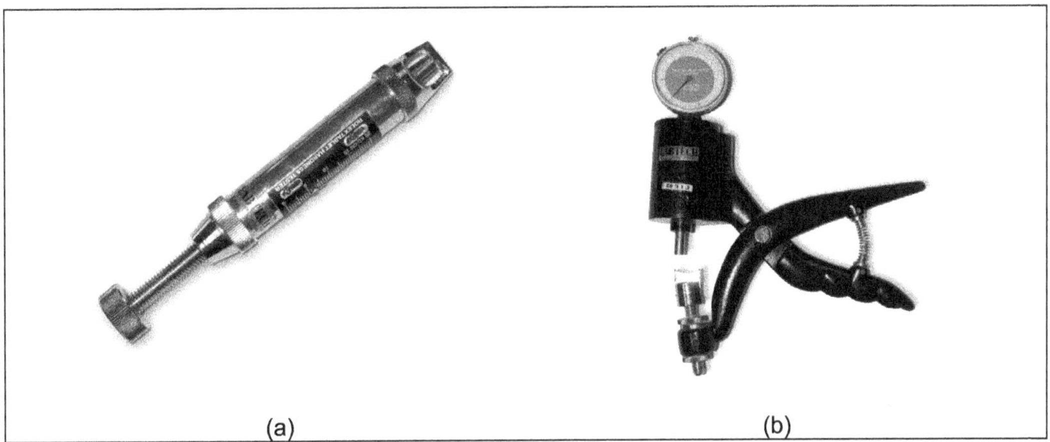

Figure 2.3 Hardness Tester, (a) Monsanto Type, (b) Pfizer Type.

Friability

This is also another measure of tablet strength to withstand both shock and abrasion during handling, packaging and shipping.

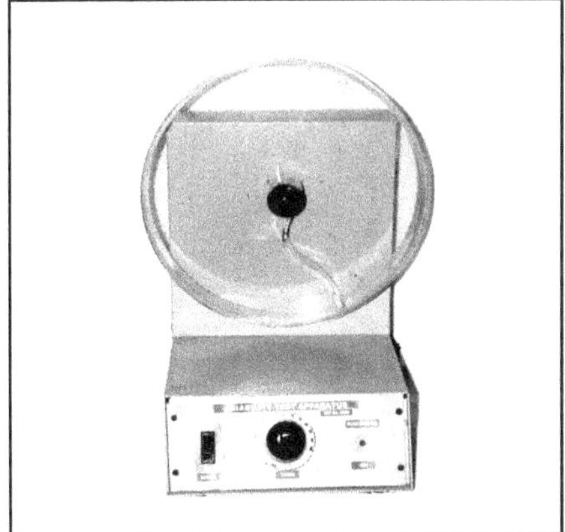

Crudely the tablets are shaken together in cupped hands for about a minute and then inspected visually whether the tablets are capped, chipped or fragmented. But, in the laboratory a friability tester, Roche Friability tester is used for this test.

Method: Take 20 or 40 tablets as per the size of the tablets, weigh accurately and place in the plastic chamber. Close the chamber with its lid.

Figure 2.4 Friability Test Apparatus.

Allow the chamber to rotate at 25 rpm. During each rotation of the chamber the tablets are dropped from a height of 6 inches. After 100 revolutions or as prescribed the tablets are removed and separated from fragments or dust and weighed again. The loss should not be more than 1% w/w.

Disintegration Test

Except the tablets for use in the mouth and modified-release tablets all the tablets should comply with this test.

Method: Use Disintegration Test Apparatus IP. Put one tablet into each of the six tubes and, if necessary, add disc to each tube. Suspend the assembly in the beaker, usually 1000 ml capacity, containing purified water maintained at $37° \pm 2°C$ unless otherwise mentioned.

Operate the apparatus for specified time maintaining the same temperature. If 1 or 2 tablets out of 6 tablets fail to disintegrate within the specified time, repeat the test on another 12 tablets and at least 16 out of 18 (6+12) tablets should disintegrate within the specified time. If the tablets adhere to the discs and fail to disintegrate, repeat the test without discs.

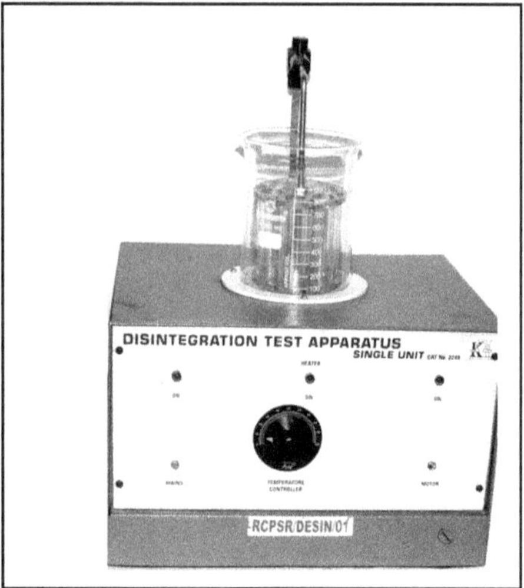

Figure 2.5 Disintegration Test.

The volume of water in the beaker should be such that when the assembly is at the highest position the wire mesh remains at least 2.5 cm below the water surface and at the lowest position of the assembly the wire mesh is at least 2.5 cm above the bottom of the beaker.

Type of tablets	Disintegration time	Disintegration medium	Temperature
Uncoated tablets	15 minutes	water, unless otherwise specified	$\pm 37°C$
Dispersible/soluble tablets	3 minutes	-do-	$25 \pm 1°C$
Film coated tablets	30 minutes	-do-	$37 \pm 2°C$
Other coated tablets	60 minutes*	-do-	-do-
Enteric coated tablets	60 minutes**	mixed phosphate buffer	-do-
Effervescent tablets	5 minutes***	water	$25° \pm 5°C$

*for repeat test use 0.1M Hydrochloric acid.

**prior to this test the tablets are subjected to disintegration test using 0.1M HCl and no tablet should disintegrate or even crack during 120 minutes.

***tablets should disintegrate without agitation.

Dissolution Test

There are two types of Dissolution Test Apparatus, Apparatus 1 and 2. Unless otherwise mentioned use Apparatus 1 consisting of a round bottom transparent vessel having 1 L. capacity and 74.5 ±0.5 mm ID (Internal Diameter). The vessel should be made of glass or inert plastic. A paddle attached to a speed regulated motor. The blade remains about 1 inch above the bottom of the vessel.

Use the dissolution medium as specified in the individual monograph. The dissolution medium should be deaerated before use and should have pH within 0.05 units of the specified pH. As per stated time limit sample solution should be drawn for analysis. The temperature of the medium should be maintained at 37°±0.5°C. Take one tablet or capsule for the test. Fix the speed of the

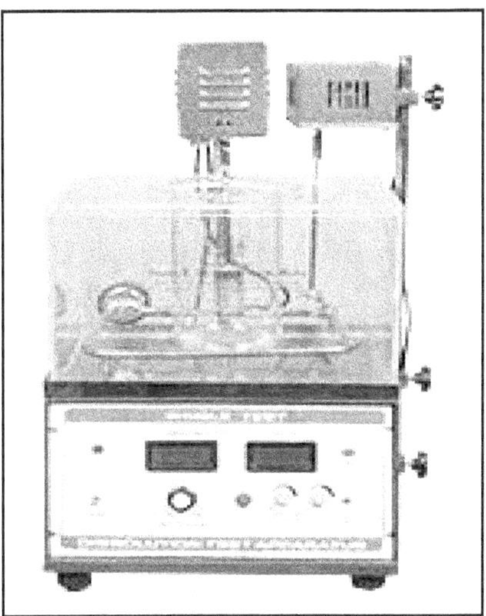

Figure 2.6 Dissolution Test Apparatus.

blade as specified in the individual monograph. Perform the test with six tablets or capsules. When two or more tablets or capsules are said to be placed together in the vessel, carry out six replicate tests.

Determine the percent of drug dissolved from each tablet or capsule (D) at the stated time.

When two or more tablets or capsules are placed, determine the percent of drug released per tablet or capsule in each test. This is stage S1. If the results do not conform to the requirements at S1 stage, repeat the test at S2 and S3 stages as indicated below:

Stage	Number of tablets to be tested	Acceptance criteria
S1	6	each unit is not less than (D + 5%) .
S2	6	average of 12 units (S1+S2) is equal to or greater than D, and no unit is less than (D – 15%) .
S3	12	average of 24 units (S1+S2+S3) is equal to or greater than D, not more than 2 units are less than (D – 15%) and no unit is less than (D – 25%) .

Formulations:

Direct Compression

Product: Methenamine Mandelate Tablets, 250 mg

Standard for drug: It contains not less than 96% of $C_6H_{12}N_4.C_8H_8O_3$ and not less than 50% of $C_8H_8O_3$ (mandelic acid) calculated on the dried basis.

Standard for tablets: Each tablet contains not less than 95% and not more than 105% of the labelled amount of $C_6H_{12}N_4.C_8H_8O_3$.

Composition:

Each Tablet contains

    Methenamine Mandelate   USP 250 mg

Use: Antibacterial (urinary tract)

Lot Size: 1000 tablets

Manufacturing Formula:

Ingredients	Specifications	Quantity per Tablet	Quantity per Lot
Methenamine Mandelate	USP, Assay-100% 12-14 mesh crystals	250 mg	250 gm

Manufacturing Method: No excipient is required.

- The drug is directly compressible, only adequate mesh size is necessary,
- The average weight of the tablets has to be fixed according to the potency of the supplied drug.

Calculation: Say, the potency of the supplied drug is 97.54%

Hence, the average weight of the tablets shall be $\dfrac{\text{label claim (mg)}}{\text{potency of the drug}}$ i.e.,

$$\frac{250}{\dfrac{97.54}{100}} = \frac{250 \times 100}{97.54} = 256.3 \text{ mg.}$$

Thus, for 1000 tablets 256.3 gm of the drug shall be required instead of 250 gm.

Product: Aspirin Tablets

Standard for drug: Aspirin contains not less than 99.5% and not more than 100.5% of $C_9H_8O_4$ on anhydrous basis.

Standard for tablet: Aspirin tablets contain not less than 95% and not more than 105% of the stated amount of aspirin, $C_9H_8O_4$.

Composition:

    Each Tablet contains

        Aspirin IP 300 mg

Use: Analgesic and antipyretic

Lot size: 1000 Tablets

Manufacturing Formula:

Ingredients	Specifications	Quantity per Tablet	Quantity Per Lot
Aspirin I.P.	Crystals of mesh size 10 – 20	300 mg (100% assay)	300 gm
Starch I.P.	Perfectly white, fine, free from black particles.	25 mg	25 gm
Talcum I.P	White, free from grittiness	10 mg	10 gm

Manufacturing Method:

- Take all the ingredients, weigh each of these and mix these thoroughly,
- Adjust the quantity of starch as per assay value of aspirin,
- Compress the mix using 10.5 mm flat die and punch,
- Fix the average weight of tablet to 335 mg,
- Calculate the quantity of aspirin as per the method shown in previous example.

Hardness: 3 – 5 kg/Sq.cm

Friability: Not more than 1%

Disintegration time: As per I.P.

Dry Granulation

Product: Vitamin B Complex Tablets NFI (Prophylactic)

Composition:

Each tablet contains

Thiamine Mononitrate, I.P	2.0 mg
Riboflavine, I.P	2.0 mg
Pyridoxine Hydrochloride, I.P	0.5 mg
Niacinamide, I.P	25.0 mg
Calcium Pantothenate, USP	1.0 mg

Use: Supplementing Vitamin

Lot Size: 1000 Tablets

Manufacturing Formula:

Ingredients	Specifications	Quantity per Tablet(mg)	Quantity required per 1000 tabs.
Thiamine Mononitrate	IP, Assay- 100%	2.0	2.0 gm*
Riboflavine	IP, Assay- 100%	2.0	2.0 gm*
Pyridoxine Hydrochloride	I.P, Assay- 100%	0.5	0.5 gm*
Niacinamide	I.P, Assay- 100%	25.0	25.0 gm*
Calcium Pantothenate	USP, Assay- 100%	1.0	1.0 gm*
Lactose	I.P, spray dried	27.0	27.0 gm
DiCalcium Phosphate	I.P, unmilled	26.0	26.0 gm
Microcrystalline Cellulose	Avicel PH101	26.0	26.0 gm
Talcum	I.P,	6.0	6.0 gm
Stearic Acid	I.P, fine, free from grittiness	3.0	3.0 gm
Magnesium Stearate	I.P, fine, free from grittiness	2.0	2.0 gm

*Quantity shall vary according to actual assay.

Manufacturing Method:

- Pass Talcum, Stearic acid and Magnesium stearate individually through 80 mesh,
- Weigh each ingredient accurately and transfer into a suitable blender,
- Blend thoroughly for 25 – 30 minutes,
- Compress into slugs using 16 mm flat punch,
- Crush the slugs and screen through 14 mesh sieve,
- Lubricate the granules with talcum and compress using 6 mm shallow concave die and punch,
- Fix the average weight of the tablet to 120 mg.

Product: Aspirin Tablets

Standard for drug: Aspirin contains not less than 99.5% and not more than 100.5% of $C_9H_8O_4$ on anhydrous basis.

Standard for tablet: Each tablet contains not less than 95% and not more than 105% of the labelled amount of $C_6H_{12}N_4.C_8H_8O_3$.

Use: Analgesic and antipyretic.

Lot size: 1000 Tablets

Manufacturing Formula:

Ingredients	Specifications	Quantity per tablet	Quantity per lot
Aspirin I.P.	Granules of mesh size 10 - 20	300 mg	300 gm
Starch I.P.	Perfectly white, fine, free from black particles.	35 mg	35 gm
Talcum I.P	White, free from grittiness	10 mg	10 gm
*Polyvinyl Pyrrolidone USNF/B.P.C	Calcium content should be minimum	*5 mg	5 gm

*PVP shall be required as dry binder if granular Aspirin is used.

Manufacturing Method: Aspirin is granular;

- Weigh the ingredients as per Batch composition, mix them thoroughly with 50% of talcum as mentioned in the batch composition,
- Adjust the quantity of starch as per assay value of Aspirin,
- Compress the mix into flat tablets (slug) of 22 mm,
- Crush the slugs to make granules of 10 mesh,
- Mix the granules with rest of talcum,
- Compress the final mix into tablets using 10 mm flat die and punch,
- Fix the average weight to 350 mg per tablet,
- Adjust the hardness to 3 – 5 kg/sq.cm.

Wet Granulation

Product: Chlorpheniramine Maleate Tablets

Standard for drug: It contains not less than 98% and not more than 101% of $C_{16}H_{19}ClN_2,C_4H_4O_4$; calculated on dried basis.

Standard for product: Chlorpheniramine Tablets contain not less than 95% and not more than 105% of the stated amount of $C_{16}H_{19}ClN_2,C_4H_4O_4$.

Use: Antihistaminic.

Lot size: 1000 Tablets

Manufacturing Formula:

Sl. No.	Ingredients	Specifications	Use	Quantity Per tablet	Quantity per lot
1.	Chlorpheniramine Maleate.	I.P	Drug	4 mg	*4 gm
2.	Lactose	I.P	Diluent	45 mg	45 gm
3.	Starch	I.P	Do	15 mg	15 gm
4.	Starch	I.P	Binder	2 mg	2 gm
5.	Methyl Paraben	I.P	Preservative	0.1 mg	0.1 gm
6.	Propyl Paraben	I.P	Do	0.02 mg	0.02 gm
7.	D.M.Water		Solvent	0.2 ml	200 ml
8.	Talcum	I.P	Lubricant	2 mg	2 gm
9.	Magnesium Stearate	B.P	Do	2.5 mg	2.5 gm
10.	Starch	I.P	Disintegrant	5.5 mg	5.5 gm

*Calculate the actual quantity of the drug required on the basis of assay value.

Manufacturing Method:

- Sieve each of the ingredients through 40 mesh separately,
- Weigh the ingredients as per the batch composition,
- Prepare the starch paste (10%) with the items no.4, 5, 6 and 7,
- Allow it to cool to room temperature,
- Mix items no.1, 2, and 3 thoroughly,
- Add the paste to the powder mix and mix thoroughly to produce a wet mass,
- Pass the wet mass through 12 mesh screen,
- Dry the wet granules at 50 °C,
- Pass the dried granules through a screen of 16 mesh and weigh,
- Add the ingredients no. 8, 9, 10 to the granules and mix thoroughly,
- Draw a sample of the final mix and test for loss on drying and assay,
- Fix the average weight and compress into tablets using 6 mm flat die-punch.

Product: Paracetamol Tablets

Standard for drug: Paracetamol contains not less than 99% and not more than 101% of $C_8H_9NO_2$ on dried basis.

Standard for product: Paracetamol tablets contain not less than 95% and not more than 105% of the stated amount of paracetamol, $C_8H_9NO_2$ on dried basis.

Composition:

Each tablet contains

Paracetamol IP 500 mg

Use: Antipyretic, analgesic

Lot size: 1000 Tablets

Manufacturing Formula:

Sl. No.	Ingredients	Specifications	Use	Quantity per tablet	Quantity per lot
1.	Paracetamol	I.P	Drug	500 mg	500 gm*
2.	DiCalcium Phosphate		Diluent	40 mg	40 gm
3.	Starch	I.P, white, free from black particles	Do	40 mg	40 gm
4.	Starch	Do	Binder	20 mg	20 gm
5.	Gelatin	I.P	Binder	11 mg	11 gm
6.	Methyl Paraben	I.P	Preservative	1 mg	1 gm
7.	Propyl Paraben	I.P	Do	0.2 mg	0.2 gm
8.	Glycerin	I.P	Excipient	8 mg	8 gm
9.	Starch	Do	Disintegrant	25 mg	25 gm
10.	Talcum	I.P, white, free from Grittiness	Lubricant	6 mg	6 gm
11.	DM water		Solvent	0.23 ml	230 ml

*Calculate the actual quantity of the drug on the basis of its assay value.

Manufacturing Method:

- Sieve each of the solid ingredients through 40 mesh and weigh accurately as per lot size,
- Prepare starch-gelatin paste (binder) according to the method described in general,
- procedure using ingredients no. 4, 5, 6, 7, 8 and 11. Cool the paste to room temperature,
- Mix the ingredients no.1, 2 and 3 thoroughly,
- Add the paste to the powder mix and mix thoroughly until a wet mass is obtained,
- Pass the mass through a screen of 8 mesh,
- Dry the granules at 60±5°C,
- Pass the dried granules through mesh 12,
- Weigh the granules, mix thoroughly with ingredients no. 9 and 10 for 15 – 20 minutes,

- Test a sample from the final mix for loss on drying and assay,

- On the basis of the assay value fix the average weight of the tablets and compress the granules using 12 mm flat die-punch.

Paracetamol Tablets I.P.

Each uncoated tablet contains

Paracetamol IP 500 mg

Dose: 1 to 2 tablets thrice daily or as directed by the physician. Overdose may be injurious to liver.

Storage: Protect from light.

Mfg. Lic.

Manufactured in India by   B.No. 5642

MNC Pharmaceuticals   Mfd. MM YYYY

Kohka Kurud Road, Bhilai, C.G.   Exp. MM YYYY

                                           M.R.P. Rs.

Coating of Tablets

The reasons for coating of a dosage form are;

- To protect the drug from its environmental conditions,- air, moisture and light, i.e. to improve the stability of the drug,

- To mask the unpleasant odour and taste of the drug,

- To improve the patient's acceptability, so that a patient can easily swallow the product,

- To make a product easily identifiable both to the manufacturer and to the patient,

- To protect the drug from cross contamination during handling,

- To make the product resistant to abrasion, attrition during handling,

- To reduce the risk of interaction between the components that are physico-chemically incompatible,

- The release of the drug can be modified – sustained release product, enteric coated product, etc.

For coating of solid dosage forms, there are four methods usually employed. They are, sugar coating, film coating, microencapsulation and compression coating. The most commonly used processes are sugar coating and film coating.

Sugar Coating of Tablets

Coating process is the last critical step in the tablet production cycle. Sugar coating process involves several steps, the duration of which ranges from a few hours to a few days. The quality of the product depends on the skill of the coating operator. Sugar coating increases the tablet weight by 50% to 100%. Since sugar coating is a long and vigorous process, the core tablets should be resistant to breakage, chipping and abrasion. The shape of the tablet cores should be deep to shallow concave with thin rounded edges to facilitate sugar coating.

The process is done in 6 steps, - seal coat, sub-coat, smooth coat, plain syrup coat, colour coat and polishing.

***Step*-I: *Seal coating*:** This coating is done to resist penetration of moisture into the tablet core.

Seal coating is done with a solution of shellac in isopropyl alcohol or alcohol. Care should be taken during use of inflammable solvent. The tablets should be free from dust, granules or broken tablets.

Place the tablets in the pan, start the pan to rotate with exhaust on. Allow the tablets to roll, apply required quantity of the shellac solution (approximately 1.0 L/lac of tablets) rapidly and spread the solution over the rolling tablets by hand using a glove. Allow the tablets to roll until they become tacky. Dust the tablets with little talcum by sprinkling over the tablets to make them separated from one another. Let the tablets to roll for about 3-5 minutes. Stop the pan to rotate and start for a quick roll, stop it again. This is just to prevent the tablets from adhering. This sort of job should be done for 40 mins at 3 mins interval. During this process hot air and exhaust should be kept on for drying the tablets for 30 mins and during last 10 mins cold air should be blown with exhaust on.

Repeat the same process of coating for another 3-4 times using lesser quantity of shellac solution, 800 ml, 600 ml, 400 ml per lac of tablets. Remove the tablets from the pan. Wash the pan thoroughly.

***Shellac solution*:**

Shellac (Blonde type) 33 g

Isopropyl alcohol q.s to make 100 ml.

Take required quantity of shellac in a clean, dry conical flask; add 70% of required quantity of isopropyl alcohol, soak it for about one hour. Attach an air condenser to the flask and place the flask over a boiling water bath with occasional shaking. Continue heating till a clear solution is obtained. Make up the volume with isopropyl alcohol. Stopper the flask tightly.

***Step*-II: Sub-coating:** Sub coating is done to build up the tablet shape and to round up the edges.

Once the shellac coat is over, the tablets are to be dedusted and put in the clean pan. Allow the tablets to roll keeping the exhaust on. Add quickly adequate quantity of the warm sub-coating solution (500mL/lac) to wet the tablets. For uniform spreading/wetting the tablets should be stirred by hand covered with a glove. When the tablets show the sign of tackyness, a little amount of dusting powder is to be sprinkled over the tablets just to make the tablets rolling freely. Allow the tablets to roll for 15-20 mins to set sub-coat over the surfaces. No excess dust should remain in the pan. If it is there, it should be removed. Dry the tablets for 30 mins by blowing hot air over the tablet bed.

Repeat the process for 8-9 times. The last coat should be done only with plain syrup and no dusting powder should be used. Unload the tablets and dry in hot air oven for 4 hrs at 40°C.

Sub-coating solution:

Sucrose	100 g
Gelatin	39 g
Gum Acacia	39 g
Purified water	72 mL

Take gelatin and gum acacia in a 100 mL beaker, add 3.5 mL of purified water to soak, see that no lump is formed. Heat the mixture over a boiling water bath with stirring until a clear solution/mucilage is obtained. Add the sucrose, stir and boil for 5 mins. Remove the scum. Make up the volume to 100 mL with purified water. Filter the solution through a clean muslin cloth and keep in a clean beaker.

Dusting Powder:

Sucrose powder, 80 mesh	32.5 g
Calcium carbonate, 80 mesh	32.5 g
Gum Acacia, 80 mesh	3.0 g
Talcum, 80 mesh	32.0 g

Powder sucrose, pass through 80 mesh, weigh the required amount. Pass other three items individually through 80 mesh and weigh as the formula. Mix all the items thoroughly and keep in a clean, dry container with lid.

***Step*-III: Smooth coating:** This is done to fill in the imperfections in the tablet surface caused by sub coating step so that the tablet surface becomes smooth.

The dust free sub-coated tablets are to be removed from the drier and put in the clean and dry pan. Keep the exhaust and hot air (50°C) on. Add required quantity of smooth coating suspension (approx. 500mL/lac) in a thin stream over the tablet bed. Stir the tablet bed by hand to spread the suspension uniformly over the tablet surfaces till occurrence of dryness.

Allow the tablets to roll continuously under hot air and exhaust on till dust just start appearing over the tablet bed. This takes usually less than 5 mins. As soon as the tablets are just dried next coat is to be applied and the process is to be repeated until the tablet surfaces are reasonably smooth. Maximum of 12-15 coats are required to complete this process. Dry the tablets at 40 °C for 6 hrs.

***Smooth coating syrup*:**

Sucrose	66.7 g
Talcum	25 g
Purified water	34 mL

Take sucrose in a beaker, add purified water and heat with continuous stirring, boil the solution for 10-15 minutes, remove the scum and filter through a clean muslin cloth. Add talcum slowly with continuous stirring.

***Step*-IV: *Plain Syrup coating*:** This coating finally imparts the desired smoothness of the surface before coating with colour.

Transfer the dried tablets into the pan and continue coating the tablets as per the method described under smooth coating using plain syrup as the coating material. Usually 9-10 coats are to be applied depending on the surface finish. The surface of the tablets should be satisfactorily smooth.

***Plain syrup*:**

Sucrose	80 g
Purified water	40 mL

Take sucrose in a 150 mL beaker, add purified water, stir and heat till the solution is complete. Boil the solution for 15-20 mins. Remove the scum, filter the solution through a clean muslin cloth.

***Step*-V: *Colour coating*:** When the plain syrup coating is completed, the tablets are to be removed from the pan and the pan is to be washed and dried. The tablets are to be put inside the pan with reduced air exhaust. Keep rolling the tablets and pour a required amount of coloured syrup solution in a stream over the rolling tablets. The tablets are to be stirred by hand for uniform spreading of coloured syrup. The tablets are to be allowed to roll till drying of the solution. The tablets should neither be tacky nor dusty. Repeat the colour coating till the

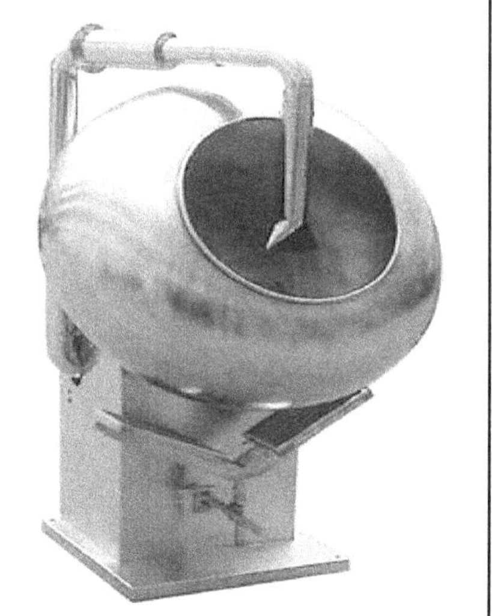

Figure 2.7 Tablet Coating Pan.

desired colour shade is obtained. Each colour coat should be applied as soon as the tablets show a frosted appearance.

The concentration of the colour in syrup should be increased gradually. Initially 25%, then 50% and finally 100%. The colour syrup coats are to be repeated rapidly 3 - 4 times. After last coat the pan is to be jogged one forth of a turn every few minutes for 4 – 5 times.

Keep the tablets in the pan closed with lid for not less than 8 hours without exhaust and no air is to be blown. The last coat of syrup can be applied without colorant, this gives depth to the colour and enhances the elegance of coat.

***Step* VI: *Polishing*:** Transfer the colour-coated tablets into a canvas polishing pan. Keep both air and exhaust shut off. Allow the tablets to roll, pour half of the polishing solution in a stream over the rolling tablets. Spread the solution by stirring the tablets by hand. Let the tablets to roll till there is no smellable odour of the solvent. Repeat the polishing twice with remaining solution and continue rolling till the odour of the solvent goes away completely and the tablets show the desired glossiness.

***Polishing solution*:**

Carnauba wax	2.5 g
Beeswax	2.5 g

Isopropyl alcohol q.s to make 100 mL.

Take the required quantity of the waxes in 90 ml of isopropyl alcohol in a steel or glass container, warm it over a boiling water bath with continuous stirring till the waxes are completely dissolved. Cool the solution to room temperature, make the volume with isopropyl alcohol, cover the container tightly.

***Film Coating*:**

The film coating technology was developed in early 1950s as a substitute of sugar coating. In this method a thin film is uniformly deposited over the surface of a core materials – powders, granules, non-pareils, capsules and tablets. This broad range of substrates makes it different from sugar coating. The solution of film forming materials are sprayed over the moving materials continuously either manually or by automated equipment.

The advantages of film coating are:

- Increase in weight of core material is minimum, in case of tablet weight increase is about 2 – 3% only,
- Processing time is less,
- Efficiency and output of the process is more,
- Range of core materials (types of substrate) is more,
- Occurrence of chipping of the coating is less.

Formerly, volatile solvents were used for quick drying and the solvents were highly inflammable, toxic, costly and causing environmental pollution. With the development of process technology and equipment, the problems have been reduced to a great extent. Presently, even water can be used as a solvent for film coating. Thus, two types of film coating solutions are used, - aqueous and non aqueous.

***Film coating materials*:**

Composition of coating solution varies with the type of solution- aqueous and non aqueous.

The general composition of an aqueous film coating and non-aqueous film coating solution is given below in the Table 2.11.

TABLE 2.11

The list of ingredients used for aqueous and non aqueous film coating of tablets.

Type of ingredient & use	for Aqueous film coating	for Non aqueous film coating
Film former – to produce smooth, thin films. concentration - 5 to 20%.	methyl cellulose, hydroxyl propyl cellulose, hydroxyl propyl methylcellulose	ethylcellulose, cellulose acetate phthalate.
Plasticizer – to make the film flexible and elastic. Concentration - 0.5 – 2%.	glycerin, propylene glycol, polyethylene glycol, dibutyl sub-acetate,diethyl phthalate.	castor oil, diethyl phthalate
Opacifier and colourant – to develop opacity to colour of the product. concentration - 2 – 8%.	food grade lake colours, iron oxide pigment.	food grade colour, Titanium dioxide as opacifier.
Glossant – to provide a glossy appearance.		Beeswax
Surfactant – to enhance spreadability,		polyoxyethylene sorbitans.
Alloying substance – to make water soluble, or increase permeability to body fluids, i.e. to enhance bioavailability.		polyethylene glycol
Sweetener, flavour		saccharins, aspartame as artificial sweetener with suitable flavour, e.g. vanillin.

Film coating can be done by using conventional pan coating method and the film coating solution is either poured or sprayed over the rolling tablets or other substrate. The solution can be sprayed either manually operated spray gun or by using automated spray gun.

Dental Cones

These tablets are smaller in size and administered over the socket following tooth extraction to prevent bacterial proliferation or to check bleeding at the extraction site.

These contain active ingredients like antibacterial, astringent or coagulant. Commonly used ingredients are sodium bicarbonate, sodium chloride or an amino acid; but not any material that can accentuate bacterial growth.

Troches and Lozenges

These are another type of solid dosage form. Troches, lozenges and pastilles are synonymous and come under same category. These are usually discoid-shaped solids having the active ingredient (medicinal substance) in a suitably flavoured base. Commonly sugar candy or glycerinated gelatin is used as base. Sometimes a mixture of sugar and adequate amount of mucilage is used as base. These are intended to be sucked by holding in the mouth so that the medicament is released slowly to result a local effect in the mouth or throat. They are usually used for throat sore or cough. The active ingredients in these forms are antiseptic, antibacterial, local anaesthetic, demulcent, astringent or antitussive in nature. These do not disintegrate, but either erode slowly or dissolve on sucking. They also contain colouring agent, flavouring agent and sweetening agents. In early days, the troches and lozenges are prepared manually and dispensed. Water is added gradually to a mixture of powdered drug, sugar and a suitable gum until a pliable mass is formed. The wet mass is either rolled out and cut into pieces by a cutter or rolled into a cylinder and cut into pieces of desired sizes. Each piece is suitably shaped and dried. About 7% of gum acacia would be sufficient for making the troches. The other gums used are gum tragacanth, guar gum, etc.

When the drug is heat stable, the lozenges are prepared either by candy-moulding method or by fusion. The moulded lozenges can be prepared by using candy base. The drug is added to a concentrated hot syrup and mixed thoroughly. To the homogeneous, warm mixture colour and flavour are added and mixed well. The warm paste like mass is then moulded by using a mould of suitable size and shape or the mixture is rolled into a pipe of suitable diameter and then cut into suitable size. The lozenges thus formed, are then dried at moderate temperature. On cooling these become hard and candy.

When the drug is not stable at higher temperature, these are prepared by compression. The troches are prepared by compression like other tablets. These tablets are harder than usual tablets so that these can dissolve or erode slowly in the mouth. The ingredients which can promote slow disintegration are only selected. As this method involves a compression machine, the productivity and accuracy of the dose is more, and the method is preferred one. When the holes are to be impinged in the troches or compressed lozenges, the core-rod tooling is used. The lower punch carries the rod in its centre and the upper punch carries the hole in its centre to allow the rod to enter into it.

Standard for Moulded Lozenges

Uniformity of weight: Randomly sampled 20 numbers of lozenges are taken for the test. Determine the average weight and weigh individually also.

The individual weight of not more than 2 lozenges can deviate by more than 10% from the average weight and none of the individual weights can deviate by more than 15%.

If 10 lozenges are taken for the test, not more than one weight can deviate by more than 10% from the average weight and none of the weights can deviate by 15%.

Content of active ingredient: If limits for content of active ingredient are specified in the monograph, it includes all permissible allowances for variations due to manufacturing methods and purity of the active ingredient.

Unless otherwise specified, the limits are applicable only if 20 lozenges are taken as sample for the test.

In case 20 lozenges are not available, at least 10 lozenges are to be taken for the test and permitted allowances shall increase by ± 5%.

Compressed lozenges

These are prepared as per the method of preparing tablet using a heavy duty compression machine and the hardness should ensure slow disintegration in the mouth.

Formulations

Product: Liquorice Lozenges

Composition:

Each lozenge contains

Liquorice Extract	200 mg
Anise Oil	0.03 ml
In a flavoured and coloured basis	

Use: Demulcent

Lot size: 50 lozenges

Manufacturing Formula:

Liquorice Extract	1.0 g
Anise Oil	1.5 ml
Acacia, fine powder	3.5 g
Sucrose, fine powder	100 g
Colour, Tartrazine	0.05 mg
Purified water	q.s

Manufacturing Method:

- Screen the powders through mesh 60,
- Weigh accurately the powders and mix anise oil with sucrose powder thoroughly,
- Add acacia powder and mix them uniformly,
- Add measured volume of liquorice extract and mix,
- Take 10 ml of purified water, add the colour and make a solution,
- Add the colour solution to powder mix and granulate, if required add purified water in small quantities until a lump is prepared,
- Put the lump into moulds of 1 gm lozenges, mould properly and dry the moulded lozenges at a temperature below 60°C for 2 hrs, allow it to cool,
- Pack the dried lozenges in suitable container and carry out the appropriate tests,
- Label the product.

Capsules

Among the oral dosage forms capsule is one of the preferred dosage forms because, these are easy to carry, identify and convenient to administer a correct dose independently.

The advantages of capsule dosage form are;

- A drug having unpleasant odour and taste can be easily administered through it,
- It itself has no taste and its physical appearance is elegant,
- It can protect the stability of a drug provided it is stored properly,
- It can be easily swallowed,
- The shells are inert and absorbable in the system,
- For encapsulation much of additives are not necessary to be mixed with the drug,
- The manufacturing procedure is simple and faster,
- During manufacture many machines or equipment are not required,

- Shipment is economic, very little or no damage during transportation,
- It is commonly used carrier in clinical trials of new drug,
- In special circumstances it can be opened and the contents either as a whole or in portion can be dispensed with food or drink by a pharmacist without compromising the quality or therapeutic efficacy of the drug.

The principal constituent of capsule shell is gelatin which is obtained from partial hydrolysis of collagen. The sources of collagen are skin, white connective tissues and bones of animals. Depending on the composition the gelatin shells may be hard or soft.

Hard Gelatin Capsule

The main constituents of hard gelatin shells are gelatin, sucrose and water. The moisture content of hard gelatin capsules within 12 – 16% and with this moisture these are stable and have rigid shape. In cold water gelatin is insoluble but it can absorb moisture up to 10 times of its weight. Hence, if these are stored in humid area additional moisture can be absorbed resulting to the loss of shape and microbial growth over the capsules.

The shells may be colourless and transparent. Usually to improve its look and protective ability opaquant like titanium dioxide, permitted colour and anti-microbial preservative are incorporated into the shells. Sometimes sweetening agent and flavouring agents are also added.

They have two parts- body and cap with cylindrical shape. They are manufactured in different sizes ranging from 000 to 5. Each size has a definite filling volume.

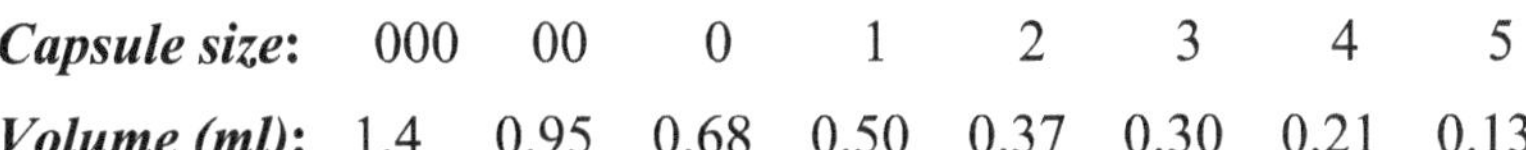

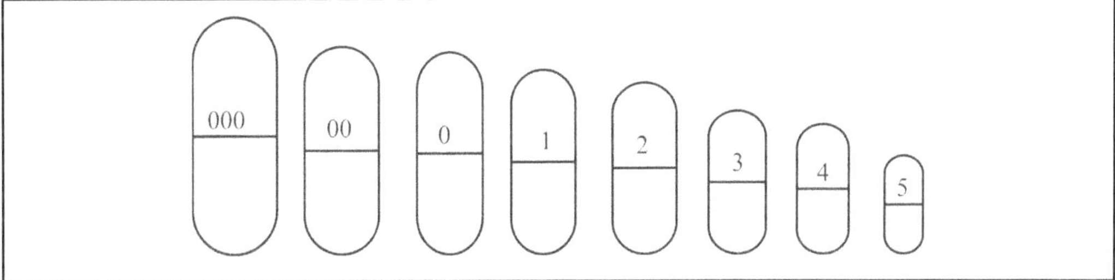

Figure 2.8 Hard Gelatin Capsules of Different Sizes.

Both the parts of shells may be grooved near their rims (snap-fit capsules) so that the halves can be locked after filling.

Although the shells act as packaging material it is treated as pharmaceutical ingredient as per the Drugs & Cosmetic Act, 1948, since it goes into the body along with the drug enclosed. Accordingly there is a separate monograph for Hard Gelatin Capsule Shells in the IP.

Hence, the hard gelatin capsules should meet the standards mentioned in the monograph of the IP.

The optimum moisture content of empty capsules (12 – 16%) depends on the storage condition.

- at very low humidity it looses its moisture and become brittle,
- at high humidity it becomes flaccid and lose its shape,
- high temperature has also adverse effects on capsules.

The best storage conditions for capsules are at temperature, $20° – 25°C$ and with humidity 35 – 40 %.

Formulation considerations

There are five basic steps for manufacturing capsule dosage form with the purpose of providing stable dosage form, correct dose, desired bioavailability, consistent quality and ease of production.

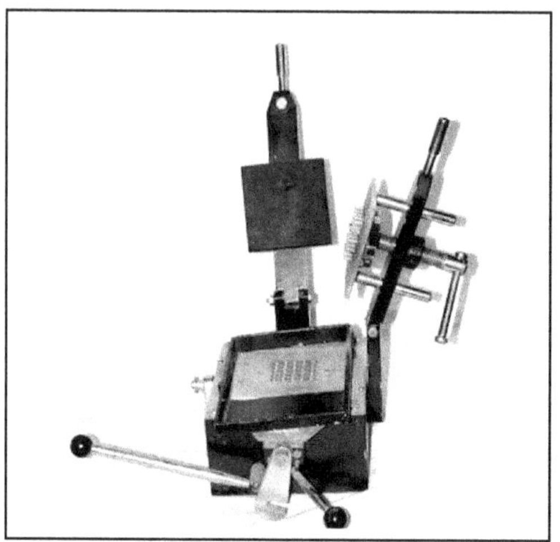

Figure 2.9 Hand Operated Gard Gelatin Capsule Filling Machine.

- Development of formulation,
- Selection of capsule size,
- Filling and sealing of capsules,
- Cleaning and polishing of filled capsules,
- Packaging of filled capsules.

While developing a formulation the following activities need to be carried out.

- Determine the tapped density and flow property (angle of repose) of the drug(s) to be encapsulated,
- Check the quantity of the drug(s), as per the strength of the dosage form, with the capacity of the capsule (size) apparently selected,
- See whether the bulk density of the drug needs to be increased by compaction and granulation or to be reduced by milling,
- Select the diluent/filler to be mixed and their proportion also,

- According to flow property of the powders, select a suitable lubricant and minimum quantity to be mixed to get desired flowability,
- Mix all the items thoroughly and fill in at least 10 capsules(trial lot),
- determine the disintegration time and dissolution rate of the filled capsules,
- If required add sufficient quantity of a suitable disintegrating agent in the formulation,
- Finally check the total amount of the powders to be filled and volume of the capsule selected, if necessary adjust the quantity of the filler/diluent or size of the capsule,
- Once all these activities are satisfactorily completed and the trial product satisfies all standards, proceed for final filling of the capsules.
- Remove the powders adhered on outer surface of the filled capsules by rubbing with a clean cloth,
- Carry out in-process control tests as desired.

Example: Selection of capsule size for Ampicillin Capsules, 250 mg

The mol. wt. of Ampicillin = 349.4, and the mol.wt. of Ampicillin Trihydrate = 403.45

So, 349.4 g of Ampicillin ≈ 403.45 g of Ampicillin Trihydrate.

Say, Tapped density of Ampicillin trihydrate is 790 mg/mL which is supplied,

So, 250 mg of Ampicillin ≈ $403.45 \times \dfrac{250}{349.4}$ = 288.67 mg of Ampicillin Trihydrate, IP

the volume to be occupied by 288.7 mg of Ampicillin Trihydrate = $\dfrac{288.7}{790}$ = 0.365 mL, nearest to the volume of size 2 capsule which is 0.37 ml, shall be required.

Thus, $0.365 \times \dfrac{100}{0.37}$ = 98.65% of the capsule volume shall be occupied by the drug itself and 1.35% space can be left for other excipients.

Commonly used additives in capsule formulations are mentioned below in the Table 2.12.

TABLE 2.12

Additives commonly used in capsule formulations

Diluent / Filler	Disintegrant/wetting agent	Lubricant / Glidant
Microcrystalline cellulose,	Sodium starch glycolate,	Magnesium stearate,
Lactose,	Pregelatinized starch, Croscarmillose,	Talcum,
Starch, etc.	Dried starch,	Stearic acid,
	Sodium lauryl sulphate, etc.	Silicon dioxide, Starch, etc.

Colour is normally used in sustained release formulations and coloured granules are filled in transparent capsule shells.

Process Control Tests: The tests to be carried out during manufacture of capsule formulation are presented below in the Table 2.13.

TABLE 2.13

In-process control tests to be carried out

Manufacturing step	Tests to be carried out
Filling	Average weight, Individual weight variation, Loss on drying of the capsule contents, Drug content, Disintegration test, if necessary, Dissolution rate.
Strip Packing	Leak test.

Soft Gelatin Capsules

Soft gelatin capsules are prepared with varied proportion of gelatin, glycerin or sorbitol and water. These contain more moisture than hard gelatin capsules and thus, a suitable preservative, e.g. methylparaben or propylparaben is incorporated in these.

The shape of soft gelatin capsule may be oblong, oval or round. These may be of single colour or multi colour, transparent or opaque, plain or printed.

These are prepared mainly by two methods – (a) plate method, and (b) rotary or reciprocating die method.

In the first method a warm sheet of gelatin is placed at the bottom plate of the mould, the preparation is evenly poured on it. Then another sheet is carefully placed on the top of the preparation, the top plate of the mould is put and the mould is pressed to form, fill and seal the capsules. The capsules are removed and washed with a suitable inert solvent.

In the second method the capsules are formed, filled and sealed in a continuous operation. Between the set of vertical dies the gelatin ribbons of controlled thickness are fed, through oil lubricating bath over the guide rolls, down the wedge and die rolls. Material to be capsulated is fed by positive displacement pump which measures the material into the gelatin ribbons between the die rolls. Bottom of wedge contains small orifices lined up with die pockets of the die rolls. Capsule is half sealed when the pressure of pumped material forces the gelatin into the die pockets. The capsule gets simultaneously filled, shaped, hermetically sealed and cut from the gelatin ribbons. Sealing of capsules is then achieved by mechanical pressure on die rolls heated to 37° - 40°C. Capsules are conveyed through Naphtha wash unit which removes mineral oil lubricant and then manually air dried on trays.

Soft gelatin capsules are used to encapsulate water-immiscible volatile and non-volatile liquids, water-miscible non-volatile liquids, suspensions, semi solids, and even dry powders. Water or any liquid which migrate through the gelatin shell cannot be filled in these capsules.

Various shapes of soft gelatin capsules are shown in Fig. 2.10 below.

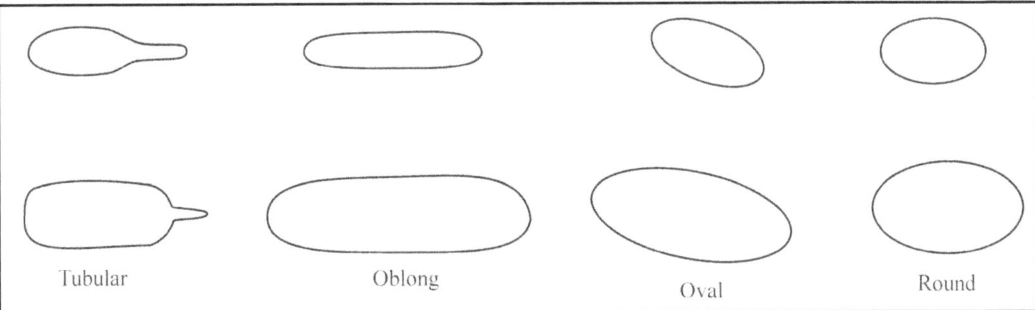

Figure 2.10 Soft gelatin capsules of different shapes.

Difference between hard gelatin capsules and soft gelatin capsule

Hard gelatin capsules	Soft gelatin capsules
The shells are of thin walled.	The shells are thick walled.
These are of cylindrical shape only.	These may be of various shapes; e.g. oval, oblong, tubular, round, etc.
The shell is combination of two parts- body and cap, which can be opened even after filling.	The shell is of single piece, hermetically sealed.
These are alternatively called as Dry Filled Capsules (DFC) as they are used to fill only dry materials; like powders, granules, small compressed tablets etc.	These are used to fill liquid and semisolid materials; e.g. solution, dispersion, ointment containing solvent that does not dissolve the capsule shell.
Shells are hard and hygroscopic. In moist environment can absorb moisture, become soft and lose their shape. In hot environment loose moisture and become more hard and brittle. These require special environment, 20-25°C with 40-45% RH for proper storage.	The shells remain soft throughout their storage. Of course these are required to be stored properly after formulation.
These have fixed volume and are classified into 8 sizes, from 5-000 with average filling volumes ranging from 0.13-1.36 mL. The smallest size capsule bears the number 5 and the largest 000.	The size can be varied according to the need. Usually ranges from 0.1 to 30 mL.

Contd...

Hard gelatin capsules	Soft gelatin capsules
These are less flexible, containing plasticizer up to 5%.	These are more flexible as they contain plasticizer up to 20 – 40%.
Encapsulation is a multi-step process. Separation of body and cap of empty capsule → placing of body in cavity → filling of drug in a single time or multi-times → putting of cap over the body → mechanical sealing of body and cap.	Encapsulation is a single process; as it is formed, filled and sealed simultaneously.
Uniformity of content depends on flow of powders or granules from hopper to capsule body cavity and uniformity of drug content depends on mixing efficiency of powder or granules before encapsulation.	Uniformity of drug content is better because, the drug in dissolved or in uniformly dispersed state is volumetrically filled into the capsules.
Bioavailability depends on disintegration of capsules. Sometimes the filled powders become lump which lately disintegrate.	As the drug is present in solution or dispersion state, the bioavailability of the drug is better.

Minimum Fill Volume

This is calculated from the specific gravity of liquid, if the liquid is packed by weight. The nearest die size and shape is usually chosen. The size of the die can be increased if dilution is desired. The aim is to establish the smallest possible size, consistent and uniform capsule content with maximum physical stability. Solids which are not sufficiently soluble are filled as suspensions. In such cases, the minimum fill volume is calculated by a tool known as "base adsorption."

Base adsorption (BA) is expressed as the number of grams of liquid base required to produce a capsulatable mixture when mixed with one gram of solid(s). Base adsorption of solid is influenced by solid's particle size, shape, physical state, its density, its moisture content and its hydrophobic nature.

$$\text{Base adsorption} = \frac{\text{weight of base}}{\text{weight of solid}}$$

Base adsorption mixture is milled and deaerated, and specific gravity is taken. The specific gravity is the weight of mixture(w) per cubic cm or per 16.23 minims(v). Base adsorption is used to determine the "minims per gram" factor (M/g) of the solids. The M/g factor is the volume in minims that is occupied by one gram of the solid(s) of the solid plus the weight of the liquid base (BA) required to make a capsulatable mixture.

$$M/g = \frac{(BA + S)V}{W}$$

BA and M/g data need not to be obtained on any material that is to be capsulated alone at concentration of 50.0 mg or less. M/g factors are additive in nature and hence, making multivitamin formulation is easy.

The usual shape and Fill-volume of soft gelatin capsules are given below in the Table 2.14.

TABLE 2.14

Fill-volume with respect to soft gelatin capsule shape

Shape	Fill-volume (ml)
Round	0.05 – 6
Oval	0.05 – 6.5
Oblong	0.15 – 25
Tube	0.15 – 30

Modified-release Capsules

Modified-release or sustained release capsules are hard or soft gelatin capsules whose contents are specially prepared or shells or both are specially processed so that the release of the drug contained in them are modified or sustained.

Enteric Capsules

These are either hard or soft gelatin capsules prepared in such a way that the shell does not disintegrate in stomach but disintegrate when reaches the intestine. By coating with cellulose acetate phthalate the soft gelatin capsules may be made enteric coated.

General Standards

Content of active ingredients

Determine the content of drug per capsule using the method mentioned in the individual monograph. The results should remain within the stated range, if 20 capsules are taken for assay, the range depends on the number of samples taken for assay, as shown below in the Table 2.15.

TABLE 2.15

Sample size with respect to the quantity of drug per capsule

Quantity of drug per capsule	Subtract from the lower limit if the nos. samples taken are			Add to the upper limit if the nos. of sample taken are		
	15	10	5	15	10	5
120 mg or less	0.2	0.7	1.5	0.3	0.8	1.8
More than 120 mg but less than 300 mg	0.2	0.5	1.2	0.3	0.6	
300 mg or more	0.1	0.2	0.8	0.2	0.4	1.0

Uniformity of weight

20 capsules are to be taken for the test. Each capsule is weighed individually, the contents are removed as completely as possible and the shell is weighed. The difference in two weights is the weight of the content of that capsule. Repeat the same with remaining 19 capsules.

In case of soft gelatin capsules, weigh individual capsule, then wash with ether or other suitable solvent to remove the contents. After washing allow the shell to stand for complete removal of the solvent. Then weigh. The difference in two weights is the weight of the content of that capsule. Carry out this test with 20 capsules.

Determine the average weight in both the cases.

Interpretation of the results: Not more than 2 individual weights can deviate from the average weight beyond the limits shown below and none of the weights can deviate by twice that limit.

Average weight	Limit for weight variation
Less than 300 mg	± 10 % of av. wt.
300 mg or more	± 7.5 % of av. wt.

Note: Where the test for Uniformity of content is performed, this test is not necessary.

Uniformity of content

This test should be carried out when the capsules contain less than 10 mg or less than 10% of the active ingredient. If the capsules contain more than one drug the content of each drug should be determined and should comply with the requirement.

The test should be carried out on each of the 10 capsules collected randomly, after completion of the individual assay find out the average value (av. content).

$$\downarrow$$

The capsules shall pass the test if

$$\downarrow$$

not more than one individual value is beyond the limits of ± 15 % of the average value, & if none is beyond the limits of ± 25% of the average value

$$\downarrow$$

2 or more values cross the limits of ± 15 % of the average value then, the test should be repeated with 20 nos. of capsules and the results shall be interpreted on 30 values.

The capsules shall now pass the test if,

$$\downarrow$$

not more than 3 individual values cross the limits of $\pm 15\%$ of the average value, and if none is beyond the limits of $\pm 25\%$ of the average value, the lot is considered to pass the test.

Note: *This test need not to be carried out on the capsules containing multivitamins.*

Disintegration test

This test shall not apply to (a) modified-release capsules, and (b) the capsules whose dissolution tests are to be performed.

Perform the test as per the method given in IP for tablets and capsules. Unless otherwise mentioned use water as the medium and operate the apparatus for 30 minutes for hard capsules and 60 minutes for soft capsules.

If the capsules float, use disc and if they adhere to the disc, replace the disc with a removable stainless steel woven gauze having mesh aperture of 2 mm.

Enteric Capsules: Follow the method described as Disintegration test for tablets and capsules in IP. The Table 2.16 presents the type of capsule, disintegration time limits, disintegration medium and temperatures to be maintained.

1. Use 0.1M Hydrochloric acid as the medium and operate the apparatus for 2 hours.

    * there shall be no sign of disintegration or rupture on any of the 6 capsules.

2. Replace the medium with mixed phosphate buffer pH 6.8 and continue the test for 1 hour. The product shall pass the test, if

    * there is no residue on the screen or on the bottom-side of the disc.

    * any residue is found, it should be either fragments of shell, no soft mass of unmoistened core.

TABLE 2.16

Type of capsule, disintegration time limits, disintegration medium and temperatures

Type of capsules	Time limit for disintegration	Disintegration medium	Temperature (°C)
	30 minutes	Water(unless otherwise mentioned)	37 ± 2
	60 minutes	- do -	- do -
	60 minutes*	Mixed Phosphate Buffer pH 6.8	- do -

*Prior to phosphate buffer the capsules are subjected to the test for two hours using 0.1M Hydrochloric acid as the medium and no capsule show any sign for disintegration or rupture allowing the contents to escape.

Containers

The capsules should be packed either in strips of aluminium foils or in blister pack. The strips should be air-tight.

In case of bulk packing the capsules should be packed in amber glass bottles, jars, or vials, in amber or opaque plastic containers, or in aluminium containers coated internally with a suitable lacquer or lined with paper. The containers should be closed with lacquered or lined screw-caps, preferably each container should contain a packet of silica to protect from moisture.

Storage: Capsules should be stored in cool place.

Formulations:

Product: Ampicillin Capsules

Standards for drug: It contains not less than 96% and not more than 100.5% of Ampicillin calculated as $C_{16}H_{19}N_3O_4S$ on dried basis.

Standards for product: It should contain not less than 92.5% and not more than 107.5% of the stated amount of Ampicillin calculated as $C_{16}H_{19}N3O_4S$.

Strength: 250 mg

Composition:

Each Capsule contains

Ampicillin Trihydrate IP equivalent to

Ampicillin IP 250 mg.

Use: Antibacterial

Lot size: 50 Capsules

Manufacturing Formula:

Sl. No.	Ingredients	Specifications	Quantity per capsule	Quantity per Lot
1.	Ampicillin Trihydrate	IP, Compacted	288 mg*	14.4 g*
2.	Lactose	IP, Anhydrous	250 mg	12.5 g

*Calculate the quantity on the basis of assay of the supplied material.

Manufacturing Method:

- Weigh accurately the ingredients and mix thoroughly for 30 mins.,
- Fill the powders into size 1 capsules using a suitable capsule filling machine,
- Carry out the tests, fill the filled capsules in a clean, dry amber bottle, seal with a cap properly,
- Label the bottle properly.

Product: Amoxycillin Trihydrate Capsules

Standard for drug: It contains not less than 95% and not more than 100.5% of Amoxycillin calculated as $C_{16}H_{19}N_3O_5S$ on dried basis.

Standard for product: It should contain not less than 90% and not more than 110% of the stated amount of Amoxycillin calculated as $C_{16}H_{19}N_3O_5S$.

Strength: 250 mg

Composition:

Each Capsule contains

Amoxycillin Trihydrate IP equivalent to

Amoxycillin IP 250 mg.

Use: Antibacterial

Lot size: 50 Capsules

Manufacturing Formula:

Sl. No.	Ingredients	Specifications	Quantity per capsule	Quantity per lot
1.	Amoxycillin Trihydrate	IP, Compacted	288 mg*	14.4 g*

*Calculate the quantity on the basis of assay of the supplied material.

Manufacturing Method:

- Weigh accurately the required quantity of the drug,
- Fill uniformly in size-1 hard gelatin capsules with a suitable capsule filling machine,
- Carry out the process control tests specified for capsules,
- Fill the capsule in a suitable amber glass bottle, put a silica bag inside and seal with a screw cap,
- Label properly.

Product: Tetracycline Capsules

Standard for drug: It should have a potency not less than 950 µg of Tetracycline Hydrochloride, calculated as C22H24N2O8, HCl on dried basis.

Standard for product: It should contain not less than 90% and not more than 120% of the stated amount of Tetracycline Hydrochloride, calculated as C22H24N2O8, HCl.

Strength: 250 mg

Composition:

Each Capsule contains

Tetracycline Hydrochloride IP 250 mg

Use: Antibacterial

Lot size: 50 Capsules

Manufacturing Formula:

Sl. No.	Ingredients	Specifications	Quantity per capsule	Quantity per lot
1.	Tetracycline Hydrochloride	IP, LOD < 1%	250 mg	12.5 g*
2.	Talcum	IP	10 mg	500 mg

*Calculate the quantity on the basis of assay of the supplied material.

Warning: Metronidazole has been shown to be carcinogenic in mice and rats. Unnecessary use of the drug should be avoided.

R_x

Amoxicillin Capsules I.P.

Each capsule contains
Amoxicillin Trihydrate IP
equivalent to Amoxicillin   250 mg
Approved colour used in empty hard
gelatin capsules.

SCHRDULE H DRUG
Warning: To be sold by retail on the prescription of a
Registered Medical Practitioner only.

Dosage: As directed by the physician . Store in a cool, dry place, Protected from light. Mfg. Lic. xxxxx

Manufactured in India by
XYZ Pharmaceuticals
Kohka-Kurud road, Bhilai

B. No. 1234
Mfd. MM.YYYY
Exp. MM.YYYY

Manufacturing Method:

- Weigh accurately the required quantity of the drug,
- Fill uniformly in size-2 hard gelatin capsules with a suitable capsule filling machine,
- Carry out the process control tests specified for capsules,
- Fill the capsule in a suitable amber glass bottle, put a silica bag inside and seal with a screw cap,
- Label properly.

Product: Chloramphenicol Capsules

Standard drug: It contains not less than 98% and not more than 102.0% of $C_{11}H_{12}Cl_2N_2O_5$.

Standard product: It should contain not less than 92.5% and not more than 107.5% of the stated amount of chloramphenicol calculated as C11H12Cl2N2O5.

Strength: 250 mg

Composition:

Each Capsule contains

Chloramphenicol, IP   250 mg

Use: Antibacterial

Lot size: 50 Capsules

Manufacturing Formula:

Sl.No.	Ingredients	Specifications	Quantity/Capsule	Quantity/Lot
1.	Chloramphenicol	IP	250 mg	12.5 g*
2.	Lactose	IP	50 mg	2.5 g**

*Calculate the quantity on the basis of assay of the supplied material.
**Calculate the quantity on the basis of bulk density, quantity of the drug to be filled and fill-volume of the capsule size.

Manufacturing Method:

- Weigh accurately the required quantity of the drug,
- Fill uniformly in size-2 hard gelatin capsules with a suitable capsule filling machine,
- Carry out the process control tests specified for capsules,
- Fill the capsule in a suitable amber glass bottle, put a silica bag inside and seal with a screw cap,
- Label properly.

Product: Vitamin B-Complex Capsules

Composition:

Each Capsule contains

Thiamine Mononitrate IP	4.5 mg
Riboflavine IP	5.0 mg
Pyridoxine Hydrochloride IP	1.5 mg
Cyanocobalamine IP	5.0 mcg
Niacinamide IP	45.0 mg
Calcium D-Pantothenate USP	5.0 mg

Use: Supplementing vitamins

Lot size: 50 capsules

Manufacturing Formula:

Sl. No.	Ingredients	Specification	Quantity/ Cap.	Quantity/ Lot	Overage (%)
1	Thiamine Mononitrate	IP	4.95 mg	247.5 mg*	10
2	Riboflavine	IP	5.5 mg	275 mg*	10
3	Pyridoxine Hydrochloride	IP	1.725 mg	86.25 mg*	15
4	Cyanocobalamine	IP	1.0 mcg	50 mcg*	100
5	Niacinamide	IP	49.5 mg	2.475 g*	10
6	Calcium D-Pantothenate	USP	6.0 mg	300 mg*	20
7	Lactose	IP	15 mg	750 mg	
8	Thiourea	IP	0.15 mg	7.5 mg	
9	Aerosil	IP	0.10 mg	5.0 mg	

* Calculate the quantity on the basis of assay of the supplied material.

Manufacturing Method:

- Weigh accurately each of the vitamins and other ingredients as per the formula,
- Mix item No.4 (cyanocobalamine) with lactose uniformly, add thiourea and aerosol to the mixture and mix thoroughly,
- Mix item Nos. 1, 2, 6 and 5 thoroughly, mix this with previous mixture, add other ingredients to the bulk and mix the whole once again to make an uniform mixture.
- Carry out the process control tests,
- Fill the powder mix into suitable hard gelatin capsules,
- Carry out the tests as the monograph and fill the capsules in an amber colour bottle, put a silica bag inside and seal with screw cap,
- Label the bottle properly.

Evaluation of Tablets, Lozenges, Dental cones and Capsules (Hard Gelatin) etc

Common tests to be employed for evaluation of tablets.

1. Physical Tests
    1.1 Description - Colour, Shape, Odour and Taste
    1.2 Hardness
    1.3 Diameter and Thickness
    1.4 Friability
    1.5 Average weight
    1.6 Individual weight variation (uniformity of weights)
    1.7 Disintegration time
    1.8 Dissolution rate, if desired or directed
    1.9 Loss on drying
2. Chemical Tests
    2.1 Identification tests
    2.2 Assay
    2.3 Uniformity of contents
3. Biological Tests
    3.1 Microbiological assay, if applicable
    3.2 Microbial contamination, if applicable

Powders and Granules

Introduction

The powders, the finely divided solids, are one of the oldest dosage form. Originally the crude drugs had been made powder and mixed with other ingredients, then the mix was divided into single dose packets and dispensed. These became obsolete because of certain limitations, like-

- inconvenience to the patients to take or administer,
- difficulty in dispensing of an accurate dose of a potent drug in this form, and
- less ability to mask the unpleasant odour and taste of the drug,

However, the drugs whose dose is 500 mg or more, slight variation in the dose size does not make any appreciable difference or which are externally used, they are still formulated as powder or granule dosage forms.

Definition: Usually the term *powder* is used to describe a mixture of two or more powdered medicaments, with or without auxiliary substances, intended for internal administration. Otherwise there are other powders which are externally used. To avoid confusion the former is described as *oral powder* in the British Pharmacopoeia.

The granules that are used as a dosage form are prepared from powders which are subsequently made aggregated into larger particles.

Types: The powders or granules may be dispensed as

- bulk (multiple doses) for internal use,
- divided (single dose) for internal use,
- dusting powders for external application,
- insufflations for ear, nose and throat use,
- antibiotic syrup to be reconstituted before use,
- powders to be reconstituted before injection.

However, there are some products which are manufactured as powder but, dispensed as either an oral liquid preparation by adding sufficient purified water (suspension) or an injection by adding sufficient sterile water for injection.

Powders may be classified on the basis of particle size as follows;

Coarse powder: A powder of which all the particles pass through mesh no. 10 and not more than 40% pass through mesh no. 44.

Moderately Coarse powder: A powder of which all the particles pass through a mesh no. 22 and not more than 40% pass through a mesh no. 60.

Moderately Fine powder: A powder of which all the particles pass through a mesh no.44 and not more than 40% pass through a mesh no. 85.

Fine powder: A powder of which all the particles pass through a mesh no. 85.

Very Fine powder: A powder of which all the particles pass through a mesh no. 120.

Each mesh has a definite aperture, called as sieve size. The Table 2.17 presents the sieve size with respect to mesh no.

TABLE 2.17

The sieve size with respect to mesh no.

Mesh No.	Sieve size	Mesh No.	Sieve size
4	4.00 mm	60	250 μm
5	3.35 mm	85	180 μm
6	2.80 mm	100	150 μm
10	1.70 mm	120	125 μm
22	710 μm	150	106 μm
30	500 μm	200	75 μm
44	355 μm		

Oral Powders or Granules

The ingredients, medicament(s) and auxiliary substances, if directed in the form of powders are mixed thoroughly and packed as such in a suitable container, preferably in a wide mouth jar, or the powder mix is converted to granular form and then packed.

The drug with a large dose can also be formulated in this form. The powders may be soluble or insoluble in water. Oral powders may be prepared as single dose or multiple dose and contain flavouring and colouring agents, if specified. The single dose can be packed in a sachet or a small vial. For multi-dose powders, it is necessary to provide a suitable measuring device for delivery of required/prescribed quantity of the powder.

Effervescent oral powders need to be dissolved or dispersed before administration.

Antacid or laxative powders are sometimes administered in this way.

Storage: These should be stored in tightly-closed containers and usually in a cool dry place.

TABLE 2.18

Additives used for powders and granules

Diluent
Sweetening agent (for oral powders)
Colour   ,,
Flavour   ,,
Lubricant   ,,
Granulating agent (for granules)

General Standards

Uniformity of content

1. *Applicable to single dose containers in which the active ingredient present is either 10 mg or less than 10% of the content.*
2. *Not applicable when the preparation contains multivitamins and trace elements.*
3. *If the preparation contains more than one active ingredients, the test is to be carried out for each active ingredient.*

- Draw randomly a sample of 10 containers or packets.
- Open and empty each container and remove the contents as completely as possible.
- Determine the content of active ingredient(s) in each of 10 containers.
- Calculate the average content of ingredient(s).

The lot or batch shall pass, if

1. Not more than one value exceeds the limits of ±15% of the average content,
2. None of the 10 values exceeds the limits of ±25% of the average contents.

If the lot or batch deviates from the above limits, repeat the test with another 20 containers. Calculate the average value for 30 containers.

The lot will pass, if

1. Not more than 3 individual values exceed the limits of ±15% of the average content,
2. Not more than 1 individual value exceeds the limits of ±25% of the average content.

Uniformity of weight: This test is not applicable, if uniformity of content is carried out.

Draw 20 numbers of pessaries or suppositories randomly. Weigh each one and calculate the av. weight. The lot or batch shall pass, if

- Not more than 2 individual weights deviate from the av. weight by ± 5% of the av. weight.
- None deviates by ± 10%.

Formulations

Product: Compound Effervescent Powder

Composition:

> Each packet No.1 contains
>> Sodium Potassium Tartrate 7.5 g
>> Sodium Bicarbonate　　　　2.5 g
>
> Each packet No. 2 contains
>> Tartaric acid　　　　　　　2.5 g

Standard Mixture of packet No.1, content of sodium potassium tartrate: 73 – 77%, calculated as $C_4H_4KNaO_6$, $4H_2O$ and sodium bicarbonate: 24 – 26%, calculated as $NaHCO_3$

Use: Antacid

Lot size: 30 g

Manufacturing Formula:

> Sodium Potassium Tartrate　　　　18.0 g
> Sodium Bicarbonate　　　　　　　6.0 g
> Tartaric acid　　　　　　　　　　6.0 g

Manufacturing Method:

- Sift the powders individually through mesh No.60, check for black particles,
- Dry sodium bicarbonate at about 100°C for 2 hrs., allow to cool,
- Weigh accurately the required quantity of sodium bicarbonate and sodium potassium tartrate, mix thoroughly,
- Determine their contents in the mixture,
- Pack 10 g of this mixture suitably in an air-tight container/poly pack, seal,
- Pack 2.5 g of sodium bicarbonate in suitable container/poly pack, seal,
- Label the product appropriately with the *direction of use*.

Storage: Store in cool, dry place.

Product: Compound Magnesium Trisilicate Powder

Standard

Content of sodium bicarbonate: 23.7 – 26.3%, calculated as $NaHCO_3$

Content of silica: 11.0 – 15.2%, calculated as SiO_2

Composition:

Each gram of the powders contains

Magnesium trisilicates	250 mg
Chalk, in powder	250 mg
Magnesium carbonate, Heavy	250 mg
Sodium bicarbonate	250 mg

Use: Antacid

Lot size: 10 g

Manufacturing Formula:

Magnesium trisilicate	2.50 g
Chalk, in powder	2.50 g
Magnesium carbonate, Heavy	2.50 g
Sodium bicarbonate	2.50 g

Manufacturing Method:

- Sift the powders individually through mesh No.60, check for black particles,
- Dry all ingredients at about 100°C for 2 hrs., allow to cool,
- Weigh accurately the required quantity of each item, mix thoroughly,

- Determine their contents of sodium bicarbonate and silica in the mixture,
- Test for identification of magnesium and calcium in the mixture,
- Pack 10 x 1g of this mixture suitably in an air-tight container/poly pack, seal,
- Label the product appropriately with the *direction of use.*

***Storage*:** Store in cool, dry place.

Product: Calcium Carbonate Powder, Compound.

***Standard*:**   Acid-insoluble matter: 11.7 – 13.1%

Content of Magnesium: 2.99 – 3.56%, calculated as Mg;

Content of Calcium carbonate: 34.7 – 39.6%, calculated as $CaCO_3$

Content of Sodium bicarbonate: 35.3 – 39.8%, calculated as $NaHCO_3$

***Composition*:**

Each gram of powder contains

Calcium Carbonate	37.5 mg
Light Kaolin or Light Kaolin natural	12.5 mg
Magnesium Carbonate, Heavy	12.5 mg
Sodium Bicarbonate	37.5 mg

***Use*:** Antacid

***Lot size*:** 10 g

***Manufacturing Formula*:**

Calcium Carbonate	37.5 mg
Light Kaolin or Light Kaolin natural	12.5 mg
Magnesium Carbonate, Heavy	12.5 mg
Sodium Bicarbonate	37.5 mg

***Manufacturing Method*:**

- Sift the powders individually through mesh No.60, check for black particles,
- Dry all ingredients at about 100°C for 2 hrs., allow to cool,
- Weigh accurately the required quantity of each item, mix thoroughly,
- Determine their contents of ingredients as mentioned under standards of the product,

- Pack 10 × 1g of this mixture suitably in an air-tight container/poly pack, seal,

- Label the product appropriately with the *direction of use*.

Storage: Store in cool, dry place.

Product: Oral Rehydration Salts IP (ORS-A)

Standard: It contains not less than 90% and not more than 110% of the stated amount of each ingredient. ORS may contain suitable flavouring agents and, if necessary, suitable flow agent in minimum quantity required to improve powder flow. It should not contain any artificial sweetening agent like saccharine, aspartame, etc.

Composition:

Each packet contains

Dextrose, Anhydrous	27.0 g
Sodium chloride	1.25 g
Potassium chloride	1.5 g
Sodium citrate	2.9 g

Use: Diarrhoeal rehydration

Lot size: 40 g

Manufacturing Formula:

Dextrose, Anhydrous	33.10 g
Sodium chloride	1.52 g
Potassium chloride	1.84 g
Sodium citrate	3.54 g
Aerosil	0.04 g
Flavour q.s	

Manufacturing Method:

- Dry sodium chloride, potassium chloride and dextrose at about 80°C for 2 hrs. allow it to cool,

- Weigh accurately each of the ingredients including sodium citrate and aerosol as per the formula, mix these thoroughly,

- Determine the content of each ingredient,

- Mix the required amount of dry flavours uniformly,

- Calculate the average weight of the product and pack in suitable container/poly pack, seal properly,

- Carry out the mixing and filling under cool and dry area, at a temperature below 25°C and relative humidity not more than 45%,
- Label the product with a direction of use. The label should also mention the contents of Na^+, K^+, Cl^-, $C_6H_5O_7^{-3}$ and dextrose in m Eq. g.

Storage: Store in cool, dry place.

Oral Rehydration Salts I.P.

O R S   **33 g**

W.H.O RECOMMENDED FORMULA

Each pack of 33 gm contains

Dextrose, Anhydrous	IP	27.0 g
Sodium chloride	IP	1.25 g
Potassium chloride	IP	1.5 g
Sodium citrate	IP	2.9 g
Excipients		q.s

Concentration in mOsmol per litre

Sodium	41.45	Potassium	20.0
Chloride	65.0	Citrate	10.0

Dextrose 150.0

Total Osmolarity 286.45

Store in a dry place.

Dosage: Depending upon age and severity of dehydration.

Infants and Children: 1-2 litres(5-10 glasses) over a period of 24 hours.

Adults: 2-4 litres (10-20 glasses) over a period of 24 hours. Continue treatment until diarrhoea stops/dehydration is corrected. **Solution to be used within 24 hours.**

Mfg. Lic. No. WERT

Manufactured by

QAZ Pharmaceuticals	B.No. 7886
Kohka Kurud Road	Mfd. MM YYYY
Bhilai, CG	Exp. MM YYYY
M.R.P. Rs.	

Caution: Use with caution in impaired renal function or intestinal obstruction. Close tightly after every use and keep away from moisture.

Evaluation of Oral Powders

Common tests to be employed for evaluation of oral powders

1. Physical Tests

    1.1   Description - Colour, Odour, Taste

    1.2   Clarity of solution of powders

    1.3   pH

    1.4   Average weight

    1.5   Individual weight variation (uniformity of weights)

    1.6   Dissolution rate, if desired or directed

    1.7   Loss on drying

2. Chemical Tests

    2.1   Identification tests

    2.2   Assay

    2.3   Uniformity of contents

3. Biological Tests

    3.1   Microbiological assay, if applicable

    3.2   Microbial contamination, if applicable

Dusting Powders

These are nontoxic preparations, intended for local application, and usually contain mixture of two or more substances in finely powdered form. These should be free from grittiness. The fineness of these powders make these more effective and less irritant. The powder mixtures are passed through sieve No 80 or 100. These do not have any systemic effect. Dusting powders are applied to various parts of the body for their protective, absorbent, antipruritic, antiseptic, antibromhidrotic, astringent, and antiperspirant effects. Talcum, kaolin, starch and other natural minerals are commonly used excipients of this type of preparation and are susceptible to contamination with bacteria like Cl. tetani, Cl. welchii, B.anthracis, etc. Hence, before use, these materials should be properly sterilised by heating at 160 °C for at least 2 hrs. However, if the final product needs to be sterilised, pre-sterilisation is not necessary. Dusting powders are usually nontoxic. Use of preparation containing boric acid to large areas of abraded skin of infant can cause toxic reactions. Inhalation of powders containing zinc stearate by infants can cause pulmonary inflammation also. Dusting powders should not be applied to open wounds or to raw surfaces of large area.

Containers

Extemporaneous preparations are dispensed in sifter-top containers or pressure aerosols. The pressure aerosol packages are expensive than others, but with such packaging the preparation can be protected better from air, moisture and contamination. These are also convenient to use. Foot powders and talcum powders are available as pressure aerosols. However, these are usually packed in suitable coloured glass or plastic jars, preferably fitted with a reclosable perforated lid, unless otherwise specified in the individual monograph.

Labelling

Along with all relevant information the label should mention clearly, *For external use only.*

Formulations

Product: Chlorhexidine Dusting Powder

Composition:

Each gram of powder contains,

Chlorhexidine Hydrochloride	5 mg
Sterilised Maize Starch	995 mg

Standard: Content of Chlorhexidine Hydrochloride: 0.45 – 0.55%,

Sterility: It should comply with the test for sterility.

Use: Antiseptic

Lot size: 5 g

Manufacturing Formula:

Chlorhexidine Hydrochloride	25 mg
Sterilised Maize Starch	4.975 g

Manufacturing Method:

- Take about 6 g of starch, free from gritty particles. Dry at 160°C for 2 hrs,
- Allow to cool,
- Weigh accurately 25 mg of chlorhexidine hydrochloride and 4.97 g of dried starch,
- Transfer the chlorhexidine hydrochloride into a clean, dry mortar, add little starch and mix with a spatula,
- Add starch in portions and continue mixing till entire starch is consumed,
- Mix well to get uniform mixture,
- Determine the content of chlorhexidine HCl,
- Pack the powders in suitable container,
- Label properly.

Product: Talc. Dusting Powder

Composition:

Each gram of powder contains,

Purified Talc, sterilised	900 mg
Starch powder	100 mg

Use: Absorbent

Lot size: 5 g

Manufacturing Formula:

Purified Talc, sterilised	4.5 g
Starch powder	0.5 g

Manufacturing Method:

- Take about 6 g of talcum powder and about 1 g of starch separately, dry at 160°C for 2 hrs., allow these to cool, screen separately through a mesh No. 120,
- Weigh accurately each of these, as per formula. Transfer these into a clean, dry mortar, mix well with a spatula to make a uniform mixture,
- Pack the powder in a suitable container, seal and label properly.

Product: Zinc, Starch and Talc Dusting Powder

Standard product: Content of zinc oxide: 23.3 – 26.4 % calculated as ZnO

Acid-insoluble matter: 46.1 – 52.5%

Composition:

Each gram of powder contains,

Zinc Oxide	250 mg
Starch powder	250 mg
Purified Talc, sterilised	500 mg

Use: Astringent, absorbent

Lot size: 5 g

Manufacturing Formula:

Zinc Oxide	1.25 g
Starch powder	1.25 g
Purified Talc, sterilised	2.5 g

Manufacturing Method:

- Take about 4 g of talcum powder, dry at 160 °C for 2 hrs., allow to cool,
- Take zinc oxide and starch separately and dry at about 105 °C for 2 hrs., cool,

- Weigh each of the ingredients according to the formula, transfer into a clean, dry mortar, mix thoroughly with a spatula until uniformly mixed,
- Determine the content of zinc oxide and acid-insoluble matter,
- Pack the powder in a suitable container, seal and label.

Douche Powders

These are water soluble powders. The solutions of these powders are intended to be used as antiseptics or cleaning agents for body cavity, mostly for vaginal cavity. They may also be prepared for nasal, optic or ophthalmic use. Usually these preparations contain aromatic oils, for which the powders may agglomerate and form lumps. To eliminate the lumps these are screened through a sieve No 40 or 60. By screening through sieve the mixing can also be made more uniform.

These preparations are dispensed in wide-mouth glass containers. Glass containers protect the powders from air and moisture. Also the loss of volatile materials can be prevented. Moreover, the users can easily use the material, if packed in glass containers.

Triturations

These are mixtures of a potent drug and a suitable diluent at a definite ratio. When a potent drug is to be diluted in solid state, the drug is mixed uniformly with a suitable nontoxic, inert diluent in a definite proportion by weight, so that the drug content in the diluted mixture remains uniform within the allowable limits. Hence, the dilution should be properly done. Earlier, these were official preparations for dilution of drug from 1 to 10 times. As the name indicates these are prepared by triturating the drug with successive portions of diluent till the drug is mixed with the entire quantity of diluent.

The best method to prepare a trituration is,

- Calculate the weight proportion of drug and diluent,
- Weigh the required amount of diluent, sieve it through a mesh No 40, and keep it separately,
- Weigh the drug accurately, transfer it into a clean, dry mortar pestle,
- Powder the drug to a moderate fine state,
- Add almost equal quantity of the diluent and mix thoroughly by triturating in the mortar,
- Add portions of the diluent successively with continuous trituration,
- Continue the process until entire quantity of the diluent is mixed,
- Earlier, the dispensing pharmacist used to prepare the trituration of a poisonous substance like atropine using lactose as the diluent.

Caution*: The entire quantity of diluent should never be mixed at a time, mixing shall be gradual.*

Insufflations

These are mixtures of micronized powders intended for introduction into the body cavity, e.g. nose, throat, tooth-sockets, ear, vagina.

To ensure administration of uniform dose of the drug an efficient insufflator (powder blower) or an aero haler is used. It is very difficult to administer a uniform dose and for this reason the preparation could not become a popular dosage form.

However, specialised equipments like Aero haler Cartridge, Spin haler, Pressure aerosols, etc., have been developed to administer micronized powders of potent drugs. For example, Aero haler Cartridge of Norisodrine sulphate has been developed and marketed by Abott. This aero haler contains a ball inside the pack. When inhaled, the ball strikes the cartridge and shakes the proper amount of powder and is made free to come out of the cartridge for inhalation. Spin haler is a propeller-driven equipment designed to deposit a mixture of lactose and micronized cromolyn sodium into the lung for treatment of bronchial asthma. The pressure aerosol is the best device for administration of insufflations of potent drugs. This has metered valve which ensures controlled dose delivery.

Cachets

These are one type of unit solid dosage form. These also provide a convenient method of administering a drug having unpleasant odour and taste. Cachets are alternatively called wafer capsules. The cachet shells are prepared from rice flour. The flour is mixed with sufficient purified water to make a wet mass and the wet mass is then moulded to different shapes and sizes. The sheets are prepared by passing the wet mass between two hot rollers.

Commonly the shells are of two types:

- the slip-over or dry seal type, with dome or without dome and
- the flanged type or wet seal type.

The latter type is closed by moistening the edges and pressing the two halves together in a machine.

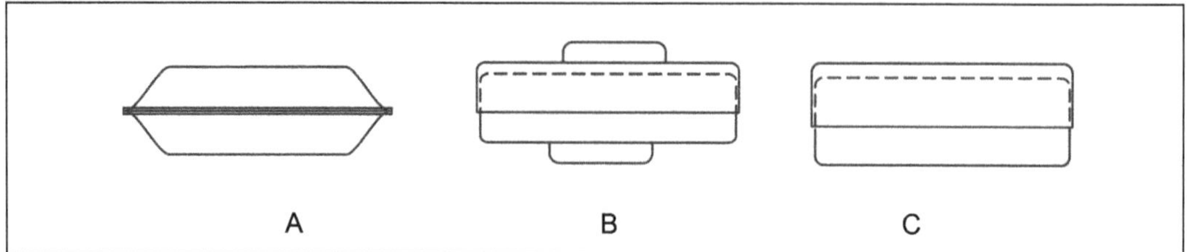

Figure 2.11 Different types of cachets, A-Wet-seal, B-Dry-seal with dome, and C- Dry-seal without dome.

There are various sizes of cachets which can contain 0.2 to 1.5 gram of powder having medium density.

The drug substance with a dose size 60 mg or less are triturated with sufficient lactose to make about 200 mg and then filled into the cachet and sealed. Cachets are not suitable for hygroscopic materials.

For administration, the cachets are dipped in water for few seconds, then placed over the tongue and with a little water swallowed.

The advantages of cachets are,

- The manufacture of cachets are simple and does not require any complicated machinery,
- Dispensing of a drug through cachet is also simple,
- Disintegration of the shell and release of drug is faster,
- Drug being released as powder form its absorption is also expected to be faster,
- Large doses of a drug can be administered and swallowed comfortably.

These have certain **limitations** also,

- These are quite hard and cannot be swallowed directly, a
- Before swallowing these need to be softened by immersing in water for few seconds,
- If dipped in water for longer period, these may become indispensable,
- These are brittle and can be damaged easily,
- The protection of drug from light and moisture in cachets is poor,
- As the shells are brittle the powders cannot be compressed,
- Large scale manufacturing of cachets is difficult,
- Compared to capsules or tablets, cachets occupy more space.

However, cachets are rarely used now a days.

Containers: Cachets should be packed in wide-mouth glass or plastic containers which can adequately protect the preparation from moisture and stress. If aluminium containers are used their inner wall should have a suitable lacquer coating or lined with a paper. Preferably screw-cap or plastic caps should be used.

Storage: Cachets should be stored in dry and cool place.

Labelling: Along with all requisite information a direction regarding administration should be given on the label.

Standards

Uniformity of weight: Draw a sample of 20 cachets randomly, remove the contents from each cachet as completely as possible and weigh individually. The average weight of 20 cachets should not deviate by 2.5% from the stated amount. Not more than 2 individual weights out of 20 can deviate by more than 5% from the average weight, and none should deviate by more than 10%.

Uniformity of content: Mix the contents of 20 cachets obtained from above test and carry out the test for assay as per the method prescribed in the individual monograph. Calculate the content of active ingredient(s) per cachet. It should remain within the limits stated in the monograph.

Formulations:

Product: Sodium Aminosalicylate Cachets

Standard for drug: It contains not less than 98% and not more than 101% of $C_7H_6NNaO_3$, calculated on anhydrous basis.

Standard for product: Each cachet should contain 95 – 105 % of the stated amount of Sodium Aminosalicylate calculated as $C_7H_6NNaO_3, 2H_2O$.

Composition:

Each Cachet contains

Sodium Aminosalicylate   USP   1.5 g

Use: Antibacterial (tuberculostatic).

Lot size: 5 cachets

Manufacturing Formula:

Sodium Aminosalicylate   USP   7.5 g

Manufacturing Method:

- Select the appropriate size of the cachet to be used for filling based on bulk density of the powder (sodium aminosalicylate) and filling volume of the cachet,

- Weigh accurately 1.5 g of sodium aminosalicylate, put it on a clean butter paper,

- Take the cachet, preferably dry seal without dome type and open the lid, fill the drug through a clean, dry funnel held over the cachet, press the powder with a thimble or wooden plunger gently,

- See that no powder falls on the rim of the cachet,

- Wet the inner sides of the top half of the cachet with a wet felt pad and place it down over the filled lower half, push gently the top and ensure firm seal,

- Repeat the process for other 4 cachets, put these filled cachets in an oven at a temperature not exceeding 50°C to dry the cachets,

- Pack the cachets suitably with a proper label.

Pessaries

Pessaries are solid preparations having a shape suitable for vaginal administration and contain medicament intended for local actions. These may be prepared by moulding, like suppositories or by compression like tablets.

Moulded pessaries are commonly conical in shape. Theobroma oil, glycerol-gelatin or hydrogenated vegetable oil may be used as base as in the case of a suppository. A base containing gelatin should be heated for one hour at 100 °C with simultaneous replacement of water lost by evaporation. Thereafter, other ingredients should be added. The base should be formulated in such a way that the pessaries prepared shall melt at or slightly below 37 °C.

For tropical or subtropical climates the amount of gelatin in glycerol pessaries can be increased to meet stability requirement at higher temperature, but not more than 18%. However, there shall be no change in the quantity of active ingredient in the product.

Compressed pessaries are generally prepared by moist granulation, dry granulation or direct compression method as appropriate for the particular drug, and contain the additives like diluents, binder, disintegrant, lubricant, etc., as required to manufacture a tablet. The compressed pessaries are the tablets having the shape of diamond, almond, wedge, disk, or any other.

Formulation considerations

The parameters to be considered for moulded pessaries are same as discussed for suppositories.

Similarly, the parameters considered for tablet formulation development should be considered for compressed pessaries also.

General Standards: Given under Suppositories

The moulded pessaries should meet the standards described under suppositories and compressed pessaries should meet the standards described under tablets or described under individual monograph. The basic standards are uniformity of weight, uniformity of content, disintegration time, etc., mentioned under suppositories.

Content of Active Ingredient: If the limits for content of active ingredient are given in the monograph, the limits include all permissible allowances, including variations due to method of manufacture and due to variation of purity of the active ingredient.

Unless otherwise mentioned the limits are applicable only when the sample of 20 compressed pessaries are taken for the test. In case of smaller sample size, like 5,10 or 15, the limits shall be wider as fixed for the tablets in the Pharmacopoeia.

If the compressed pessaries contain small amount of active ingredient, the sample size to be taken for the test, should be more than 20.

The disintegration time: See under suppositories

Containers: Moulded pessaries should be packed in partitioned boxes, in shallow lined with waxed paper, or in suitable plastic containers. The pessaries should be suitably strip packed or wrapped separately in metal foils when intended to be used in tropical or subtropical climates.

The compressed pessaries are packed in containers as mentioned for tablets.

Storage: These should be stored in cool place.

Formulations:

Product: Nystatin Pessaries

Standard for drug: It should contain not less than 2000 units per mg.

Standard for product: Content of Nystatin: 90 – 120% of the stated amount in terms of units.

Composition:

Each compressed pessaries contains

Nystatin equivalent to 1,00,000 units of Nystatin, U.S.P.

These are prepared by moist granulation and compressed as tablets.

Note: Nystatin is hygroscopic and is sensitive to light, air and moisture.

Product: Lactic Acid Pessaries

Standard for product: Content of Lactic acid: 90 - 115% w/w of the stated amount, calculated as $C_3H_6O_3$.

Composition:

Each moulded pessary contains 5% w/w of Lactic acid.

These are prepared as moulded pessaries by incorporating lactic acid in melted glycerol suppositories base. Average weight of these pessaries would be 8 g.

Suppositories

These are solid preparations of various weights, suitably shaped containing medicaments for introduction into human body cavities. Suppositories are intended for three purposes,

- local action, for example, anaesthetics like cinchocaine, benzocaine; astringents like bismuth subgallate, extract of hamamelis or tannic acid and anti-inflammatory like hydrocortisone are administered in the form of suppositories to relieve from pain and irritation of haemorrhoids in the rectum.

- evacuation of bowel, for example, laxative like glycerol and bisacodyl are used,

- systemic effect of the drug incorporated in them, for example, few drugs like aminophylline (anti-asthmatic and anti-bronchitic), indomethacin, phenylbutazone (analgesic and anti-inflammatory), etc., are administered in the form of suppositories.

Suppositories are best suited to the patients who are infants, unconscious, mentally disturbed or who cannot take medicines orally for other reasons.

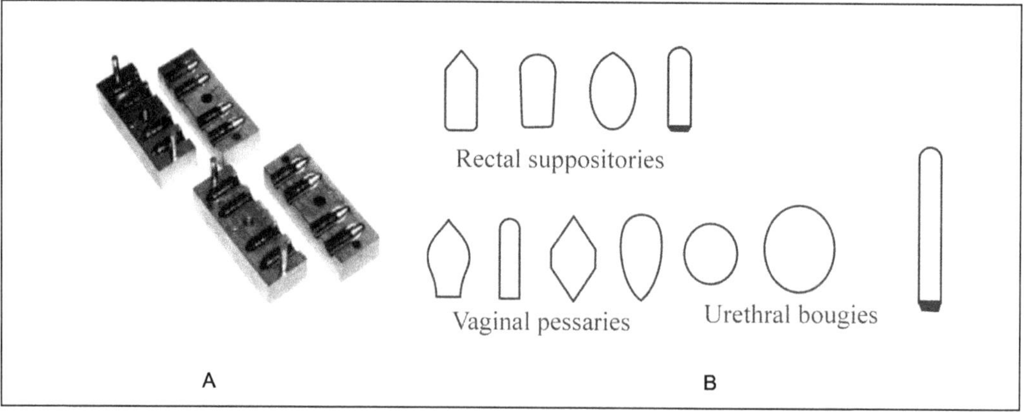

Figure 2.12 A. Suppositories Moulds, B. Different shapes of Suppositories.

Formulation Considerations

While manufacturing the powder dosage form, the compatibility with other excipients, stability studies and other physicochemical properties of the drug substance, e.g., colour, odour, taste, solubility, melting point, bulk density, flow property, etc., need to be determined.

Accordingly, the storage conditions and container are to be selected to ensure maximum stability of the product and also easy to handle. However, a standardized packing material, e.g. a sachet cannot be changed regularly to accommodate size variation from lot to lot. Hence, during purchase of raw materials, the specifications for the bulk density needs to be considered.

Similarly, during granulation the physicochemical property of the drug need to be considered, e.g. if the drug is hydrolysable or decomposable in presence of moisture, water should not be used as granulating solvent and moisture content of the product as a whole needs to be optimized.

Rectal or vaginal absorption of drug from suppositories depends mainly on,

- Physical state of the medicament,
- Partition coefficient of the drug,
- Excipient present, and
- pH of the rectal or vaginal secretions.

There are two types of suppository base,

- Fatty bases, natural and synthetic bases which melt at body temperature, and
- Water soluble and water miscible bases which either dissolve or disperse in rectal secretions.

Fatty bases may be natural, e.g., theobroma oil or synthetic, e.g., hydrolysed-hydrogenated vegetable oils. Theobroma oil has the advantages, like

- Low melting point and quick setting,
- Blandness, and
- Compatibility with many ingredients.

But, it has also disadvantages like,

- It absorbs water poorly,
- Leaks from the body,
- Deteriorates on storage,
- Not very stable in tropical climate,
- Soluble ingredients can lower the melting point,
- Adheres to mould, and
- Not very economic also.

Glycerol-gelatin also has certain limitations,

- Itself is a laxative,
- Not very easy to handle and prepare,
- Solubility depends on the quality of gelatine, and
- More important is its incompatibility with certain substances.

Macrogols have some advantages,

- By varying the proportion of the polymers physical properties of the base can be modified,
- Melting point being around 42°C suitable for tropical climate,
- Does not adhere to the mould,
- Water absorbability is high,
- Low leakage from the body, and
- Dispersion in the body is good.

But, it suffers from the following limitations,

- more hygroscopic,
- slowly release the drug,
- can cause crystal growth of certain drugs, and
- on storage may become granular and brittle.

Thus, every base has some benefits and limitations. The selection of the base should be done judiciously.

Calibration of Moulds: The volume of the mould is fixed and the nominal capacity of the mould is usually measured with respect to base. But, the volume of a formulation may vary with the density of the substance(s) mixed with the base. Thus, the nominal capacity of a mould, in terms of weight, needs to be standardised before casting the preparation. The amount of base is to be adjusted with respect to the formulation. The simple and convenient method is the use of *Displacement value* of the medicament – *the number of unit weights of a medicament which can displace one unit of base.*

Example 1: Prepare 6 suppositories, each containing 300 mg of a drug. The density of the drug is 2.8 g/ml and density of the suppository base is 0.93 g/ml. The mould has nominal capacity of 2 g.

The weight of drug required for 6 suppositories = 6 × 0.3 = 1.8 g

As per nominal capacity, the amount of base of the suppository = 2.0 g

The density ratio of drug and base = 2.8 / 0.93 = 3.01

The amount of base displaced by the drug = 2.0 / 3.01 = 0.664

Thus, the amount of base to be required for 6 suppositories $= 6 \times 2 - 0.664$
$= 12 - 0.664 = 11.336$ g

And the average weight of 6 suppositories $= \dfrac{(1.8 + 11.336)}{6} = 2.19$ g.

Example 2: Use of Displacement value.

Prepare 6 suppositories of 1 g, containing 300 mg of a drug.

Say, weight of 6 suppositories containing drug + base $= 7.2$ g

As per nominal capacity, weight of 6 suppositories of the base $= 6$ g

So, the average content of base $= 70 \times \dfrac{7.2}{100} = 5.04$

The average content of drug $= 30 \times \dfrac{7.2}{100} = 2.16$

The base displaced by 2.46 g drug $= 6 - 5.04 = 0.96$ g

Therefore, the displacement value of the drug $= \dfrac{2.16}{0.96} = 2.25$

Example 3: Use of Displacement value prepare 6 suppositories of 1g, each containing 300 mg of a drug having displacement value of 3.

For 6 suppositories, the amount of drug required $= 6 \times 300$ mg $= 1.8$ g,

The displacement value is 3, i.e., 3 g of the drug displace 1 g of the base.

So, 1.8 g of drug can displace, $1 \times 1.8/3 = 0.6$ g of the base,

So, the amount of base required for 6 suppositories of 1 g $= 6 \times 1 - 0.6 = 5.4$ g

And the amount of drug required for 6 suppositories is 1.8 g,

The total weight of 6 suppositories $= 5.4 + 1.8 = 7.2$ g and average weight will be $\dfrac{7.2}{6} = 1.2$ g.

Note: This method *can be used for preparing pessaries also.*

General Standards

Uniformity of container content: Applicable to tablets, capsules, suppositories, pessaries packed in containers.

Draw a sample of 10 containers randomly. Count the numbers of units (contents) packed in each container. The lot or batch shall pass, if

- The average number of units in the 10 containers shall not be less than the labelled numbers.

- No single container shall contain the numbers of units beyond the limits of ± 2% of the labelled numbers.

If failed, repeat the test with another sample of 10 containers. The lot or batch shall pass, if

- Not more than one out of 20 (previous 10 + present 10) deviates from the limits of ± 2% of the labelled numbers.

Uniformity of content: Applicable to pessaries, suppositories which contain less than 10 mg or less than 10% of the active ingredient.

The test should be carried out only on a pooled sample of a preparation as directed in the individual monograph.

According to IP this test is not applicable to preparations containing multivitamins and trace elements.

Uniformity of weight: This test is not applicable, if uniformity of content is carried out.

Draw 20 numbers of pessaries or suppositories randomly. Weigh each one and calculate the av. weight. The lot or batch shall pass, if

- Not more than 2 individual weights deviate from the average weight by ± 5% of the average weight.

- None deviates by ± 10%.

Disintegration Test: This test is not applicable to the pessaries or suppositories made for prolonged local action or for modified release.

The test should be carried out as per the method followed for Tablets or capsules.

The **Disintegration time limits** for Moulded pessaries/suppositories : Not more than 60 minutes.

for compressed pessaries/suppositories : Not more than 30 minutes.

for shell pessaries/suppositories : Not more than 30 minutes.

Additives used for powders and granules commonly used are shown in the Table 2.19 below.

TABLE 2.19

Additives used for powders and granules

Diluent
Sweetening agent (for oral powders)
Colour   ,,
Flavour   ,,
Lubricant   "
Granulating agent (for granules)

Formulations

Product: Compound Bismuth and Resorcin Suppositories.

Composition:

> Each suppository contains

Bismuth subgallate	200 mg
Resorcinol	60 mg
Zinc oxide	120 mg
Castor oil	60 mg

> In a suitable base.

Use: Analgesic and antipruritic.

Lot size: 6 suppositories of 1g each.

Manufacturing Formula:

Bismuth subgallate	1.2 g
Resorcinol	0.36g
Zinc oxide	0.72g
Castor oil	0.36g
Theobroma oil	4.86g*

*the amount of theobroma oil is calculated as follows;

Ingredient	Displacement value	Qty. required for 6 suppositories	Quantity of theobroma oil being displaced	
Bismuth subgallate	3	1.2 g	1.2/3	= 0.400 g
Resorcinol	1.5	0.36 g	0.36/1.5	= 0.24 g
Zinc oxide	5	0.72 g	0.72/5	= 0.144 g
Castor oil	1	0.36 g	0.36/1	= <u>0.36 g</u>
Total amount of theobroma oil will be displaced				= 1.144 g

Hence, Theobroma oil to be required for 6 suppositories will be $6 - 1.144g = 4.856$ g.

***Manufacturing Method*:**

- Weigh accurately each of bismuth subgallate, zinc oxide and resorcinol, transfer these into a clean, dry mortar pestle,
- Powder these finely, add weighed amount of castor oil and make into a smooth paste,
- Melt the weighed quantity of theobroma oil, add gradually and mix with the paste uniformly,
- Lubricate the clean, dry moulds with a tinge of talcum, pour the paste into the moulds, if necessary, warm the paste before pouring,
- Allow the suppositories to solidify,
- Once the suppositories completely solidify open the mould and carry out the tests,
- Pack these suitably by wrapping with a butter paper, label properly.

Product: Hamamelis Suppositories

***Composition*:**

Each suppository contains

Hamamelis Extract 200 mg

In a suitable base.

***Use*:** Used in internal haemorrhoids and anal fissures.

***Lot size*:** 6 suppositories of 1g each.

***Manufacturing Formula*:**

Hamamelis Dry Extract	1.2g
Theobroma oil	5.2g

***Manufacturing Method*:**

- Take 1.2 g of Hamamelis Dry Extract into a clean, dry mortar pestle, powder it finely,
- Melt the weighed quantity of theobroma oil over boiling water bath, pour a portion of it to the mortar, make a smooth paste,
- Add the rest amount of melted base and mix thoroughly,
- Pour the mixture into clean, dry and lubricated moulds, allow to stand,
- When the suppositories solidify completely, remove these from the moulds,

- Carry out the tests, pack these suitably by wrapping with butter paper,
- Label the product properly.

Exercises

Short Questions

1. (a) Name different types of tablets.
   (b) What is the time limit for disintegration of chewable tablets?
   (c) Name different types of capsules.
   (d) Write the best storage conditions for hard gelatin capsules.
   (e) Define effervescent and dispersible tablets.
   (f) Name few dosage forms inserted into body cavity.
   (g) What is an additive?
   (h) What is average weight?
   (i) What is a diluent? Name three materials used as diluent in solid dosage form.
   (j) What is displacement value?
   (k) What is minimum fill volume?
   (l) Name the methods used for manufacture of tablets.
   (m) Name different shapes of soft gelatin capsules.
   (n) Name at least two materials used as disintegrants.
   (o) Name at least three materials used as binder in wet granulation method.
   (p) How dental cones are administered?
   (q) What are various types of coating?
   (r) Which materials are suitable for filling in soft gelatin capsules?
   (s) What for the pessaries are used?
   (t) What are uses of suppositories?
   (u) What are the limits of weight variation with respect to av. weight of capsules?
   (v) Name different sizes of hard gelatin capsules.
   (w) What is the optimum moister content of empty hard gelatin capsules?
   (x) Name different steps of sugar coating of tablets.
   (y) What are compressed tablets and moulded tablets?

2. Discuss the steps of tablet manufacture using wet granulation technique.

3. Name the excipients used in tablet formulations. Mention at least two examples of each type.

4. Distinguish between hard gelatin capsules and soft gelatin capsules.

5. Write down at least three problems which may occur during tablet compression and their   solutions.

6. Describe briefly the different steps of sugar coating of tablets.

7. Make a list of tests to be carried out during process control of tablet manufacturing and capsule filling.

8. Illustrate with suitable example how the displacement value is useful to calculate the amount of base for moulding suppositories.

9. Discuss in short how the disintegration test of filled capsules are done.

10. Describe briefly the dissolution test is done for a tablet. Write down the acceptance criteria.

11. Discuss the advantages and limitations of different types of suppositories bases.

12. Make a list of tests to be carried out for evaluation of tablets.

13. Describe the method of test for Friability and Loss of tablets.

14. Explain with a suitable example how the av. weight of tablets are fixed. What do you mean by theoretical and actual av. weight.

15. Short notes on:

    (a) Buccal and Sublingual tablets,   (b)   Lozenges,
    (c) Troches,   (d)   Dispensing tablets,
    (e) Enteric coated Tablets,   (f)   Hardness Testers,
    (g) Oral powders,   (h)   Film coating,
    (i) Minimum Fill Volume,   (j)   Douche Powders,.
    (k) Cachets,   (l)   Insufflations,
    (m) Calibration of moulds,   (n)   Triturations.
    (o) Dusting Powders

3 Semi Solid Dosage Forms

Ointments

These are semi-solid preparations commonly of a medicament or mixture of medicaments either dissolved or dispersed in a suitable basis intended for application over the skin. The basis is usually non-aqueous. The common uses of ointment are to provide,

- emollient effect on the skin,
- protection of the skin, and
- local medication.

Emollient and protective ointments may contain vegetable oils, synthetic esters of fatty acids or wool fat along with an inert base, e.g. soft paraffin.

The Ointment Bases are of Four Types:

1. *Hydrocarbon Base*: These are sticky, inert, immiscible with water and are not absorbed by the skin. Hence, these act as a barrier to heat and moisture, and keep the skin soft. Soft paraffin, hard paraffin and liquid paraffin fall into this category.

   The solid accommodating capacity of this base can be improved by following method. 5 g of polyethylene of molecule weight. 21000 is mixed with sufficient liquid paraffin to make 100 g, the mixture is heated to 130 ^{O}C to dissolve the polyethylene. If the solution is then suddenly cooled, a gel will be produced which will have fairly stable consistency within a temperature ranging from 15 ^{O}C to 60 ^{O}C accommodating a large amount of solids. Such a gel can replace soft paraffin. The powders are to be incorporated only by levigation. Further heating shall change the physical characteristics of the base. However, such bases fail to incorporate all types of ingredients. By adding glyceryl monostearate during preparation of the gel water absorbability of the base can be improved. Such a base is called *plastibase*.

2. *Absorption Base* can absorb water considerably and hence, hydrophilic in nature. These bases are of two types emulsified (w/o) and non-emulsified suitable for w/o emulsions.

   Emulsified base can absorb more water than non-emulsified base. Lanolin (Hydrous Wool-fat) is most common example of this type. This is an emulsion of water and wool-fat (3:7). It is used as an ingredient as well as a base. It has good emollient activity.

Non-emulsified base can absorb water and produce w/o emulsion. This has good spreadability and also emollient effect. It helps oil-soluble drug to penetrate into the skin, but less occlusive. Anhydrous lanolin (Wool fat), wool alcohols, beeswax and cholesterol are the common examples of this category.

3. *Water-soluble Bases* are obtained from polyethylene glycols (macrogols). These are mixtures of polycondensation products of ethylene oxide and water. According to the molecular weight their physical state varies from liquid to solid, and these are known by the number respective to their molecular weight.

For example, Polyethylene glycol (PEG) 200, 300, 400 are viscous liquids,

PEG 1500 is semisolid and PEG 1540, 3000, 4000, 6000 are waxy solid.

Being water soluble also these have waxy texture. Depending on the molecular weight their solidification temperature varies from 40° to $60\ ^\circ$C. the liquid PEGs are more hygroscopic than solid PEGs. These can be sterilised by heat, solids by dry heat and liquids by moist heat. These are non-toxic and non-irritating to the skin. These non-greasy also. These type of bases are absorbed by the skin, fairly compatible with most drugs and are stable during storage (ageing effect).

4. *Water-miscible bases or Absorption Bases* are hydrophilic and can emulsify a large amount of water. But, these are greasy like and cannot be easily washed out from the skin, since these have limited water-miscibility. These are very suitable for making o/w cream or ointment. The general composition of this type of base is:

Emulsifying wax – 3 parts,

White soft paraffin – 5 parts, and

Liquid paraffin – 2 parts.

Depending on the type emulsifying agent used, the base may be anionic, cationic and non-ionic. This type of ointment base is fairly inert, miscible with secretions from lesions and possesses good cosmetic appearance. Due to the presence of an surface active agent (emulsifying agent) its skin adherence is also good.

But, this type of base has certain limitations:

- limited miscibility with water. By incorporating higher fatty alcohols, *e.g.* cetostearyl alcohol, water miscibility capacity can be increased and the texture of the base can also be improved.

- reduces antibacterial activity of certain substances, *e.g.* quaternary ammonium compounds, phenol, p-hydroxy benzoates, etc. Even some antibacterial agents become inactivated, e.g. penicillin.

- because of hygroscopic nature these are less bland than paraffins.
- Macrogol ointments should not be packed in containers made of polythene or Bakelite due to their solvent action.

Formulation Considerations

The following factors are to be considered while developing a semisolid preparation like cream, ointment, gel, paste, etc.

- the specific use of the preparation, i.e. protective, emollient or therapeutic. In the former cases the base and other additives should be selected accordingly.
- the characteristics of the skin surface on which the preparation shall be applied.
- in case of a medicated preparation, the stability of the drug in the base.
- effect of the base on the permeability, release characteristics of the drug.
- intended therapeutic action, i.e. completely localised surface action or systemic action.
- selection of the appropriate base and optimization.

Usually the epidermal barrier restricts the penetration of most of the drugs topically applied, this limits serious side effects of the drugs. When a drug applied needs to penetrate the diseased cells in the skin, some amount of drug reaches the blood stream also. In such case the drug and its metabolites are to be eliminated from the body through general pathway. Otherwise on repeated administration, accumulation of the drug and its metabolites will take place and this may cause serious side effects. Drugs may penetrate the epidermis either through keratinized cells of the horny layer or through hair follicles.

General method of manufacture of ointment: Depending on the nature of the ingredients there are two general methods,

- fusion, and
- incorporation.

Fusion: In this method the ingredients, except thermo labile (heat sensitive) and volatile substances, are first melted together with constant stirring till the mass is congealed. When the temperature of the mass comes down to about 40 °C the volatile and thermo labile substances are added and mixed thoroughly. If these contain any solid material, it should be finely powdered before mixing.

If the ointment contains ingredients to be emulsified or an emulsion base, both melting and emulsification are done to prepare the product. The oil soluble heat stable components are melted with oil and waxes over boiling water bath or in a steam bath to about 70-75 °C. Similarly, water soluble, heat stable materials are mixed required quantity of water and heated to 70-75 °C. Then, the hot aqueous solution is gradually mixed with the melted mixture with constant stirring. The temperature during stirring is initially maintained at about 70-75 °C for 5-10 minutes. Thereafter, the mixture is cooled slowly and stirring is continued till the product is congealed.

Incorporation: In this method the ointment base is prepared separately and cooled to room temperature. Other solid ingredients of the formulation are finely powdered in a mortar pestle for extemporaneous compounding. The required amount of base is taken and other ingredients in the form of powder mixture or liquid mixture or solution is incorporated into the base in portions. After each addition or incorporation, it is mixed using a spatula to make the mixture smooth and uniform. The process of incorporation is continued until entire powders are completely mixed with the base. It is always better to incorporate powders using a levigating agent like glycerine when water is the external phase and mineral oil when oils are the external phase. By this uniform mixing become possible.

Formulations

Product: Methyl Salicylate Ointment

Standard drug: It contains not less than 98%w/w of Methyl Salicylate, calculated as $C_8H_8O_3$.

Standard product: Content of methyl salicylate: 45.0-52.5% w/w, calculated as $C_8H_8O_3$.

Composition:

Each g contains

    Methyl Salicylate 500 mg in a suitable flavoured base.

Use: Local analgesic

Lot size: 10 g

Manufacturing Formula:

Methyl Salicylate	5.0 g
White Beeswax	2.5 g
Hydrous Wool Fat	2.5 g

Manufacturing Method:

- Take weighed quantity of white beeswax and wool fat in a shallow porcelain dish, place over a boiling water bath to melt,

- When the base is completely melted, remove the dish from the heat, add gradually the weighed quantity of methyl salicylate with continuous stirring till the ointment becomes cold,
- Carry out the tests,
- Fill in a suitable collapsible tube and seal properly,
- Label the preparation.

Product: Bacitracin Ointment

Standard for drug: Bacitracin should have minimum of 40 U.S.P Units per mg.

Standard for product: Content of Bacitracin: 450 – 575 Units per g.

Composition:

Each g contains

Bacitracin 1.25%w/w in a suitable non-aqueous ointment base.

Use: Antibacterial

Lot size: 5 g

Manufacturing Formula:

Bacitracin USP	75 mg
Liquid paraffin, heavy IP	125 mg
Soft paraffin, white IP	4.8 g

Manufacturing Method:

- Weigh accurately the required amount of bacitracin and transfer into a mortar pestle,
- Add liquid paraffin to the drug and levigate properly to make a smooth paste, add gradually the soft paraffin with continuous levigation until an uniform paste is obtained,
- Carry out the test, fill in a suitable collapsible tube or in a wide mouth glass bottle, seal properly and label.

Product: Paraffin Ointment

Use: Ointment base.

Lot size: 10 g

Manufacturing Formula:

Hard Paraffin	0.3 g
Soft paraffin, white	9.0 g
White Beeswax	0.2 g
Cetostearyl Alcohol	0.5 g

Manufacturing Method:

- Take the required quantities of all ingredients in a dish, place over a boiling water bath until melt,
- Levigate thoroughly until the mixture becomes cold,
- Fill the ointment base in a wide mouth glass bottle and seal.
- Label the base.

Product: Zinc oxide Ointment

Standard for drug: It contains not less than 99%w/w of ZnO.

Standard for product: Content of Zinc oxide: 18.5-21.5%w/w, calculated as ZnO.

Composition:

Each g contains

Zinc oxide 0.2%w/w in a non-aqueous ointment base.

Use: Astringent, Protective

Lot size: 10 g

Manufacturing Formula:

Zinc oxide	IP	2.0 g
Liquid Paraffin, heavy	IP	1.5 g
White wax		0.325 g
Soft paraffin, white		6.175 g

Manufacturing Method:

- Transfer weighed quantity of zinc oxide into a mortar pestle, levigate with liquid paraffin until a smooth paste is formed,
- Take weighed amounts of white wax and soft paraffin in a dish, heat on a boiling water bath until these melt, mix well,
- Add melted base gradually to the zinc oxide paste, continue to levigate until uniformly mixed and desired smoothness is attained,
- Carry out the test,
- Fill the preparation in a suitable collapsible tube or wide mouth glass bottle, seal with a cap,
- Label the preparation properly.

Product: Salicylic Acid and Sulphur Ointment

Standard drug: Salicylic Acid contains not less than 99.5 and not more than 101.05w/w of $C_7H_6O_3$, calculated on dried basis. Sulphur contains not less than 99.5%w/w of S.

Standard product: Content of Salicylic Acid: 2.85 – 3.15%w/w, calculated as $C_7H_6O_3$, and content of Sulphur: 2.85 – 3.15%w/w, calculated as S.

Composition:

Each g contains

Salicylic Acid	IP	30 mg
Sulphur	IP	30 mg

In a suitable base.

Use: Scabicide

Lot size: 10 g

Manufacturing Formula:

Salicylic Acid	IP	0.3 g
Sulphur, precipitated	IP	0.3 g
Liquid paraffin, heavy	IP	1 g
White wax		0.4 g
Soft paraffin, white		7.6 g

Manufacturing Method:

- Take weighed quantities of precipitated sulphur and salicylic acid in a mortar pestle, levigate with liquid paraffin to make a smooth paste,
- Take white wax and soft paraffin in a dish, place it over a boiling water bath and stir with a glass rod until these melt completely,
- Add the melted base to the paste gradually with continuous levigation, continue to levigate till uniform smooth ointment is obtained,
- Carry out the test and fill in a suitable collapsible tube or in a wide mouth bottle, seal the container and label properly.

<table>
<tr><td colspan="2" align="center">Salicylic Acid and Sulphur Ointment</td><td align="right">10 g</td></tr>
<tr><td colspan="3">Each g contains</td></tr>
<tr><td>Salicylic Acid IP</td><td>30 mg</td><td>Store below 25°C. Do not freeze.</td></tr>
<tr><td>Sulphur   IP</td><td>30 mg</td><td>Keep out of reach of children.</td></tr>
<tr><td colspan="2">In a suitable base.</td><td>Use as directed by the physician</td></tr>
<tr><td colspan="2"></td><td>Mfg. Lic. No. Xxxxxx</td></tr>
</table>

FOR EXTERNAL USE ONLY

Manufactured in India by :	Batch No. 1324
RCP Pharmaceuticals	Mfd. MM YYYY
Kohka Kurud Road	Exp. MM YYYY
Bhilai, CG	M.R.P. Rs.

Creams

Creams are usually intended for external use. These are viscous, homogeneous, semi-solid emulsions, may be either oil-in-water type (o/w, aqueous cream) or water-in-oil type(w/o, oily cream). Certain water miscible bases having a complex matrix-like physical structure are also known as *creams*, they are often anhydrous or contain only a small proportion of water and similar in appearance to traditional emulsion-type cream base.

Creams are used to apply solution or dispersion of medicament to the skin for therapeutic or prophylactic purpose where a highly occlusive effect is not necessary.

Bland creams may also be used for their emollient, cooling or moistening effect upon the skin.

Cream bases and raw materials: Aqueous creams are usually o/w emulsions. By the selection of anionic, cationic or non-ionic emulsifying agents it is possible to formulate aqueous creams which are compatible with most active ingredients.

The w/o emulsions, i.e., oily creams are usually used for their emollient and occlusive properties. These are formed by metallic soaps, beeswax, wool fat and its derivatives and some synthetic non-ionic substances. Non-emulsified systems having appearance and consistency of creams which are generally used as topical vehicles for corticosteroids; they usually contain a continuous solubilising phase and a solid phase. The solvent in the solubilising phase may be propylene glycol and the solid phase a mixture of a fatty acid and high molecular weight macrogols.

Material used in creams and other semisolids are;

(a) Hydrocarbons (hard, soft and liquid paraffins)

(b) Alcohols (cetostearyl, cetyl, stearyl)

(c) Glycols (glycerol, macrogols, propylene glycol)

(d) Lanolin and its derivatives, fatty acids (oleic, stearic)

(e) Beeswax, vegetable oils (almond, arachis, castor, coconut, cotton seed, maize, olive)

(f) Esters (isopropyl myristate), and

(g) Emulsifying agents.

Rheology and Stability

As emulsified creams are non-Newtonian systems their rheological properties vary with the shear force applied.

Thus, the viscosity and flow characteristics vary with the degree of homogenisation and with the amount of shear applied during processing.

o/w creams may have a visco-elastic gel network, the rigidity of which can be increased by the inclusion of higher concentration of mixed emulsifying agents, e.g. cetrimide with cetostearyl alcohol. In most emulsified systems, the overall viscosity may be increased by

- increasing the viscosity of the continuous phase,
- increasing the content of a single emulsifying agent, or
- reducing the globule size by homogenization.

Major factors which affect the stability of emulsified creams are,

- temperature,
- cohesive and gravitational forces,
- physical and surface properties of the oily substances, and
- the relative densities,
- viscosities and
- concentration of the two phases.

In formulating creams the physicochemical properties of the active ingredients must be carefully considered; for instance, anionic substances are incompatible with cationic emulsifying agents. Hydrolysis of an active substance may be enhanced if an aqueous base is used. Electrolytes can react with emulsifying agents or may induce gel formation.

Preparation of creams

Emulsified creams which contain waxes or fatty solids are prepared by heating the oil soluble or oil miscible constituents together with the emulsifying agents, if oil soluble, at $70° - 75°C$.

Water soluble or water miscible constituents dissolved in or incorporated with the aqueous phase are heated to the same temperature. The two phases are then mixed. If the dispersed phase occupies only a small volume, it is usual to add this to the continuous phase, otherwise the order of mixing is of little importance. The important factors are that the two phases should be at similar temperature and addition should be steady to avoid entrapment of air. Subsequent cooling should be slow with stirring. Sudden cooling or excessive aeration can lead to a granular product. After cooling to $30 - 40°C$, the cream can usually be homogenized. All apparatus used in preparation and the final containers should be thoroughly cleaned before use and rinsed with freshly boiled and cooled purified water before drying.

Microbial contamination

o/w type creams provide suitable environment for growth of micro-organisms. Even when a preservative is included the efficiency of the system may be impaired due to partitioning of the preservative between the oily and aqueous phases of the cream, or due to the partial inactivation of the preservative by the emulsifying agent or a hydrophilic colloid present. Increased amount of preservative may cause undesirable side effects. Consequently, the concentration of the preservative is necessarily a compromise. Thus, a high standard of cleanliness during processing and handling is essential.

Packaging of creams

Well-closed containers those can prevent evaporation and contamination should be used. The material of construction should resist absorption and diffusion of the content. Collapsible tubes of metal or flexible plastic tubes may be used for packing of creams.

If aluminium tubes or containers are used they either should have a inner lacquer coating or a mixture of 0.1% of Na_2HPO_4 and 0.2% of NaH_2PO_4 may be used as buffer in the cream, if no specific buffer is mentioned or recommended to protect aluminium from corrosion and to reduce the chance of formation of hydrogen. Particularly creams containing organic mercury compound should not be packed in uncoated aluminium tubes.

Storage: Unless otherwise specified the creams should be stored at temperature below $25°C$.

But not in a refrigerator.

Labelling: Along with other information it should mention distinctly, *For external use only*; strength of the active ingredient in terms of %w/v or w/w and in case of diluted creams, it should also mention that unless otherwise mentioned, *the diluted cream should not be used after 2 weeks after preparation.*

Difference between Ointment and Cream

Ointment	Cream
Ointments are semisolid preparations in which the active substance(s) remain either as soluble state or suspended. These are intended for external application	Creams are aqueous or oily semisolid emulsions in which the drug is generally remains in soluble state. These are also intended for external application.
These are usually gresier than the creams. The extent of greasiness depends on the type of base used.	These are less greasy and are either o/w (oil-in-water) or w/o (water-in-oil) emulsions.
These are more viscous and they exhibit plastic low with a definite yield value.	These are less viscous and pseudoplastic in nature.
Ointments are sticky and less spreadable.	These are soft and they have good spreadability.
These are protective and soothing.	Creams of w/o type are emollient, soothing and cleansing. This type is preferred for better spreadability and less greasiness. The o/w type creams due to continuous evaporation of water leave a residue on the skin after evaporation of water.
They can adhere to the skin for longer time, they are not easily removable.	These can be removed easily.
The occlusiveness depends on the type of base used. The extent of occlusion - oleaginous base>absorption base>emulsifying base>water soluble base.	The w/o type creams are less occlusive than ointment and o/w type creams are non-occlusive.
Cosmetically less attractive.	Cosmetic appeal is more. Non-medicated creams are used as cosmetics. Vanishing creams are of o/w type.
Occlusive ointments interfere with normal function of the skin.	Oil-in-water (o/w)creams have less interference with normal function of the skin.
Drug in ointments of hydrocarbon base is better absorbed.	O/w cream also promotes percutaneous absorption of drug.

Formulations:

Product: Zinc Cream

Standard for drug: It should contain not less than 99% and not more than 100.5%w/w of ZnO on dried basis.

Standard for product: Content of zinc oxide, 29.6 – 34.4%w/w, calculated as ZnO.

Composition:

It contains 32%w/w of Zinc oxide in a cream base.

Use: Astringent, protective

Lot size: 50 g

Manufacturing Formula:

Zinc oxide, finely shifted	16.0 g
Calcium hydroxide	0.022 g
Wool fat	4.0 g
Oleic acid	0.25 ml
Arachis oil	16.0 ml
Purified water, freshly boiled and cooled	16.0 ml

Manufacturing Method:

- Take zinc oxide and calcium hydroxide in a mortar pestle, triturate, add oleic acid and arachis oil, triturate to a smooth paste,
- Add wool fat, continue trituration, when a smooth paste without any grittiness is produced, add about 16 ml of purified water very slowly in a stream with continuous trituration,
- The cream should be of uniform consistency,
- Pack the cream in a clean, dry wide mouth appropriate container, seal and label properly.

Product: Aqueous Cream

Use: Cream base

Lot size: **50 g**

Manufacturing Formula:

Emulsifying ointment	15.0 g
Chlorocresol	0.05 g
Purified water, freshly boiled and cooled	35.0 ml

Manufacturing Method:

(a) *Preparation of Emulsifying ointment*, 50 g.

Emulsifying wax	15 g
White soft paraffin	25 g
Liquid Paraffin	10 g

Take all the three ingredients in a 100 ml beaker, heat gently to melt, place under an electric stirrer, until the mixture becomes cold continue stirring. Transfer the product into a suitable clean, dry container, seal and label properly.

(b) *Preparation of Emulsifying wax, 50 g*

Cetostearyl alcohol	45 g
Sodium Lauryl sulphate	5 g
Purified water	2 ml

- Take the cetostearyl alcohol in a 50 ml beaker and heat to about 80°C,
- Add sodium lauryl sulphate, stir with a glass rod to mix thoroughly.
- Add purified water, heat to 115°C.
- Continue heating at 115°C with vigorous stirring till frothing cesses, and the product becomes translucent.
- Filter the product while hot through a clean cloth, cool and pack in a suitable container.

(c) *Preparation of Aqueous Cream.*

Emulsifying ointment	15 g
Chlorocresol	0.05 g
Water q.s to make	50 g

- Dissolve chlorocresol in 35 ml of purified water with aid of heat.
- Weigh the emulsifying ointment in a 50 ml beaker, heat to melt.
- Transfer molten emulsifying ointment into a mortar pestle.
- Add warm chlorocresol solution very slowly with continuous trituration. The two phases should have same temperature while mixing.
- Gently triturate till the cream attains room temperature.
- Pack the cream in a clean, dry suitable container, seal and label properly.

Product: Buffered Cream

Standard for product: pH, 5.7 – 6.3 when determined directly on the cream.

Use: In the prevention and treatment of diaper rash, skin cream

Lot size: 50 g

Manufacturing Formula:

Citric Acid monohydrate	0.25 g
Sodium Phosphate	1.25 g
Chlorocresol	0.05 g
Emulsifying ointment	15.0 g
Purified water, freshly boiled and cooled	33.45 ml

Manufacturing Method:

- Take measured amount of purified water in a 100 ml beaker, add chlorocresol, citric acid and sodium phosphate heat to dissolve,

- In another 100 ml beaker take emulsifying ointment, heat to melt, place under a stirrer,

- See that both the phases have same temperature, add aqueous phase very slowly to the emulsifying ointment with gentle stirring. Continue stirring till the cream attains room temperature,

- Fill the product in a suitable clean, dry container, seal and label properly.

Product: Cetrimide Cream

Standard for drug: It should contain not less than 96% and not more than 101%w/w of alkyl trimethyl ammonium bromides, calculated as $C_{17}H_{38}BrN$ on dried basis.

Standard for product: Content of cetrimide: 0.44 – 0.53%w/w calculated as $C_{17}H_{38}BrN$.

Composition:

It contains Cetrimide 0.5%w/w in a water soluble cream base.

Use: Bactericide, pharmaceutical aid

Lot size: 50 g

Manufacturing Formula:

Cetrimide	0.25 g
Cetostearyl alcohol	2.50 g
Liquid Paraffin	25.00 g

Purified water, freshly boiled and cooled 22.25 ml

Manufacturing Method:

- Take the cetostearyl alcohol in a 100 ml beaker, heat gently to melt, add the liquid paraffin, mix with glass rod, heat at 45°C,

- In another 50 ml beaker take purified water, add the cetrimide and dissolve, heat it to 45°C,

- Add the warm aqueous solution gradually to the warm molten cetostearyl alcohol with constant stirring with a paddle stirrer,

- Continue stirring until the mixture attains room temperature,

- Draw a sample and determine the content of cetrimide,

- Pack the cream in a suitable clean, dry container, seal and label.

Product: Neomycin Cream

Standard for product: Content of Neomycin sulphate, not less than 85% of the stated amount.

Composition:

It contains

Neomycin sulphate	0.5%w/w
Chlorocresol	0.1%w/w
In a cream base.	

Use: Antibiotic.

Lot size: 10 g

Manufacturing Formula:

Neomycin sulphate	0.05 g
Di-sodium edetate	1.0 mg
Chlorocresol	10 mg
Cetomacrogol emulsifying ointment	5 g
Purified water, freshly boiled and cooled	6.94 ml

Manufacturing Method:

- In a 25 ml beaker take disodium edetate and chlorocresol, add 3 ml of water, gently heat to dissolve,
- In a mortar pestle take cetomacrogol, place it over boiling water bath to melt the cetomacrogol. Add the aqueous solution of disodium edentate and chlorocresol, stir to mix thoroughly,
- In the same beaker take neomycin sulphate, add 3.94 ml of purified water, dissolve and add this solution to the mortar pestle and continue stirring until the cream attains room temperature,
- Determine the content of neomycin and chlorocresol,
- Fill the cream in a suitable collapsible ointment tube, seal and label.

Product: Zinc and Ichthamol Cream

Standard for drug: Zinc oxide: It should contain not less than 99% and not more than 100.5%w/w of ZnO on dried basis.

Standard for product: Content of zinc oxide, 23.4 – 29.3%w/w, calculated as ZnO.

It contains	Zinc oxide	26.24%w/w
	Ichthamol	5.0%w/w

In a cream base.

Use: Astringent, protective

Lot size: 10 g

Manufacturing Formula:

Zinc cream	8.2 g
Ichthamol	0.5 g
Cetostearyl alcohol	0.3 g
Wool fat	1.0 g

Manufacturing Method:

- Take the zinc cream in a mortar pestle, add wool fat and cetostearyl alcohol triturate constantly until a smooth and uniform cream is obtained,
- Add ichthamol to the bulk and triturate thoroughly,
- Determine the content of zinc oxide and ichthamol,
- Fill the cream in a suitable clean collapsible ointment tube, seal and paste the label over the tube.

Product: Salicylic Acid and Sulphur Cream

Standard for drug: Salicylic acid : It should contain not less than 99% and not more than 100.5%w/w of $C_7H_6O_3$ on dried basis.

Sulphur: It should contain not less than 99.5% w/w of S on dried basis.

Standard for product: Content of Salicylic Acid: 1.8 – 2.2%w/w, calculated as ZnO.

Content of Sulphur: 1.8 – 2.2%w/w, calculated as S.

It contains Salicylic acid   IP 2%w/w

Sulphur, precipitated   IP 2%w/w

Standard for product: Content of salicylic acid, 1.80 – 2.20%w/w, calculated as $C_7H_6O_3$ and content of sulphur, 1.80 – 2.20%w/w, calculated as S.

Use: Keratolytic and scabicide

Lot size: 10 g

Manufacturing Formula:

Salicylic Acid, freshly shifted	0.2 g
Precipitated sulphur, freshly shifted	0.2 g
Aqueous cream	9.6 g

Manufacturing Method:

- Take salicylic acid and sulphur in a mortar pestle, add a portion of aqueous cream, triturate until a smooth paste is formed,
- Add gradually the remaining portions of aqueous cream with continuous trituration,
- Determine the content of salicylic acid and sulphur,
- Fill the cream in a suitable clean collapsible ointment tube, seal and paste the label over the tube.

Pastes

These are one of the types of semisolid preparations. The difference between ointment and paste is that the solid content in the latter is high even up to 50%. A large quantity of insoluble solid powder is incorporated into an ointment base for which the paste is found to be more stiff. A paste when spreaded over skin adheres in the form of a thick layer, it forms a protective and soothing coating over the inflamed and affected skin surface. With this ability pastes are useful for protecting the face and lips from the sun.

Pastes are usually less oily than the ointments and they form thick layer over the skin surface and thus their cosmetic elegance is also less. Since the solid content is high, paste of a potent medicament may produce reaction on the skin also.

Pastes are prepared by levigating the fine powder of the solid with a portion of the congealed base till uniformly mixed, then the rest portion of the base is gradually added with continuous levigation until uniform dispersion of the powders is made.

Base used for preparing paste may be hydrocarbon base, e.g. emulsifying wax, glycerol; sometimes water soluble base, e.g. macrogol base is used.

Comparison between ointment and paste:

Ointment	Paste
The ointments are soft due to less content of powders.	Pastes are stiff due to high content of powders, even up to 50%.
On application these leave a very thin layer over the area of application.	On application these leave a thick coat over the area of application.
The protective activity is less compared to paste.	The protective activity is more due to formation of thick coat over the area of application.
Ointments have very good spreadability and free from grittiness.	Pastes do not have spreadability, these are also free from grittiness.
Ointment can migrate from its area of application, Hence, a powerful drug can affect the normal and healthy skin also.	Due to thickness, paste cannot migrate from its area of application. Thus, there is no damage of the normal, healthy skin by a powerful drug.
Ointments are emollient and greasy in nature.	Pastes are emollient and less greasy.

Contd...

Ointment	Paste
Ointments being greasy, can affect perspiration through skin.	Pastes are porous due to high content of powders do not affect perspiration.
Ointment cannot absorb exudates.	Because of high content of powders, these can absorb exudates.
Ointments with hydrocarbon base are more macerating in their action.	Pastes even made with similar hydrocarbon base are less macerating the ointments.
These are cosmetically attractive.	These are cosmetically less attractive, as they leave a thick layer on the skin.
These do not require any device to apply.	These are applied either with a spatula or spread on tint or with other dressing.
These can be easily removed from the skin and can be applied on the scalp.	These are not suitable for scalp treatment, as these cannot be removed easily from the hair.
These need not to be kept on skin for long time.	Once applied, left for long period.

Packaging and storage: Pastes should be packed in glass or plastic containers fitted with screw caps having impermeable liners or with close-fitting slip-on lids to prevent the content from diffusion or absorption. alternatively these can be packed in collapsible tubes like ointments.

Formulations:

Product: Aluminium Paste, Compound

Synonym: Baltimore Paste.

Standard for product: Content of zinc oxide, 37.0– 42.0 % calculated as ZnO;

Content of aluminium, 15.8 – 20.0 % calculated as Al.

Use: Protective in burns

Lot size: 10 g

Manufacturing Formula:

Aluminium powder	2.0 g
Zinc oxide	4.0 g
Liquid Paraffin	4.0 g

Manufacturing Method:

- Take weighed quantity of aluminium powder and zinc oxide into a mortar pestle, add measured volume of liquid paraffin and triturate until a smooth paste is obtained,
- Determine the content of aluminium and zinc oxide,
- Pack the preparation in a clean, dry, wide mouth suitable glass container,
- Seal with a pilfer proof cap and label appropriately.

Product: Magnesium Sulphate Paste

Synonym: Morison's Paste.

Standard for product: Content of magnesium sulphate, 36 – 41% calculated as $MgSO_4$; content of phenol, 0.45 – 0.55% calculated as C_6H_6O.

Use: Dehydrating (drawing) boils and carbuncles

Lot size: 10 g

Manufacturing Formula:

Phenol	0.05 g
Glycerin	5.5 g
Dried Magnesium Sulphate	q.s

Manufacturing Method:

- Dry about 7 g of magnesium sulphate at 150°C for $1^1/_2$ hours or at 130°C for 4 hrs., keep it in a desiccators,
- Dry glycerin at 120°C for one hour and cool in a desiccators,
- Dissolve phenol in measured volume of glycerin,
- Weigh 4.5 g of magnesium sulphate, transfer it into a clean, dry mortar pestle,
- Add phenol solution to the powder and triturate until a smooth paste is obtained,
- Determine the content of magnesium sulphate and phenol,
- Pack in a suitable glass container and label appropriately.

Note: The label should mention, *Stir well before use.*

Product: Resorcinol and Sulphur Paste

Standard for product: Content of resorcinol, 4.75 – 5.25% calculated as C_6H_6O;

Content of sulphur, 4.75 – 5.25% calculated as S;

Content of zinc oxide, 38.0 – 42.0% calculated as ZnO.

Use: Anti-acne

Lot size: 10 g

Manufacturing Formula:

Resorcinol, finely sifted	0.5 g
Precipitated Sulphur	0.5 g
Zinc oxide, finely sifted	4.0 g
Emulsifying ointment	5.0 g

Manufacturing Method:

- Transfer the weighed quantity of zinc oxide, precipitated sulphur and resorcinol,
- Into a clean mortar pestle, triturate these with a little of emulsifying ointment,
- Until a smooth paste is obtained,
- Add gradually the remaining portion of emulsifying ointment and continue trituration,
- When an uniform, smooth paste is obtained, determine the content of zinc oxide,
- Sulphur and resorcinol,
- Fill the preparation in a suitable container, seal with a pilfer proof cap and label.

Product: Titanium Dioxide Paste

Standard for product: Content of Zinc Oxide, 23.7 – 26.3% calculated as ZnO;

Residue on ignition, 53 – 58%w/w.

Use: Sun burn protectant

Lot size: 10 g

Manufacturing Formula:

Titanium Dioxide	2.0 g
Chlorocresol	0.01 g
Red Ferric Oxide	0.2 g
Light Kaolin	1.0 g
Zinc Oxide, fine sifted	2.5 g
Glycerin	1.5 g
Purified water	q.s

Manufacturing Method:

- Transfer the weighed quantity of titanium dioxide, ferric oxide, kaolin and zinc oxide, mix thoroughly and triturate,
- Dissolve the chlorocresol in the glycerin, add 2.8 ml of purified water,
- Add the solution gradually to the powder mix and triturate until a smooth paste is obtained,
- Determine the content of zinc oxide and residue on ignition,
- Fill the preparation in a suitable container, seal with a pilfer proof cap,
- Label.

Gels

These are semisolid disperse systems containing polymers or long chain molecules in the internal phase. The long-chain molecules or the polymer cross-link and interact among themselves and form a web like structure. Within this structure the external phase is entrapped. Such a system seems to be single phase. Hydrated gelatin is a classic example of gel. Sometimes, the suspensions, milks and magmas of inorganic hydroxides and clays are called as gels as they are highly viscous. The particles of bentonite form a three dimensional structure throughout the gel. This is a real two-phase system where the particles of bentonite do not dissolve in water but only dispersed throughout the continuous phase. Reversible gels are semisolids and viscous at low temperature. These become liquids when temperature rises. Most of the aqueous and nonaqueous gels are prepared with the help of heat and high speed mixing.

Now a days, gels are one of the widely used as drug delivery systems. Gels are most commonly used for oral, topical, ophthalmological and parenteral administration. A gel can be used for prolonged action of a drug when injected intramuscularly or implanted into the body. The cosmetic preparations in the form of gels may be shampoo, skin, fragrance and hair-care preparations, dentifrices etc. The gellants are used as binders in tablet formulations, as protective colloids in suspensions, as thickening agents in oral liquids and suppository base.

Based on the nature of the colloidal phase (gellants), gels are primarily of two categories- inorganic and organic. Organic gels may be of two types,- natural and synthetic. The natural gums like acacia, xanthan, and carrageenan are anionic polysaccharides. Synthetic gellants may be cellulose derivatives, e.g. carboxymethylcellulose sodium, hydroxypropylcellulose, hydroxyethylcellulose, hydroxypropylmethyl cellulose, etc., polyethylene and its copolymers, acrylic polymers, metallic stearates and synthetic block copolymers.

Based on the nature of solvent gels may be divided into two types- aqueous (hydrogel) and nonaqueous (organogel). There is another type, xerogel. Xerogel are solid gels containing less amount of solvent. Dry gelatin, tragacanth ribbons, acacia tears are the common example of xerogel. These are frequently prepared by evaporating the solvent from the gel.

Some gels may contract on storage and the internal liquids comes out at the surface of the gel. This process, called as *syneresis*, may occur in organogels, organic and inorganic hydrogels. Mostly this is observed in gels containing less amount of polymer. The reason may be, the decrease in elastic stresses during setting of the gel, decrease in the space for the solvent, as a result the liquid is forced to come out of the gel matrix. The concentration of salts in the gel may have effect on syneresis.

Conversely, a gel may absorb liquid resulting the increase in volume. This phenomenon is called *swelling*. This is due to the penetration of solvent into the gel matrix.

When the hydration of a gellant depends on temperature, gel is formed due to change in temperature and such gel is reversible. When due to a chemical reaction, e.g. salt bridging or cross-linking, a gel is formed, it is irreversible.

The viscosity of a gel directly related to the molecular weight of the polymer (gellant). That is lesser amount of a polymer of higher molecular weight can result the desired viscosity of the gel. Gels are pseudoplastic fluids and show non-Newtonian flow characteristics.

Commonly used gelling agents in the pharmaceutical preparations are given below in the Table 3.1.

TABLE 3.1

Commonly used pharmaceutical gelling agents.

For Aqueous solution	For Non-Aqueous solution
Carbomers	Clays and organoclays
Gelatin	Colloidal silicon dioxide
Colloidal silicon dioxide	Modified cellulosics
Cellulosics	Low HLB surfactants
Natural gums (xanthans, aligns, carrageenans, pectins)	polyethylene
Non-ionic surfactants	
starches	

Formulations:

Product: Diclofenac Gel

Standard for drug: It should contain not less than 99.0% and not more than 101%w/w of Diclofenac Diethylamine, calculated as $C_{18}H_{22}Cl_2N_2O_2$ on dried basis.

Standard for product: It should contain not less than 90% and not more than 110%w/w of the Stated amount of Diclofenac, calculated as $C_{18}H_{22}Cl_2N_2O_2$ on dried basis.

Composition:

It contains

Diclofenac Diethylamine	BP	1.10%
Equivalent to Diclofenac sodium	IP	1%
Linseed oil	BP	3.0%

Methyl salicylate	IP	1.0%
Menthol	IP	5.0%
Benzyl Alcohol	IP	1.0%

in a flavoured washable gel base.

Use: Analgesic, anti-inflammatory

Lot size: 10 g

Manufacturing Formula:

Diclofenac Diethylamine	BP	0.11g
Linseed oil	BP	0.3g
Methyl salicylate	IP	1.0g
Menthol	IP	0.5g
Benzyl Alcohol	IP	0.1g
Sodium Alginate Gel Base	q.s	10 g

Manufacturing Method:

- Take Diclofenac sodium, accurately weighed, in a mortar pestle,
- Add linseed oil and make a paste,
- Add benzyl alcohol and methyl salicylate, levigate thoroughly,
- Add menthol and sufficient gel base, mix thoroughly to make a uniform gel,
- Carry out the tests, fill the preparation in a suitable collapsible tube, seal and label.

Preparation of sodium alginate gel base:

Sodium alginate	IP	1.0 g
Glycerin	IP	1.0 g
Methylparaben	IP	0.02 g
Calcium gluconate	IP	0.05 g
Purified water	IP	8.0g

- Take 8 ml of purified water in a 25 ml clean beaker, add methyl paraben and heat to dissolve, cool the solution, transfer into a clean mortar pestle,
- Add glycerin and mix,
- Add sodium alginate and levigate vigorously until a smooth slurry is formed,
- Add calcium gluconate and mix vigorously,
- Pack the gel in a clean, dry wide mouth glass bottle, seal and label.

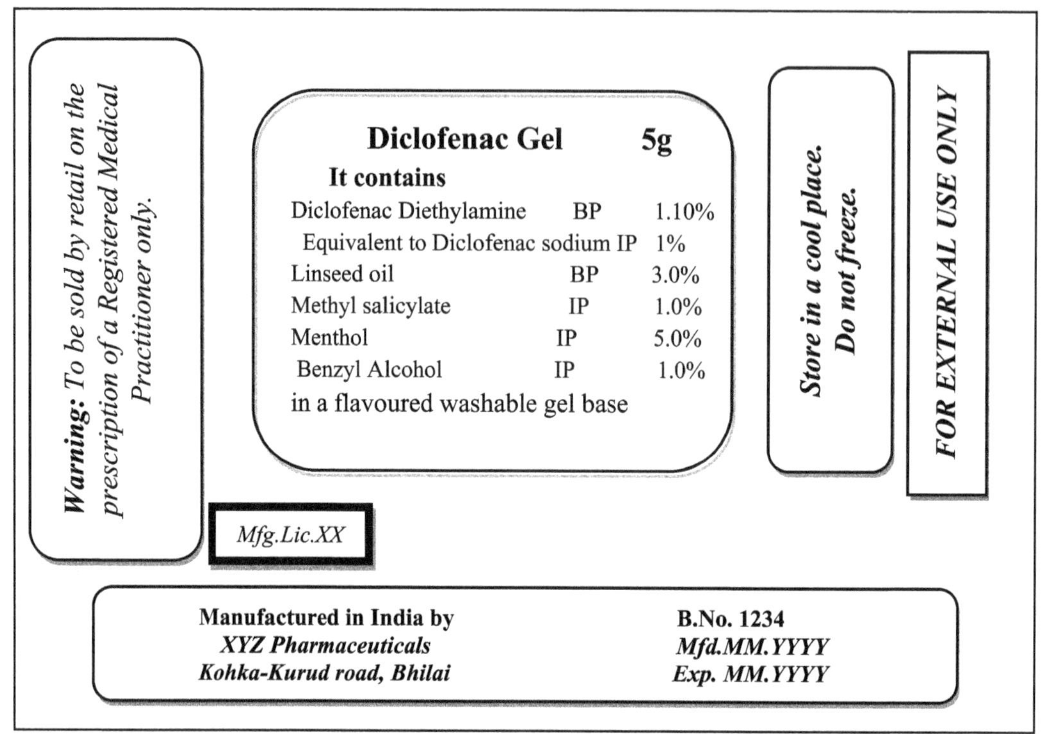

Product: Zinc oxide Gel

Composition:

> Each g contains
>
> > Zinc oxide   0.2 g
> >
> > Aqueous gel base q.s

Use: Mild astringent and topical protectant

Lot size: 5 g

Manufacturing Formula:

Zinc oxide	IP	1.0 g
Sodium hydroxide	IP	0.016 g
Carbomer 934		0.04 g
Water, purified	IP	3.9 ml

Manufacturing Method:

- Accurately weigh the carbomer 934, measure the required volume of purified water and transfer in a mortar pestle, add the carbomer to it,

- Weigh accurately 1.07 g of sodium hydroxide, dissolve in sufficient purified water to make 10 ml of solution. Pipette out 0.15 ml and add drop wise to the mortar with gentle agitation,

- Add the weighed quantity of zinc oxide slowly to the mortar with gentle stirring.

- Continue to mix slowly until a smooth, homogeneous gel is prepared. Air should not be entrapped.

- Take a sample and test for zinc oxide content.

- Fill the preparation in a 5 ml capacity collapsible tube and seal.

- Label the tube properly with a note, FOR EXTERNAL USE ONLY.

Product: Piroxicam Gel

Standard for drug: It contains not less than 97% and not more than 103%w/w of $C_{15}H_{13}N_3O_4S$, calculated on dried basis.

Standard for product: It should contain not less than 95% of the stated amount of Piroxicam IP, calculated as $C_{15}H_{13}N_3O_4S$.

Composition:

It contains

Piroxicam IP 0.5%w/w in water soluble gel base.

Use: Analgesic, anti-inflammatory

Lot size: 5 g

Manufacturing Formula:

Piroxicam	IP	25.0 mg
Methylcellulose 4000 cps		40 mg
Carbopol 934		12 mg
Propylene glycol		0.8 ml
Methylparaben		0.75 mg
Purified water		q.s

Manufacturing Method:

- Weigh accurately required quantity of piroxicam, transfer into a clean mortar pestle, crush to make fine powders,

- Weigh separately 4.975 g of gel base, add in portions to the powder and levigate thoroughly till a uniform mixture is obtained, avoid entrapment of air during levigation.

- Carry out the test, fill the gel in a clean collapsible tube and seal properly,
- Label the tube.

Preparation of 10 g of Gel base:

Methylcellulose 4000 cps	80 mg
Carbopol 934	24 mg
Propylene glycol	1.6 ml
Methylparaben	1.5 mg
Purified water q.s to make	10.0 g

Materials Method:

- Weigh accurately 120 mg of methyl paraben, dissolve in 4 ml of hot purified water,
- Pipette out 0.5ml of this solution to a 10 ml clean beaker, add another 3 ml of purified water, heat to 90°C, disperse methylcellulose, keep it in a refrigerator for overnight,
- Take another 10 ml clean beaker, pipette 3 ml of purified water, disperse carbopol,
- Adjust the pH to 7.0 by adding 2% NaOH solution, about 0.6 ml shall be required,
- Add propylene glycol and mix thoroughly,
- Mix methylcellulose and carbopol fraction thoroughly, add sufficient purified water to make 10.0 g and mix well.

Product: Ibuprofen Gel

Standard for drug: It contains not less than 98.5% and not more than 101%w/w of $C_{13}H_{18}O_2$, calculated on dried basis.

Standard for product: It should contain not less than 90% of the stated amount, calculated as $C_{13}H_{18}O_2$.

Composition:

Each g contains

Ibuprofen IP 0.02g in a gel base.

Use: Analgesic

Lot size: 10 g

Manufacturing Formula:

Ibuprofen	IP	0.2 g
Sodium alginate	IP	1.0 g

Glycerin	IP	1.0 g
Methyl Paraben	IP	0.02 g
Calcium gluconate	IP	0.05 g
Purified water	IP	8.0g

Manufacturing Method:

- Take 8 ml of purified water in a 25 ml clean beaker, add methyl paraben and heat to dissolve, cool the solution, transfer into a clean mortar pestle,
- Add glycerin and mix,
- Add sodium alginate and levigate vigorously until a smooth slurry is formed,
- Add calcium gluconate and mix vigorously.
- Add micronized ibuprofen with slow levigation until a uniform gel is obtained,
- Carry out the tests,
- Pack the gel in a clean, dry wide mouth glass bottle, seal and label.

Product: Sunscreen Gel

Composition:

Each g contains

Glyceryl-p-amino benzoate	3%
Mono isopropanolamine	0.09%
Ethanol	50 %

in a hydrous, flavoured gel base.

Use: Protection from sun burn

Lot size: 10 g

Manufacturing Formula:

Glyceryl-p-amino benzoate	0.3 g
Mono isopropanolamine	0.009g
Ethanol	5.2 ml
Carbomer 940	0.1 g
Sandal wood oil	0.01 ml
Purified water	5.0 ml

Manufacturing Method:

- Measure the required volume of alcohol and transfer into a clean and dry mortar pestle,

- Disperse the weighed quantity of carbomer940, add weighed amount of Glyceryl-p-amino benzoate and dissolve in the solution,

- Add Mono isopropanolamine to this slowly, add sandal wood oil and mix,

- Add measured volume of purified water slowly with slow stirring, care to be taken to avoid entrapment of air during stirring.

- Once the gel is formed, pack it in a suitable collapsible tube, seal well and label.

Jellies

Jelly is one type of gel with little difference in the matrix structure. The structural coherent matrix of a jelly contains large amount of liquid, usually water. These are like mucilages, with the same gum a mucilage as well as a jelly can be prepared. The difference between a mucilage and jelly lies in consistency. A mucilage does not have jelly-like consistency. A whole gum of the finest quality is better than its powdered form to make a clear preparation with uniform consistency.

The USP does not directly mention to incorporate any specific thickening agent in the official preparations. However, to increase the viscosity suitable thickening may be included in a jelly formulation.

Acacia, gelatin, tragacanth, carboxymethyl cellulose, hydroxyethyl cellulose, and similar substances can be used to prepare jellies with water.

Jellies are susceptible to microbial contamination. Hence, these require suitable preservatives, e.g. methyl-p-hydroxybenzoate, for their stabilisation.

Non-medicated jellies are used as lubricant for catheters, surgical gloves and rectal thermometers.

Lidocaine hydrochloride Jelly is used as a topical anesthetic. There are therapeutic vaginal jellies.

For contraceptive purposes some jellies like preparations are also used. These preparations contain surface active agents, which increases the spermatocidal activity of the jelly. Such preparations usually contain eucalyptol, methyl salicylate as flavouring agent.

Jellies should be stored properly, as the water may evaporate resulting the preparation dry.

Formulation

Product: Lubricating Jelly

Composition:

It contains   Methylcellulose, 0.75%

                               Carbopol 934   0.30%

Propylene glycol   16.5%

Methylparaben   0.015% in aqueous medium.

Use: Lubrication of medical devices and as vehicle

Lot size: 10 g

Manufacturing Formula:

Methylcellulose, 4000 cps	75 mg
Carbopol 934	30 mg
Propylene glycol	1.65 ml
Methylparaben	1.5 mg
Sodium hydroxide, 1% solution	q.s
Purified water	q.s

Manufacturing Method:

- Take 3.5 ml of hot (90 °C) water in a clean 10 ml beaker, disperse accurately weighed quantity of methylcellulose,, when it is completely dispersed, put the beaker inside a refrigerator for 10 hours,
- Weigh carbopol accurately and disperse in 3 ml of purified water in a clean 10 ml beaker, once the carbopol is completely dispersed, add drop wise sodium hydroxide solution (1%) to adjust the pH to 7.0,
- Weigh accurately 30 mg of methyl paraben, dissolve it in 30 ml of hot water, cool and add 1.5 ml to carbopol dispersion, mix well,
- Add 1.65ml of propylene glycol to dispersed carbopol phase, mix, then add the dispersed methylcellulose to it, mix to make uniform,
- Pack the preparation in a suitable glass container, wide mouth, seal with a pilfer proof cap and label.

Note: While mixing at any stage, care should be taken to avoid entrapment of air.

Evaluation of a semisolid preparation

Common tests to be carried out for evaluation of a semisolid preparation are,

1.   Physical Tests

1.1   Description -Colour, consistency, texture, stickiness and odour

1.2   Uniformity of mixing and smoothness

1.3   Spreadability

1.4   Viscosity

1.5   Individual weight variation(uniformity of weights)

1.6   Dissolution rate, if desired or directed

1.7   Average content

1.8   Uniformity of content

2.   Chemical Tests

2.1   Identification tests

2.2   Assay

2.3   Uniformity of contents

3.   Biological Tests

3.1   Microbiological assay, if applicable

3.2   Sterility test, if the product is claimed as sterile product

General Standards: *Applicable for ointment, cream, paste*

Uniformity of container content: *This test and specifications are applicable when the labelled amount does not exceed 100 g or 300 ml or 1000 units.*

- Draw randomly a sample of 10 filled containers.

- Remove the labels which may alter the weight while removing the contents from the containers.

- Clean and dry the outer surface of the containers.

- Weigh each container. Remove the content from each as maximum as possible.

- Weigh the empty container.

- If required, cut and open the container, wash each empty container with suitable solvent without loss of any part of the container or closure which can make error.

- Dry and weigh the empty container.

- The difference between the two weights will be the net content of each container.

- The average net weight of contents of the 10 samples shall not be less than the labelled amount and the lot or batch shall pass, if

- any single net weight does not vary from the labelled amount by ±9%, where labelled amount is 50 g or less.

- any single net weight does not vary from the labelled amount by ±4.5%, where labelled amount is more than 50 g but less than 100 g.

Exercises

Short Questions

1. (a) Why is bland cream used?
   (b) What are aqueous cream and oily cream?
   (c) Name the formulations classified as semisolid dosage form.
   (d) Name the various constituents of a cream.
   (e) Name the various ways to increase the viscosity of a cream.
   (f) Make a list of the factors that affect the stability of a cream.
   (g) What precaution to be taken if a cream is packed in an aluminium container?
   (h) What is the composition of an emulsifying wax?
   (i) What are the common uses of an ointment?
   (j) Name various bases used for manufacture of ointments.
   (k) Name the sites through which a drug can penetrate the epidermis layer of skin.
   (l) Which drugs are usually formulated as paints?
   (m) Why a paste is stiffer than an ointment?
   (n) Define syneresis.
   (o) What is swelling?
   (p) What are hydrogel and organogel?
   (q) What are gel and jelly?
   (r) How are the ointment and cream stored?
   (s) What are gel and sol?
2. Write down the general method of manufacturing of cream.
3. Differentiate between cream and ointment.
4. Discuss the characteristics of various types of ointment bases.
5. Explain the factors to be considered during development of an ointment formulation.
6. Describe the general method of manufacturing of paste.
7. Write down the general methods of manufacturing of ointment.
8. Distinguish between ointment and paste.
9. Discuss the parameters to be examined for evaluation of an ointment.
10. Describe the general method of manufacturing of gel.
11. Short notes on:
    (a) Fusion and levigation,   (b) Emulsifying ointment,
    (c) Hydrocarbon base,   (d) Absorption base,
    (e) Paste,   (f) Syneresis

4 Liquid Dosage Forms

The liquid dosage forms may be intended for oral administration (oral liquids), ophthalmic or parenteral administration (sterile liquids), or for external application (topical liquids).

These may be solution, suspension or emulsion type.

Oral liquids

These may be solutions, emulsions or suspensions of one or more medicaments in a suitable vehicle. These are administered as such or after dilution. Depending on the type, they may contain various additives, like solubilising, dispersing, emulsifying, wetting, thickening, stabilising, buffering, colouring, sweetening, and flavouring agents along with a suitable preservative system.

Elixirs, Linctuses, Mixtures, Syrups, Oral Drops, Oral Solutions, Oral Suspensions, Oral Emulsions togetherly come under this category.

Types of Oral Liquids and Definitions

Elixirs are clear, coloured and flavoured oral liquids containing active ingredient(s) dissolved in a suitable vehicle. The vehicle usually contains a high proportion of sucrose or a suitable polyhydric alcohols or alcohol (ethyl alcohol).

Linctuses are viscous, coloured and flavoured oral liquids containing active ingredients dissolved in a vehicle that usually contains a high proportion of sucrose, other sugars or a suitable polyhydric alcohol or alcohol (ethyl alcohol). They are usually prepared for use in the treatment of or relief of cough. These are commonly sipped or swallowed slowly without addition of water.

Syrups are usually coloured, flavoured and viscous preparations may or may not contain active ingredients (drug). The vehicle contains a high proportion of sucrose or other sugars with certain polyhydric alcohols to inhibit crystallisation or to modify solubilisation, taste and other physical properties of the product. Sugar may be replaced by other suitable sweetening and thickening agents. Syrups may contain alcohol as preservative or as a co-solvent. The syrups also contain a suitable antimicrobial preservative.

Oral Drops are meant for administration in small volumes through a dropper. These are generally prepared for paediatric and elderly use.

Oral emulsions are stabilised oil-in-water dispersions of active ingredient(s). Either or both phases may contain dissolved solids. Solids may also be suspended in suitable oral emulsion system. Emulsion may show phase separation which should be easily reformed on shaking.

Mixtures contain one or more active ingredients dissolved, dispersed or suspended in a suitable palatable, elegant vehicle. The suspended or dispersed preparations should be shaken well before administration to ensure dispensing of the correct dose.

Oral Suspensions contain active ingredient(s) suspended in a suitable vehicle. The suspended solids may deposit on storage but these should be easily redispersed on shaking; so that, the correct dose can be dispensed. These contain suitable colour and flavour to improve organoleptic property of the preparation.

Containers

The oral liquids may be packed in single dose or multiple doses containers. The mouth of the container used for suspension or emulsion should be sufficiently wide to facilitate the flow of the product from the bottle. A suitable dispensing device either a dropper or measuring cup marked at 5, 10, 15 ml without handling with bare hands should be provided with the container.

Storage

Oral liquids or powders and granules for preparation of oral liquids should be stored in well-closed containers, commonly glass or suitable plastic bottles. The storage temperature should not exceed $30^{\circ}C$ and no oral liquid should be stored if it is diluted.

Labelling

If the oral liquid is administered as drops and the dose is stated in volume, the label should state the number of drops per g or per ml.
If the preparation is a powder or granule and is to be constituted before use, the label should state

- That the contents are meant for preparation of an oral liquid,
- The direction for preparing the oral liquid including the nature and quantity of the liquid to be used,
- Storage condition of the constituted preparation,
- Shelf-life of the constituted preparation according to the manufacturer's recommendations,

- Strength in terms of the active ingredient(s) in a suitable dose-volume of the constituted preparation.

While formulating an oral liquid preparation whether a solution or a suspension the following criteria have to be maintained;

1. The unpleasant odour or taste of the drug, if present, has to be masked and the preparation should be made palatable.
2. Both physical and chemical stability of the product,
3. The elegance of the product should be acceptable.

Formulation Considerations

Keeping in view of the three essential criteria of an oral solution product, i.e. palatability, stability and elegance, the formulation development programme should be designed as follows;

Criterion	Studies
Palatability (in case of oral solution)	Know the taste and odour of the drug, Select some suitable taste and odour masking agents and formulate and select the best one.
Elegance	Based on the flavour used, select the suitable colorant, container and other packaging material, e.g. label design, carton, etc.
Stability	Based on the physicochemical properties of the drug, select suitable solvent system that is co-solvent(s) for an insoluble or slightly soluble drugs; e.g. a mixture of alcohol, propylene glycol and glycerin is used for paracetamol syrup, appropriate pH range, preservative system, stabilizer.

Preservatives commonly used in liquid preparations are given in the Table 4.1 below for ready reference.

TABLE 4.1

Preservatives commonly used in liquid preparations

Sl. No.	Preservative	Usual Concentration	Effectiveness
1	Benzoic acid and Sodium Benzoate	0.1 – 0.2%	Effective at pH below 5.0
2	Methyl parahydroxy benzoate and its Sodium salt (Nipazin sodium)	0.20%	Less effective at pH above 8.0
3	Propyl parahydroxy benzoate and its Sodium salt.	0.02%	Less effective at pH above 8.0, Mixture of 2 and 3 are more effective at pH 4.0 – 6.0

Flavours useful for masking of taste are shown below in the Table 4.2.

TABLE 4.2

Flavours used for taste masking

Taste	Flavour(s) used
Bitter	Anise, Chocolate, Mint, Wild cherry.
Sweet	Vanilla, Berries, Fruit.
Sour	Citrous fruits, Liquorice, Raspberry.
Salty	Butterscotch, Liquorice, Peach, Vanilla.

Stabilisation of Liquid Dosage Form

The stability of liquid dosage forms may be affected by decomposition due to oxidation, which may be checked by;

- Filling in container under vacuum or with inert gas,

- Storage of the well-closed filled containers at lower temperature,

- Incorporating a suitable reducing agent or antioxidant in the formulation.

Cause of oxidation	Remedy
Atmospheric oxygen	use of an antioxidant
Oxidising agent agent present in formulation	use of a reducing agent
Microbial contamination	use of antimicrobial preservative

Examples of some common **stabilising agents** are shown below in the Table 4.3.

TABLE 4.3

Commonly used stabilising agents

Reducing agents	Common use
Sodium sulphite	Antioxidant and antimicrobial preservative in alkaline preparations.
Sodium metabisulphite	Food and pharmaceuticals containing easily oxidisable substances.
Sodium thiosulphate	Food and pharmaceuticals
Sulphurous acid	Food (fruit) products and pharmaceuticals
Sulphur dioxide	Food (fruit) products and some injections
Dextrose	Food and pharmaceuticals

Antioxidants	Common use
Catechol	Products containing oils and fats
Gallic acid	- do -
Pyrogallol	- do -

Table 4.3 Contd...

Ethyl Gallate	Products of oils, fats, food, cosmetic and perfumes.
Propyl gallate	- do -
Octyl Gallate	- do -
Dodecyl Gallate	- do -
Nordihydroguaiaretic acid (NDGA)	Products of oils and fats
Hydroquinone	- do -
Tocopherols	Food products
Butylated hydroxyl anisole (BHA)	Cosmetics and pharmaceuticals containing oils and fats.
Amino and Hydroxy derivative of $\Box$-phenylamine diamine	- do -
Diphenylamines	- do -
Caseine and Edestine	- do -
Cysteine hydrochloride	- do -
Monohydric phenol	- do -

Synergists: These are the substances when used with suitable antioxidant, enhance the activity of antioxidants. Hence they are called synergists. These may be water soluble or oil soluble. The names of some synergists are given below in the Table 4.4.

TABLE 4.4

List of some synergists

Water soluble	Oil soluble
Citric acid	*Ascorbyl palmitate*
Tartaric acid	*Monostearyl citrate*
Phosphoric acid	*Mono-isopropyl citrate*
Ascorbic acid	*Palmityl phosphate*
Carboxymethyl mercapto succinic acid	

Natural colorants: The source of natural colours may be mineral, plant and animal. Examples of some natural colours are given in the Table 4.5.

TABLE 4.5

Example of natural colours

A. *Mineral origin (pigments)*	Colour	Common use
Red ferric oxide	Red	In lotions, cosmetics and in some topical preparations.
Yellow ferric oxide	yellow	- do -
Titanium dioxide	white	- do -
Carbon black	black	- do -

Table 4.5 Contd...

B. Plant origin

Chlorophyll	green	- do -
Anattenes (from annatto seeds)	yellow orange	- do -
Betacarotene (from carrots)	yellow	used in margarine and food products
Alizarin (from madder plants)	reddish yellow	- do -
Indigo (from indigo plants)	blue	- do -
Flavone(riboflavine, hesperidin,Quercetin)	yellow	- do -
Saffron	yellow	- do -

C. Animal origin

Tyran purple(from secretion of a snail, Murex brandaris)	purple	
Cochineal(from an insect, coccus cacti)	red	not being used due to contamination of salmonella
Carbon black(from carbon)	black	pharmaceuticals and food products
Caramel (from burnt sugar)	dark brown	- do -

Synthetic Colorants

A. Coal Tar Dyes

Common Name	Colour	Common use
Quinazarine Gress	green	pharmaceuticals and food products
Alizarin Cyanine	green	- do -
Fast Green FCF	green	- do -
Green S	green	- do -
Tartrazine	yellow	- do -
Sunset Yellow FCF	yellow	- do -
Quinoline Yellow WS	yellow	- do -
Amaranth	Red	- do -
Erythrosine	Red	- do -
Eosine Ys/Eosine G	Red	- do -
Toney Red/ Sudan III	Red	- do -

Liquid preparations are made palatable by use of suitable flavouring agent. The Table 4.6 shows a list of flavours and their solubility in different solvents.

TABLE 4.6

Flavouring agents commonly used

Name	Solubility	Used in
Ajowan oil, BPC'34	soluble in alcohol, in fixed oils	Carminative and antispasmodic preparations.
Amber oil, BPC'49	soluble in alcohol, in fixed oils	Liniments.
Anethole USNF	very slightly soluble in water, soluble (1 in 2) in alcohol	Lozenges, carminative mixtures

Table 4.6 Contd...

Name	Solubility	Used in
Anise oil BP/USNF	Soluble (1 in 3) in alcohol (90%),	- do -
Bay oil BPC'49	soluble in glacial acetic acid, in alcohol.	Hair lotion, After shave lotion
Caraway oil BP	Soluble (1 in 8) in alcohol (80%)	Carminatives
Cardamom oil BP	Soluble (1 in 6) in alcohol (70%)	- do -
Chamomile oil BPC'49	Soluble (1 in 6) in alcohol (70%), Soluble (1 in 2) in alcohol (90%), soluble in propylene glycol.	- do -
Cineole BPC'73	Soluble (1 in 2) in alcohol (90%), soluble in alcohol, in glacial acetic acid, in light liquid paraffin, and in fixed and volatile oils.	Dentifrices
Cinnamon oil BP	Soluble (1 in 3) in alcohol (70%), Soluble (1 in 0.3) in alcohol (90%), soluble in propylene glycol and in fixed oils.	Carminatives
Clove oil BP	soluble in alcohol, in glacial acetic acid, soluble(1 in 2) in alcohol (70%).	Antispasmodic, Carminative, and in dentifrices
Coriander oil BP	soluble freely in alcohol (90%) and in alcohol (70%).	Carminatives
Dill oil BP	Soluble (1 in 1) in alcohol (90%), soluble (1 in 10) in alcohol (80%), soluble in propylene glycol.	- do -
Eugenol BP	Soluble (1 in 2) in alcohol (70%), soluble in alcohol, miscible with fixed oils, glacial acetic acid and with alkali hydroxide solutions.	Dentifrices
Fennel oil BPC'49	soluble(1 in 1) in alcohol(90%).	Carminatives
Geranium oil BPC'59	Soluble (1 in 3) in alcohol (70%) may be with slight opalescence.	Dentifrices and in cosmetics
Lemon Grass oil BPC'59 (Indian)	Soluble (1 in 3) in alcohol(70%), soluble in mineral oil, freely soluble in propylene glycol.	Carminatives and in cosmetics.
Lemon oil BP	Soluble (1 in 2) in alcohol (90%) with a slight opalescence, miscible with glacial acetic acid.	Carminatives and other preparations
Nutmeg oil BP	Soluble (1 in 4) in alcohol (90%)	Carminative preparations.
Orange oil	Soluble (1 in 7) in alcohol (90%), and in glacial acetic acid.	Oral preparations
Peppermint oil BP	Soluble (1 in 4) in alcohol (70%) with a slight opalescence, soluble (1 in 0.5) in alcohol(90%).	Carminatives, dentifrices, and Oral preparations.
Spearmint oil BP	Soluble (1 in 1) in alcohol (80%)	- do -
Thyme oil BPC'49	Soluble (1 in 2) in alcohol (80%)	Carminative and Cough preparations.

Process control tests: The tests which need to be carried out during manufacture of a liquid preparation are presented in the form a table below. The type of test will vary with the step of manufacturing

Manufacturing Step	Test to be carried out for Liquid Preparations, on solutions & suspension
Mixing	Taste, odour, pH, weight/ml, drug content and alcohol content, if present. Sedimentation (for a suspension),
Filtration (solution)	Clarity
Filling & sealing	Filled volume/transfer volume, seal test, Clarity (for solution), *For Liquid extracts, Tinctures, spirit*
Extraction	Odour, total solids, weight/ml, alcohol content, drug content, clarity (for clear preparations).

Standards as per IP

Uniformity of content: Unless otherwise specified, single dose product, packed in single dose container, containing less than 10 mg or 10% of active ingredient shall comply with the following test. When more than one ingredient are present, each ingredient should be tested for compliance. Remove the contents from each container as completely as possible and determine the content (assay) of each ingredient. The test for uniformity of content should be carried out on a pooled sample of the preparation, not less than 10 containers, sampled randomly.

The preparation complies with the test,

- if the individual values thus obtained lie between 85 – 115% of the average value.
- If more than one individual value remains outside the limits, or if any one value remains outside the limit 75 – 125% of the average value, the preparation is declared as **fail.**
- If one individual value found outside the limit 85 – 115%, but inside the limit 75 – 125%; the test is to be repeated on a poled sample of 20 containers.
- if not more than 3 individual values out of 30 are outside the limit
- 85 – 115% and not more than one out of 30 is outside the limit 75
- 125% of the average value, the sample will **pass** the test.

Uniformity of weight/volume: Unless otherwise specified, oral liquids comply with the test for *contents of packaged dosage forms,* as per IP.

Solutions

Solution preparations contain one or more chemical substances usually dissolved in aqueous vehicle. The solutes are usually non-volatile. For specific therapeutic action of the solute(s) the solution is used. These may vary in terms of composition, method of manufacture, strength, mode of administration and dosage.

The method of manufacture of solution may be,

(i) **Simple solution**, e.g Merbromine solution BPC is a simple solution containing 2 g of merbromine in 100 ml of purified water, or Gentian violet lotion NFI is prepared by dissolving 1 g of gentian violet (crystal violet) in a mixture of 10 ml alcohol (95%) and 90 ml of purified water. *These are mostly intended for external use only.*

Oral solutions are solutions of drug(s) in a palatable base suitably buffered, coloured and sweetened, e.g. Syrups, Elixirs, Linctuses.

Parenteral solutions are sterile solutions and prepared specially under aseptic environment.

Ophthalmic solutions are iso-osmotic, sterile solutions and also prepared under aseptic environment.

(ii) **Solution by chemical reaction**, e.g. Aluminium acetate solution is prepared by the reaction between aluminium sulphate and acetic acid in presence of tartaric acid.

(iii) **Extraction,** e.g. Tinctures, Extracts.

Evaluation of Solution Formulations

Usually the following tests are to be performed for evaluation of a solution formulation.

1. Physical Tests

    1.1   General Description – clarity, colour, odour and taste.

    1.2   pH

    1.3   Weight/ml at 25 °C or at any other temperature specified in the individual monograph.

2. Chemical Tests

    2.1   Identification tests for active ingredients and other ingredients as directed in the individual   monograph.

    2.2   Estimation of active ingredients and other ingredients as directed in the individual monograph.

3. Biological Tests.

   3.1 Microbiological test, if applicable

Syrups

Syrups may be medicated or non medicated. The non medicated syrups containing flavouring agent, sometimes colouring agent also, are used as vehicle to prepare medicated oral liquid preparations which may be solution or suspension depending on the solubility and other physicochemical properties of the drug(s). The drugs which are water soluble and stable in the solution state can only be formulated in this form. The non medicated syrups are also used as drink after diluting with adequate amount of water.

Usually medicated syrups are prepared commercially by mixing all components of the formulation including sucrose. Mostly such a syrup contain preservatives, buffers, flavours and colours, in addition to sucrose. Some syrups contain stabilizing, thickening, solubilising agents. When a flavoured syrup is used as a vehicle, care should be taken for selection. Since, some medicated syrup are acidic, some are neutral or slightly basic. The drug should be stable in the chosen syrup.

The major and common constituent of a syrup is sucrose. As syrups can contain up to 85% of sugars, they are capable of resisting bacterial growth by virtue of their osmotic effect. They may contain lower concentration of sugars. But, in some cases, other glycogenetic substances (converted to glucose in the body) like sorbitol, glycerin, propylene glycol, etc. are used to replace sucrose partly or fully. Which can maintain a high osmotic gradient. These can also act as cosolvents for maintaining solubility of the ingredients and also for prevention of crystallisations. Sometimes, neither sucrose nor any glycogenetic material is used, a suitable cellulose derivative, e.g. methyl cellulose or hydroxyethylcellulose along with artificial sweetener is used to maintain desired consistency with sweetness. Such syrups are commonly meant for diabetic patients. In fact, these celluloses of required viscosity grade can act as excellent substitute of sucrose.

Artificial sweetening agents are sodium saccharine and aspartame, which are about 300 to 200 times sweeter than sucrose respectively. Sodium saccharine has bitter after-taste and beyond certain concentration it gives bitter taste. The use of saccharine is presently restricted because of its toxic effect.

The main advantages of syrups are

- An unpleasant or disagreeable drug can be administered orally. When a required volume syrup is swallowed, a portion of the dissolved drug can come in contact with taste buds and rest passes down the throat concealing the taste. A simple solution cannot do this.

- Infants, children, elderly patient and any other who cannot swallow a solid dosage form, can swallow a liquid.
- Usually syrup contains little or no alcohol, so it can be safely administered to infants.

Additives

The common additives of a syrup are

- Preservatives to protect the preparation from microbial growth,
- Buffers to stabilise the dissolved drug,
- Colouring and flavouring agents to enhance the organoleptic properties of the product for better acceptability.

The list of preservatives, buffers, colouring and flavouring agents have been presented earlier of this chapter.

Problems encountered and their solutions

1. **Surface dilution:** It occurs in a closed container as a result of solvent evaporation that condenses on the upper internal surface of the container and then flows back on the surface of the product, thereby produces a diluted layer which provides ideal medium for microbial growth.

    Solution:

    (a) By incorporating a sufficient concentration of preservative, so that a diluted sample of a product resists microorganisms to grow,

    (b) Adding 5 – 10% of alcohol. The vapour pressure of alcohol is greater than that of water and normally vaporises to the surface of the liquid and the cap area. This minimises the potential for microbial growth.

2. **Crystallization:** Crystallization of sugar occurs on storage and during use, within the screw cap used to seal the container.

    Solution:

    (a) This can be avoided by adding polyhydric alcohol,

    (b) By using invert syrup (mixture of glucose and fructose) in place of simple syrup.

Formulations:

Product: Citric Acid Syrup

Composition:

Each 100 ml contains

Lemon tincture	1.0 ml
Citric acid, hydrous	1.0 g
In syrup base.	

Use: Flavoured vehicle

Lot size: 25 ml

Manufacturing Formula:

Lemon Tincture USP	0.25 ml
Citric Acid, Hydrous USP	0.25 g
Purified water USP	0.25 ml
Simple Syrup USP	q.s

Manufacturing Method:

- Take weighed quantity of citric acid in a clean, 50 ml measuring cylinder,
- Add purified water, shake to dissolve,
- Add lemon tincture through a pipette, shake to mix,
- Make up the volume with simple syrup, mix with a glass rod,
- Filter through G_4 sintered glass crucible under vacuum,
- Determine alcohol content, it should not be less than 1%,
- Fill in glass bottle, seal with pilfer proof cap,
- Label properly, store at a temperature below 25°C.

Product: Disodium Hydrogen Citrate Syrup

Standard for product: Content of Disodium hydrogen citrate; 97 – 105% of the label claim.

Composition:

Each 5 ml contains

Disodium Hydrogen Citrate IP 1.4 g

In a flavoured syrup base

Use: Systemic alkaliser

Lot size: 25 ml

Manufacturing Formula:

Citric Acid Monohydrate	IP	6.23 g
Sodium Bicarbonate	IP	4.98
Sugar	IP	3.2 g
Liquid Glucose		3.5 g
Methyl paraben sodium	IP	0.025 g
Propyl paraben sodium	IP	0.0025 g
Essence Pineapple		0.025 ml
Tartrazine		0.0025 g
Purified water	IP	q.s.

Manufacturing Method:

- Take 5 ml of hot purified water in a clean 50 ml beaker, add weighed quantity of sodium bicarbonate, stir with a glass rod till it is dissolved, allow it to cool,
- Dissolve the weighed quantity of sugar and citric acid in 10 ml of purified water, add this solution slowly to the solution of sodium bicarbonate with continuous stirring,
- Add liquid glucose to the bulk solution,
- Dissolve methyl paraben sodium and propyl paraben sodium in 5 ml of hot purified water,
- Add this solution to the bulk and mix well,
- Make up the volume with purified water, stir well,
- Check the pH, it should be within 4.5 – 4.7 and specific gravity within 1.236 – 1.250,
- Estimate the content of disodium hydrogen citrate,
- Add weighed quantity of colour and flavour, mix well, allow it stand for overnight,
- Filter through G_4 sintered glass crucible under vacuum, if the solution is not clear,
- add 0.5 g of talcum powder, mix thoroughly and filter again,
- Fill the solution in bottle and seal with pilfer proof cap and label properly.

Note:

- While mixing sodium bicarbonate and citric acid solutions effervescence shall take place, care should be taken so that no material is lost,
- Instead of preparing, directly disodium hydrogen citrate can be used,

Product: Chloroquine Syrup

Standard: *Standard for the Drug-* It contains not less than 98.5% and not more than 101% of $C_{18}H_{26}ClN_3,2H_3PO_4$; calculated on dried basis.

Standard Product: Chloroquine syrup contains Chloroquine Phosphate or Chloroquine Sulphate equivalent to Chloroquine, $C_{18}H_{26}ClN_3$, not less than 95% and not more than 105% of the stated amount.

Composition:

Each 5 ml contains

Chloroquine Phosphate	125 mg
(equivalent to chloroquine base	78 mg)
In a flavoured syrupy base.	
Colour used- sunset yellow.	

Use: Anti-malarial

Lot size: 25 ml

Manufacturing Formula:

Chloroquine Phosphate	IP	625.0 mg*
Citric Acid	IP	312.5 mg
Glycerin	IP	1.25 ml
Saccharine sodium	IP	1.0 mg
Simple Syrup	IP	1.25 ml
Methyl paraben sodium salt	IP	25 mg
Propyl paraben sodium salt	IP	10 mg
Sorbitol solution (70%)	USP	0.5 ml
Soluble essence of wild cherry		0.05 ml
Sunset Yellow		0.5 mg
Purified water	IP	q.s

*Calculate the quantity of supplied chloroquine phosphate on the basis of its assay value.

Manufacturing Method:

- Take 10 ml of purified water in a 25 ml beaker, heat to about 90°C, add methyl paraben, propyl paraben and citric acid, stir till dissolve glycerin, saccharine sodium, simple syrup add and sorbitol solution (70%) to it, mix thoroughly (solution-1),

- Weigh accurately the required quantity of chloroquine phosphate and transfer into a 50 ml clean beaker, add about 10 ml of purified water heat to dissolve over a boiling water bath (solution-2),

- Add the solution-1 to the solution-2, mix well,

- Make up the volume with purified water, determine the pH, weight/ml and estimate the drug content as per IP,

- Dissolve the colour in a small quantity of the preparation, add this to the bulk, mix, filter the solution through G_4 sintered glass crucible under vacuum, add the flavour and mix thoroughly,

- Fill the preparation in a clean, dry bottle, seal with pilfer proof cap, label properly,

Product: Acacia Syrup

Composition:

Each 100 ml contains

Acacia	IP	10 g

In a flavoured base

Use: Flavoured vehicle

Lot size: 25 ml

Manufacturing Formula:

Acacia	IP	2.5 g
Sodium Benzoate	IP	0.025 g
Sucrose	IP	20.0 g
Vanilla Tincture	BPC	0.125 ml
(Alcohol content 38-42%)		
Purified water	IP	q.s

Manufacturing Method:

- Weigh accurately the required quantity of acacia, sodium benzoate and sucrose, transfer into a 50 ml beaker, add 20 ml of purified water, mix, heat over a boiling water bath, stir frequently until these dissolve completely,

- Allow the solution to cool, remove the froth, if any,

- Filter through a clean cloth, add vanilla tincture and mix well,

- Fill in a clean bottle, seal with a pilfer proof cap and label properly.

Product: Orange Syrup

Standard: Alcohol content 2 – 5%

Composition:

Each 100 ml contains

Sweet Orange Peel Tincture 5 ml

In syrup base

Use: Flavoured vehicle

Lot size: 50 ml

Manufacturing Formula:

Sweet Orange Peel Tincture		2.5 ml
(Alcohol content 62 – 72%)		
Citric Acid	IP	0.25 g
Sucrose	IP	0.41 g
Purified water	IP	q.s

Manufacturing Method:

- Weigh accurately citric acid and sucrose, transfer these into a 50 ml clean beaker, add 40 ml of purified water, stir with a glass rod till dissolve,
- Add measured volume of sweet orange peel tincture, stir well; add 1 g of talcum powder and thoroughly,
- Filter the solution through G_4 sintered glass crucible under vacuum, repeat the filtration till a clear filtrate is obtained,
- Make up the volume with purified water, mix thoroughly,
- Determine the alcohol content, weight per ml,
- Fill in a clean, dry bottle, seal with pilfer proof cap, label properly.

Product: Cough Syrup

Standard for drug: Chlorpheniramine Maleate - It contains not less than 98% of $C_{16}H_{19}ClN_2,C_4H_4O_4$; calculated on dried basis.

Sodium Citrate: It contains not less than 99% of $C_6H_5Na_3O_7$, calculated on dried basis.

Ammonium Chloride: It contains not less than 99% and not more than 100.5% of NH_4Cl, calculated on dried basis.

Standard for product: It should contain not less than 90% and not more than 110% of the stated amount of Chlorpheniramine Maleate, calculated as

C16H19ClN2,C4H4O4; not less than 90% and not more than 110% of the stated amount of Sodium Citrate, calculated as NH4Cl and not less than 90% and not more than 110% of the stated amount of Sodium Citrate, calculated as $C_6H_5Na_3O_7$.

Composition:

Each 5 ml contains

Chlorpheniramine Maleate	IP	2.5 mg
Sodium Citrate	IP	55.0 mg
Ammonium Chloride	IP	125.0 mg
Menthol	IP	1.15 mg

In a flavoured vehicle.

Colour used- Sunset yellow.

Use: Antitussive and Expectorant

Lot size: 25 ml

Manufacturing Formula:

Chlorpheniramine Maleate	IP	12.5 mg
Sodium Citrate	IP	0.275 g
Ammonium Chloride	IP	0.625 g
Menthol	IP	5.75 mg
Simple Syrup	IP	15.5 ml
Methyl paraben	IP	0.027 g
Propyl paraben	IP	0.003 g
Saccharine sodium		0.025 g
Disodium Edetate	IP	0.023 g
Sunset Yellow	FCF	0.011 g
Soluble Essence of Pineapple		0.11 ml
Chloroform	IP	1.5 ml
Purified water	IP	q.s

Manufacturing Method:

- Weigh accurately sodium citrate, ammonium chloride and disodium edetate, transfer these into a 50 ml clean beaker, add 8 ml of purified water, heat on a boiling water bath with stirring,

- Continue heating till the solids get dissolved. when a clear solution is obtained,

- Add measured volume of syrup to the solution, stir to mix,

- Add weighed quantity of chlorpheniramine maleate, methyl paraben, propylparben and saccharine sodium to the bulk solution, stir well till these dissolve,
- Take weighed quantity of sunset yellow mix with the bulk solution, allow the solution to cool,
- Dissolve menthol in chloroform, add to the bulk solution and mix thoroughly,
- Filter the solution through G4 sintered glass crucible under vacuum, make up the volume with purified water, mix well again,
- Evaluate the product completely, add the essence of pineapple and mix well,
- Fill the product in a clean, dry bottle and seal with pilfer proof cap,
- Label correctly.

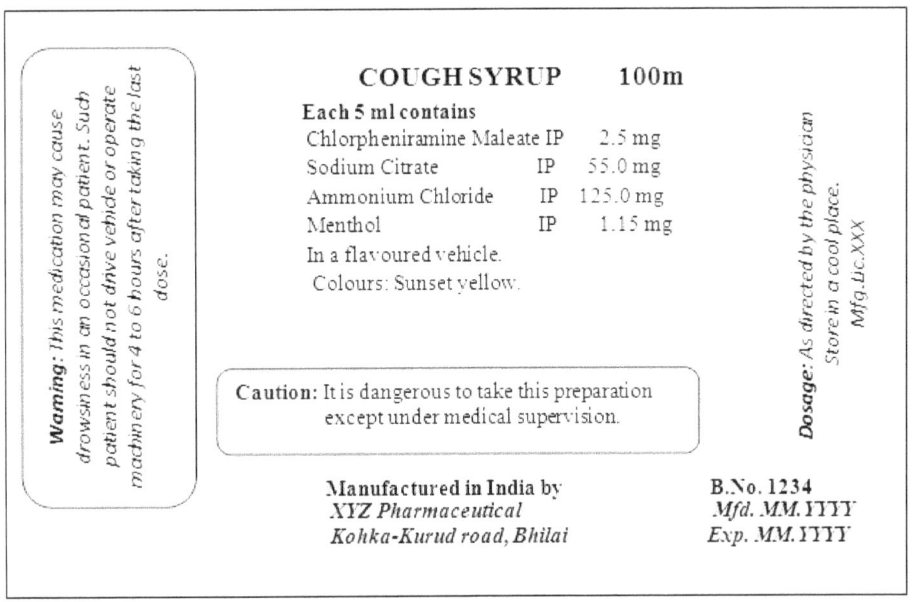

Elixirs

Elixirs are clear liquid preparations of potent or sometimes nauseous drugs in pleasantly flavoured, palatable hydroalcoholic base. The drugs may be antibiotics, antihistaminics, sedatives, etc. the vehicle usually contains high proportions of glycerin, propylene glycol, syrup, etc. in addition to other adjuvants, e.g. flavouring and colouring agents, preservatives, chemical stabilisers, etc. In fact, there is no sharp distinction between elixirs and syrups on the basis of alcohol content. The alcohol content in elixirs may vary from 3-43%.

Elixirs are usually stable preparations when packed in air-tight, light-resistant containers and if these are not diluted or mixed with other preparation. Of course, some elixirs are there such as chloral elixir a paediatric preparation, which must be prepared just before the use because of their poor stability and even some are so unstable that these are supplied in the form of granules or powders and at the time of dispensing adequate solvent is added to prepare the elixir. An appropriate warning regarding the limited shelf-life should be given on the label. For example, elixirs of phenethicillin and phenoxy methylpenicillin.

Elixirs as such usually do not favour the growth of micro-organisms; but as they contain higher quantity of syrup, glycerol or sorbitol, on dilution may become suitable medium for microbial growth. Therefore, for dispensing a prescribed dose of the drug if an elixir needs to be diluted with a suitable or prescribed vehicle, the diluted elixir must be freshly prepared and should be consumed within two weeks time unless otherwise mentioned in the individual monograph.

A clear instruction in this regard should be given to the patient.

Some of the elixirs are described in the official monographs are commercially available under the title syrup, sometimes these terms have been used synonymously.

Labelling

The label of an elixir prepared and supplied by a manufacturer should contains all informations as per general requirements for labelling of the product.

If an elixir is to be prepared before issue to the patient, the label on the container of granules or powder should state,

- the name of the preparation in form of Granules or Powder for the Elixir, as mentioned in the individual monograph,
- the name and concentration of the active ingredient in the elixir when prepared as per the directions given by the manufacturer,
- direction for storage,
- the date after which the preparation should not be used.

However, the manufacturer either through the label on the container or through a leaflet, inserted inside the pack, should state,

- the direction for preparing the elixir,
- storage conditions, and
- shelf-life of the prepared formulation.

Formulations:

Product : Aromatic Elixir

Standard: Alcohol content 21 – 23%v/v.

Composition:

Each 100 ml contains

Compound Orange Spirit USP	1.2 ml
Simple Syrup USP	37.5 ml
Alcohol(95%v/v) USP	23.8 ml
Purified water	q.s

Use: As a flavoured vehicle

Lot size: 50 ml

Manufacturing Formula:

Compound Orange Spirit USP	0.6 ml
Simple Syrup USP	18.8 ml
Alcohol (95%v/v) USP	11.9 ml
Purified water	q.s.

Manufacturing Method:

- Transfer simple syrup into a 100 ml measuring cylinder through a 10 ml graduated pipette,
- Transfer compound orange spirit through a 1 ml graduated pipette, mix by swirling,
- Add alcohol (95%) to the mixture and mix well,
- Add required amount of purified water gradually with continuous swirling the cylinder to make up the volume 25 ml,
- Mix well, add 1 g of talcum powder, mix thoroughly,
- Filter through Whatman No.1 filter paper, soaked with alcohol, refilter the solution till a clear filtrate is obtained,
- Estimate the alcohol content and fill the product in an amber bottle, seal with pilfer proof cap and label properly.

Note:

- Talcum has been used as adsorbent to clarify the solution, the solution can be filtered under vacuum through G4 sintered crucible.
- All the glass wares to be used should be clean and dry.

Product: Diphenhydramine Hydrochloride Elixir

Standard for drug: It should contain not less than 99% and not more than 101% of $C_{17}H_{21}NO,HCl$, calculated on dried basis.

Standard for product: It should contain $C_{17}H_{21}NO,HCl$ within 94 – 110% of the label claim.

Composition:

Each 5 ml contains;

Diphenhydramine Hydrochloride,	IP	12.5 mg

In a flavoured syrup base.

Colour used; Amaranth.

Use: Antihistaminic(Histamine H_1-receptor antagonist)

Lot size: 25 ml

Manufacturing Formula:

Diphenhydramine HCl, USP	62.5 mg
Orange oil	0.006 ml
Cinnamon oil	0.003 ml
Clove oil	0.002 ml
Coriander oil	0.00075 ml
Anethole	0.00075 ml
Colour Amaranth	10.0 mg
Alcohol (85%)	4.2 ml
Simple Syrup USP	9.00 ml
Purified water	q.s.

Manufacturing Method:

Preparation of solution of flavours:

- Take a clean and dry 50 ml stopper measuring cylinder,

- Transfer 34 ml of alcohol (95%) add sufficient purified water to make 40 ml, mix well. The prepared alcohol is of 85%.

- Take three clean, dry test tubes, marked 1, 2, 3. Transfer accurately required volume of flavour and alcohol (85%) into the test tubes, as indicated below, mix. Take 1.0 ml of the diluted flavour from test tube-3 for the preparation.

Test tube-1	**Test tube-2**	**Test tube-3**

Flavour + alcohol $\rightarrow$ dil.flavour + alcohol $\rightarrow$ dil.flavour + alcohol

Orange oil, 0.1 ml + 4.9 ml$\rightarrow$1.0 ml + 1.0 ml $\rightarrow$ 1.2 ml + 0.8 ml

Cinnamon oil, 0.1 ml + 4.9 ml $\rightarrow$ 1.0 ml + 1.0 ml $\rightarrow$ 0.6 ml + 1.4 ml

Coriander oil, 0.15 ml + 1.85 ml $\rightarrow$ 0.1 ml + 0.9 ml $\rightarrow$ 0.5 ml + 4.5 ml

- Take a clean, dry 25 ml measuring cylinder, transfer 10 ml of purified water,
- Add weighed amount Diphenhydramine HCl, shake well to dissolve, add weighed quantity of Colour Amaranth and shake again till a clear solution is obtained.
- Add 4.2 ml of the solution of flavours slowly and stir with a glass rod.
- Add slowly the measured volume of simple syrup and stir with glass rod, make up the volume with purified water.
- Take out the glass rod, stopper the cylinder and mix well.
- Check pH of the product, pH should be 4.5 ±0.2,
- Estimate the drug content,
- Filter the solution through G_4 sintered glass crucible under vacuum, fill in a clean, dry amber bottle, seal with pilfer proof cap.
- Label the bottle properly.

Product: Piperazine Citrate Elixir

Standard drug: It contains not less than 98%w/w of $(C_4H_{10}N_2)_3 \cdot 2C_6H_8O_7$, calculated on dried basis.

Standard product: Content of piperazine citrate, 15.1 – 17.8%w/v calculated as $C_{24}H_{46}N_6O_{14}$.

Weight/per ml at 20°C : 1.24 – 1.26 g

Composition:

Each 5 ml contains

Piperazine citrate 37.5 mg.

In a coloured, flavoured palatable syrupy base.

Colour: Green S and Tartrazine.

Use: Anthelmintic

Lot size: 25 ml

Manufacturing Formula:

Piperazine Citrate		4.6 g
Peppermint Spirit	BPC	0.125 ml

Green S and Tartrazine Solution	BPC	0.375 ml
Glycerin	IP	2.5 ml
Syrup	IP	12.5 ml
Purified Water	IP	q.s

***Manufacturing Method*:**

- Dissolve the required amount of piperazine citrate in 10 ml of purified water in a 50 ml beaker, marked at 25 ml,
- Add green S and tartrazine solution, glycerin, syrup and peppermint spirit gradually with constant stirring,
- Make up the volume with purified water and mix thoroughly,
- Carry out the tests,
- Transfer the preparation into a 25 ml amber bottle and seal with a pilfer proof cap,
- Label the bottle properly.

***Green S and Tartrazine Solution BPC*:** Mixture (1:1) of 0.5% w/v solution of green S and 0.5%w/v of tartrazine in purified water.

***Peppermint Spirit*:** A 10%v/v solution of peppermint oil in alcohol (90%).

Product: Chloral Elixir, Paediatric. BPC

***Standard drug*:** It contains not less than 99.5% and not more than 102.5% of chloral hydrate, calculated as $C_2H_3Cl_3O_2$.

***Standard product*:** Content of chloral hydrate, 3.80 – 4.20%w/v calculated as $C_2H_3Cl_3O_2$.

Weight per ml at 20°C, 1.32 – 1.33 g.

***Composition*:**

Each 5 ml contains, Chloral hydrate	USP	200 mg
In a flavoured, palatable base.		

***Use*:** Sedative

***Lot size*:** 25 ml

***Manufacturing Formula*:**

Chloral Hydrate		1.0 g
Black Currant Syrup	BPC	0.5 ml
Purified Water	IP	5.0 ml
Syrup	IP	q.s

Manufacturing Method:

- Dissolve required quantity of chloral hydrate in 5 ml of purified water in a clean, 50 ml beaker marked at 25 ml,
- Add black currant syrup, mix thoroughly,
- Make up the volume with syrup and mix well,
- Carry out the tests,
- Transfer the product into a clean, dry amber bottle, seal with a pilfer proof cap,
- Label properly,

Product: Ephedrine Hydrochloride Elixir

Standard for drug: It should contain not less than 99% and not more than 101%w/w of $C_{10}H_{15}NO,HCl$ calculated on dried basis.

Standard for product: Content of Ephedrine hydrochloride, 0.27 – 0.33%w/v calculated as $C_{10}H_{15}NO,HCl$.

Weight per ml at $20^{\circ}C$, 1.30 – 1.33 g. Alcohol content, 11 – 13%v/v

Composition:

     Each 5 ml contains

     Ephedrine hydrochloride IP 15 mg

     In a coloured, flavoured palatable syrupy base.

     Colour: Tartrazine.

Use: Sympathomimetic

Lot size: 25 ml

Manufacturing Formula:

Ephedrine Hydrochloride	IP	75 mg
Lemon Oil, soluble		0.05 ml
Tartrazine		2.0 mg
Glycerin	IP	5.0 ml
Invert syrup		5.0 ml
Purified water	IP	1.5 ml
Alcohol	IP	3.5 ml
Syrup	IP	q.s

Manufacturing Method:

- Transfer required quantity of ephedrine hydrochloride into a 50 ml beaker, marked at 25 ml, add purified water and stir to dissolve,

- Add glycerin and invert syrup with constant stirring,
- Add tartrazine and mix well,
- Add alcohol and lemon oil, mix thoroughly,
- Make up the volume with syrup, stir continuously,
- Carry out the tests,
- Fill the product in a clean, dry amber bottle, seal with a pilfer proof cap,
- Label properly.

Product: Glycyrrhiza Elixir

Standard for product: Alcohol content 21 – 23%

Composition:

Each 100 ml contains

Glycyrrhiza Fluid Extract	12.5 ml
Aromatic Elixir	87.5 ml

Use: Flavoured vehicle.

Lot size: 50 ml

Manufacturing Formula:

Glycyrrhiza Fluid Extract	USP	6.25 ml
(Alcohol content 21 – 24%)		
Aromatic Elixir	USP	43.75 ml
(Alcohol content 21 – 23%)		

Manufacturing Method:

- Measure accurately required volumes of Glycyrrhiza Fluid Extract and Aromatic Elixir, transfer into a clean, dry 25 ml stopper measuring cylinder, mix these thoroughly,
- Filter the solution through cloth, determine the alcohol content,
- Fill the product in a bottle, seal with pilfer proof cap and label properly.

Product: Low Alcoholic Elixir

Standard for product: Alcohol content 8 – 10%

Composition:

Each 100 ml contains

Compound Orange Spirit	USP	1.0 ml

Glycerin	IP	20.0 ml

In a flavoured syrup base.

Use: Flavoured vehicle

Lot size: 50 ml

Manufacturing Formula:

Compound Orange Spirit	USP	0.5 ml
Glycerin	IP	10.0 ml
Syrup	IP	10.0 ml
Alcohol	IP	5.0 ml
Purified water	IP	q.s

Manufacturing Method:

- Measure accurately required volume of compound orange spirit, glycerin and alcohol, transfer into a 100 ml stopper cylinder, stir with a glass rod, add about 20 ml of purified water and stir to mix well,
- Stopper the cylinder and keep it for 24 hrs,
- Filter the solution through G4 sintered glass crucible under vacuum, add syrup and mix well,
- Make up the volume with purified water and mix well,
- Determine the alcohol content, fill in a clean, dry bottle and seal with pilfer proof cap, label properly.

Product: Elixir Terpin Hydrate

Standard for product: Alcohol content 39 – 40%

Composition:

Each 5 ml contains

Terpin Hydrate	85 mg
Benzaldehyde	0.0025 ml

In a coloured palatable base.

Colour: Erythrosine.

Use: Expectorant

Lot size: 50 ml

Manufacturing Formula:

Terpin Hydrate		0.85 g
Orange oil	USP	0.05 ml

Benzaldehyde		0.025 ml
Sorbitol solution (70%)	USP	5.0 ml
Propylene Glycol	USP	20.0 ml
Alcohol	IP	21.5 ml
Erythrosine		0.0025 g
Purified water	IP	q.s

Manufacturing Method:

- Transfer the measured volumes of propylene glycol and sorbitol solution into a 100 ml clean beaker, heat to about 50°C, add the required quantity of terpin hydrate and stir until dissolve, allow to cool to room temperature,

- Take required volume of alcohol in a 50 ml clean beaker, add measured volumes of orange oil and benzaldehyde, mix thoroughly, add this solution to the bulk, stir well,

- Add sufficient purified water to make up the volume, mix thoroughly,

- Determine the alcohol content, pH and weight per ml,

- Filter the solution through G_4 sintered glass crucible under vacuum,

- Fill the solution in a bottle, seal with pilfer proof cap and label it properly.

Linctuses

As defined earlier, linctuses are liquid preparations of higher consistency. They usually contain sucrose and other viscous liquids along with drug substances. Commonly linctuses contain demulcent, expectorant, or sedative drugs. Out of these the most common is expectorant for relief of cough. In doses of small volume these are administered and these should be either sipped or swallowed slowly without any water.

Dilution of linctuses are done when a dose prescribed is less than or not a multiple of 5 ml according to the recommendation, if given by the individual monograph and the dose should be 5 ml or multiple thereof. Diluted linctus should always be freshly prepared and used within two weeks from the date of dilution, unless otherwise mentioned in the individual monograph.

Formulations:

Product: Noscapine Linctus

Standard for drug: It should contain not less than 98.5% and not more than 100.5%w/w of $C_{22}H_{23}NO_7$, calculated on dried basis.

Standard for product: It should contain not less than 90% and not more than 110%w/w of the stated amount of noscapine, $C_{22}H_{23}NO_7$.

Weight/ml at 20°C : 1.26 g – 1.28 g

Composition:

> Each 5 ml contains
>
> Noscapine IP 15 mg
>
> In a suitable flavoured, palatable base,
>
> Colour: Tartrazine.

Use: Cough suppressant

Lot size: 20 ml.

Manufacturing Formula:

Noscapine	IP		60 mg
Citric Acid	IP		200 mg
Orange G solution 0.015%			1.5 ml
Tartrazine solution 0.005%			1.5 ml
Alcohol 95%	IP		1.5 ml
Purified water, freshly boiled and cooled			2.75 ml
Syrup	IP	q.s	20.0 ml

Manufacturing Method:

- Take weighed quantity of noscapine and citric acid into a clean 25 ml beaker,
- Add measured volume of purified water, place over a boiling water bath and stir with a glass rod,
- Add the measured volume of colour solutions, stir with the glass rod to dissolve,
- Transfer the solution into a 25 ml measuring cylinder,
- Rinse the beaker with aliquots of syrup and add to the bulk, allow to cool,
- Add the measured volume of alcohol, mix with the glass rod,
- Make up the volume with syrup, mix thoroughly,
- Carry out the tests,
- Transfer the preparation into a clean, dry amber bottle of suitable size, seal with a pilfer proof cap and label properly.

Product: Codeine Linctus

Standard for drug: It should contain not less than 98.5% and not more than 100.5%w/w of $C_{18}H_{21}NO_3$, H_3PO_4, calculated on dried basis.

Standard for product: It should contain not less than 90% and not more than 110%w/w of the stated amount of codeine phosphate, calculated as $C_{18}H_{21}NO_3$, H_3PO_4, $\frac{1}{2}H_2O$

Weight/ml at $20^{\circ}C$: 1.30 g – 1.32 g

Composition:

Each 5 ml contains

Codeine phosphate IP 15 mg

In a suitable flavoured, palatable base,

Colour: Erythrosine.

Use: Analgesic, cough depressant

Lot size: 20 ml

Manufacturing Formula:

Codeine Phosphate	IP		60 mg
Lemon syrup			4 ml
Benzoic acid	IP		30 mg
Propylene glycol			0.3 ml
Alcohol 95%	IP		0.3 ml
Purified water, freshly boiled and cooled			0.7 ml
Erythrosine solution, 0.015%			1.5 ml
Syrup	IP	q.s	20 ml

Manufacturing Method:

- Weigh accurately the required amount of codeine phosphate and transfer into a 25 ml beaker, add measured volume of purified water and erythrosine solution, stir with a glass rod,

- If necessary, place the beaker over a boiling water bath, add weighed quantity of benzoic acid and stir until codeine phosphate and benzoic acid are dissolved,

- Add lemon syrup, mix and transfer the solution into a 25 ml measuring cylinder,

- Rinse the beaker with syrup and add to the bulk, mix thoroughly and allow to cool,

- Add measured volume of alcohol and mix, make up the volume with syrup and mix well,

- Carry out the tests,

- Transfer the preparation into a suitable size clean and dry amber colour bottle, seal with a pilfer proof cap and label properly.

Product: Tolu Linctus, Compound, Paediatric

Standard for product: Weight per ml at 20°C, 1.30 – 1.32 g

Total Acidity, 0.57 – 0.70%w/v, calculated as citric acid, $C_6H_8O_7,H_2O$.

Composition:

> Each 5 ml contains
>
> | Tolu Balsam | | 14.75 mg |
> |---|---|---|
> | Citric Acid | IP | 30.0 mg |
>
> In a suitable flavoured, palatable base,
>
> Colour: Tartrazine.

Use: As vehicle, flavouring agent and as stimulant in expectorant syrup

Lot size: 20 ml

Manufacturing Formula:

Citric Acid	IP	120 mg
Glycerin	IP	4 ml
Tartrazine solution, 0.015%		1.5 ml
Inverted Syrup		4 ml
Benzaldehyde Spirit		0.04 ml
Tolu Syrup	q.s.	

Manufacturing Method:

- Weigh accurately the required quantity of citric acid and transfer into a clean 25 ml beaker, add tartrazine solution, heat to dissolve and stir, allow to cool,
- Add glycerin and invert syrup to the solution, mix well,
- Transfer the solution into a clean 25 ml measuring cylinder, add benzaldehyde solution, mix well,
- Rinse the beaker with aliquots of tolu syrup and add to the bulk solution,
- Make up the volume with tolu syrup and mix thoroughly,
- Carry out the tests,
- Fill the preparation into a clean, dry amber, suitable size bottle, seal with a pilfer proof cap and label properly.

Note:

- The preparation should be recently prepared.

Product: Simple Linctus.

Standard for product: Content of free acid 2.24 – 2.65%w/v calculated as $C_8H_8O_7,H_2O$.

Weight /per ml at 20 °C : 1.27 – 1.31 g

Composition:

       Each 100 ml contains

Citric acid	IP	2.5 g
Concentrated Anise water		1.0 ml

       In a palatable syrup base.

       Colour: Amaranth.

Use: Diluting base

Lot size: 20 ml

Manufacturing Formula:

Citric acid	IP	0.5 g
Concentrated Anise water	BPC	0.2 ml
Amaranth solution, 0.1% in chloroform water		0.3 ml
Alcohol, 95%	IP	0.6 ml
Syrup	IP q.s	20.0 ml

Manufacturing Method:

- Weigh accurately the required quantity of citric acid, transfer into a clean, dry 25 ml beaker, add amaranth solution and place it over a boiling water bath,
- Stir with a glass rod until the acid is dissolved, cool the solution,
- Add concentrated anise water and alcohol, mix well,
- Add 5 ml of syrup, mix well and transfer the solution into a clean, dry 25 ml measuring cylinder,
- Rinse the beaker with aliquots of syrup and add to the bulk,
- Make up the volume with syrup, mix thoroughly,
- Carry out the tests, fill the preparation in a clean, dry, amber colour bottle, seal with a pilfer proof cap and label.

Extracts

These are concentrated preparations of animal or vegetable drugs. These are manufactured by separating the active constituents of the respective drug with a suitable solvent (*menstruum*), evaporating all or most of the solvent and finally adjusting the residue to prescribed standard. *The process of separation of the active principles from the drug by use of solvent is called **extraction***. The insoluble matter of the crude drug left out after extraction is called *marc*. The crude drugs may be organised or unorganised.

The **organised drugs** are cellular; that is, the active principles are present in the cells. On drying the tissues become tough with mosaic structure. Within the cellular network the active constituent remains entrapped. Hence, packing of the cellular network determine the penetration of the solvent and separation of the active principle. The separation of active constituent from cellular network takes place through diffusion process. The rate of diffusion depends on few factors, (1) concentration difference between the solutions within the cell and outside of the cell, (2) penetrating power of the solvent, (3) solubility of the active constituent in the solvent, (4) thickness and packing structure of the diffusion layer. Thus, the extraction process depends on these above factors plus extent of removal of menstruum from the marc.

Unorganised drugs are not cellular, these are resinous or oleoresinous. As the active principles are not entrapped within any compact cellular network, their separation by the menstruum is easier and hence, the rate of extraction is faster.

Irrespective of the type of drug the rate of extraction depends on the following factors;

- *Size of the crude drug.* If the size of the crude drug is reduced by cutting or milling the thickness of the diffusion layer is reduced, the solvent can penetrate easily. However, too much powdering can cause problem in separation of menstruum from the crude drug. Coarse powder is best suited for extraction.

- *Characteristics of the crude drug.* The selection of the process suitable for extraction mainly depends on the pharmacognostic character of the crude drug. For example, infusion is best suited for soft, spongy drug in which the solvent can easily penetrate. Peels of fruit like orange, lemon, etc can not be powdered, so maceration is suitable for these. Nux vomica,belladonna, etc which are hard, powderable are suitable for percolation.

- *Property of the active constituent.* During extraction many other ingredients along with active constituent may dissolve in the solvent. The selection of solvent should be made in such a way that the dissolution of unwanted materials can be avoided as far as possible and there is no problem during any step. The process is selected on the basis of the stability, cost, and other properties of the active constituent present.

- *Moistening or wetting of the drug.* The powdered drug needs to be wetted properly to remove air from the surface and to make a direct contact between the solvent and active constituent. This wetting will facilitate penetration of the solvent before start of extraction. Usually water, alcohol or mixture of water and alcohol is used for this purpose.

- *Temperature.* As the temperature increases solubility, the rate of extraction will increase with increase of temperature. This is possible only when the constituent is heat stable. Otherwise cold extraction is the only method.

- *Agitation.* Frequent shaking or agitation helps extraction. Because, it changes the concentration of solution at diffusion layer through movement of the solvent and saturated solution is replaced by fresh solvent or unsaturated solution. Thus, the extraction process is facilitated by constant flow of solvent rather than stagnant solvent.

- *Solvent.* The rate of extraction process also depends on the nature of the solvent being used. For example, at higher concentration of alcohol (more than 50%), gums and proteins precipitate out. Hence, for these if hydroalcohol is used, it should be of lower concentration.

An **ideal solvent** should be,

- non-toxic and inert,
- economic and easily available,
- specific solvent activity for desired constituent,
- should not be too volatile,
- low viscosity,
- does not facilitate the microbial growth.

Accordingly there are **different processes of extraction** - infusion, decoction, maceration and percolation. Further these processes can be classified as indicated below.

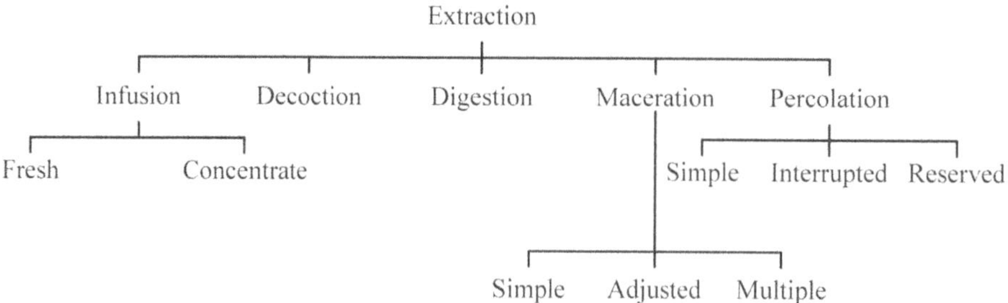

Processes of Extraction

Infusion

This is a process of extraction used when the constituents in the crude drugs is readily soluble in the solvent. The process is of short duration and the extract is a dilute solution. Either water or a mixture of water and alcohol is used as solvent and the solvent may be hot or cold. The duration of extraction ranges from 3 – 20 minutes.

Other than the potent tinctures most of the tinctures contain 20 g of the respective drug in each 100 ml tincture.

Tincture may be simple type, e.g. of a single drug and compound type, i.e. a mixture of drugs of drugs.

Normally, the tinctures are prepared from dry powdered drugs, but, there are few tinctures which are prepared from fresh substance, e.g. lemon tincture, sweet orange peel tincture. Unlike other tinctures, Tincture lemon and tincture Sweet Orange Peel contain 50 g of drug in 100 ml of tincture. Tinctures should be packed in light-resistant, air-tight containers. These should be kept away from heat.

Fresh Infusions

These are prepared by first moistening the sliced or bruised drugs with minimum required solvent in a closed container. Then rest amount of solvent is added and kept for required time with occasional agitation. The extract is strained, not pressed, and the marc is washed with small amount of fresh solvent; washing is mixed with extract to make up the volume. Usually drug: menstruum is 1 : 20.

These are sometimes prepared by diluting concentrated infusions 8-10 times with fresh solvent. Fresh infusions are susceptible to microbial growth. Thus, a fresh infusion should be used within 12 hours from its preparation.

Concentrated Infusions

As mentioned earlier these are 8-10 times more concentrated than fresh infusions. Hence, ideally the drug : solvent ratio should be 1 : 2-2.5. At this ratio extraction is not possible. Use of alcohol has one more advantage that it acts as preservative at a concentration of 10% and above. The concentrated infusion is prepared by concentrating the infusion thus prepared or by multiple maceration or reserved percolation technique. Whatever method is used some amount of menstruum is removed to bring about the required strength of the final product.

In multiple maceration technique the menstruum is divided into 2-3 portions and the drug is macerated 2-3 times with fresh menstruum. The period of maceration may be 24-48 hours. After each extraction the extract is reserved in a single container, after 12-14 days from last extraction the volume of extract is adjusted as per required strength and then filtered through suitable filter.

Decoction

Decoction is one of the oldest and common process of extraction. Water is the solvent of common choice. In this method crushed drug is put in water and boiled for at least 15 minutes. The water soluble components are extracted. After extraction the mixture is cooled and strained. The residue is washed with portions of cold water and washings are added to the bulk till the volume is made. This process is applied to drugs whose components are heat resistant. Tea leaves when boiled with water is an example of decoction. In fact, tea leaves should be put in boiling water for 2-3 minutes, this is infusion.

Digestion

This is similar to the maceration process in which extraction is done by applying heat. When the extractable matter does not degrade on heating, the process of digestion is used for extraction. Due to heat the extracting efficiency of the solvent also increases.

Maceration

In this process the required quantity of crude drug in the form of coarse powder is taken in a stopper container. The adequate volume of extracting solvent or mixture of solvents is added to soak the powders completely. Then sufficient volume of solvent is added, so that the powders are immersed in the solvent system. Usually 75% of the final volume of the preparation. The container is then closed and agitated. The mixture of crude drug and solvent is kept for 3-7 days with occasional shaking depending on the time required to dissolve the soluble constituent(s), i.e. to complete the extraction.

The mixture is filtered through an appropriate filtering medium, when most of the liquid is drained, the residue on the filtering medium is washed with portions of solvent and combined with the bulk filtrate. Finally the volume is made up. Maceration may be of three types:- simple, adjusted and multiple.

Simple Maceration

In this process the crude drug is crushed and the organised drug is put into a suitable container and required amount of menstruum is added, then the container is closed properly. Duration of maceration may continue up to 7 days and during maceration the mixture of drug and menstruum is to be agitated occasionally to facilitate extraction. After extraction the extract is strained and the marc is pressed. The pressed liquid is mixed with strained extract and filtered. The final volume is adjusted based on desired concentration of the final extract.

Adjusted Maceration or Maceration with Adjustment

In this method usually unorganised drug is used. The crushed drug is macerated with about 80% of the menstruum in a closed container with occasional agitation. The duration of extraction is less than that required for simple maceration. After due period the extract is strained and the marc is washed with remaining 20% of menstruum twice or thrice. The washings are added to main extract. In this method the marc is not pressed. The extract is then filtered, evaluated and stored in suitable container.

Multiple Maceration

In this method the drug is successively extracted with fresh solvent. Depending on the type of drug the number of extraction may be two or three. The total menstruum is accordingly divided into portions. When the drug is put in contact with first portion for a definite period, the solvent penetrate the drug completely and the soluble constituents dissolve in the solvent. After straining and pressing the concentrated extract comes out. The second portion of the solvent then added to the marc and macerated for required time. The fresh solvent dissolves the residual constituents. Thus, by successive macerations the efficiency of the extraction process is increased. Due to pressing of the marc some undissolved material comes out with the liquid. Hence, all the extracts are mixed and allowed to stand for sufficient time to settle the suspended material present in the extract. Finally the extract is filtered and stored in suitable container.

Percolation

The extraction will be more effective if the process is dynamic or continuous. In maceration both drug and menstruum remain mostly stationary during the extraction period. Because, the first layer of the menstruum in contact with the drug after dissolving constituents become saturated and an equilibrium results, while the interior layers remains free to dissolve. Unless the first layer is displaced or diluted further dissolution will not take place satisfactorily. To make it efficient frequent agitation is required. Hence, maceration is mostly a stationary process.

In percolation, the menstruum is mobile and thus, the process of extraction is more effective. Compared to maceration the total time required for extraction is less. However, in percolation the drug is initially macerated with the menstruum for some time. The damp mass is kept covered for at least 15 minutes, and then transferred to a clean percolator, a conical extracting apparatus. The percolator should be packed with a thin layer of glass wool or jute tow at the bottom so that no solid particle can escape from the percolator. Then the damp mass is transferred into the percolator and packed, during packing of the mass it is necessary to take care that no air is entrapped inside the mass. After completion of packing sufficient solvent or as prescribed, is poured in the percolator and the outlet nozzle is kept open. When the menstruum is about to drain through outlet nozzle, the nozzle is closed. In this process the menstruum over the column of drug flows downward to the outlet nozzle under the force of gravity. The percolator is then covered and kept standing for 24 hrs or for the time specified. Thereafter the extract, called percolate, is allowed to drain slowly at a specified rate and collected in a container placed below the percolator. Once almost entire solvent is drained out, further quantity of fresh solvent is poured into the percolator and according to specification the process is continued till extraction is completed, which can be ascertained by testing the last portion of the percolate for presence of a particular constituent.

As mentioned earlier, percolation may be of four types; simple, reserve, interrupted and hot continuous.

Simple percolation

It involves six main steps:

- Preparation of drug - the crude drug is coarsely powdered, so that the percolator can be packed conveniently without any problem of air entrapment and the surface area of the is sufficient for smooth and complete extraction.

- Preparation of percolator - usually conical type percolator is used. It should have an air tight cover and an outlet valve. The inner bottom of the percolator is to be plugged with a porous material, moistened glass wool or jute tow to avoid chocking. The drug is soaked with adequate menstruum in another container and the soaked drug is then packed into the percolator. There should no lump, packing should be uniform under moderate pressure without any air entrapment, so that the menstruum can easily flow within the packed layer. Usually two-third of the percolator is packed with drug and the upper layer is covered with a piece of filter paper. Then sufficient quantity of menstruum is added to saturate the drug.

- Maceration - according to the type of percolation, simple or multiple, and final volume of the extract, the volume of menstruum is calculated. Usually the ratio of the drug and menstruum is 1g : 4ml. Adequate amount of solvent is first added to the drug for complete saturation, then the outlet of the percolator is kept open to allow the menstruum to flow. Once the menstruum starts coming out of the outlet valve, the valve is closed and the solvent is poured till the level of the menstruum remains about 2cm above the upper surface of the packed column. The percolator is closed with the lid and allowed to stand for 24 hours for maceration.

- Percolation - this process starts on the following day of maceration. The lid of the percolator is removed and the outlet valve is opened to collect the extract at a moderate rate. About 70-75% of the extract is collected without drying of the upper layer of the packed drug. Completeness of the extraction is determined by performing the test for the desired constituent in the last portion of the extract.

- Recovery of menstruum – after complete percolation, the marc is removed from the percolator and pressed in a tincture press to collect absorbed menstruum as far as possible.

- Volume adjustment – the extract and pressed liquid are mixed, filtered and tested for strength. On the basis of the strength of the product the volume is adjusted.

Interrupted percolation

This is a method for preparing concentrated extract. In this method maceration and percolation processes are alternatively performed for 2-3 times. By doing so the concentration of the extract can be increased considerably with less amount of solvent. Otherwise the extract prepared by maceration or percolation is dilute and these methods are used commonly to prepare tinctures. The concentration of this extract is increased by evaporating the solvent. Hence, this method can be used for the drugs which are heat stable. For thermo-labile constituent interrupted percolation method is suitable.

Continuous hot percolation

In this method, the solvent is boiled, the vapours pass through the packed column of crude drug and condense there. Once the solvent level exceeds certain height above the drug column, most of the percolate returns back to the bulk solvent. By this the drug remains in contact with hot solvent and its vapour and extracts the constituent. In other words, the hot fresh solvent continuously passes through the drug and percolates. This process continues till the extraction is complete. Hence, this process is called continuous hot percolation.

This method is effective when the constituent of a drug is not readily soluble in the solvent, difficult to be extracted by maceration or percolation and is non-volatile and heat-stable. This requires less amount of solvent also. For this process a special apparatus, usually made of glass, called Soxhlet apparatus is used. This apparatus consists of three parts,

1. Round bottom flask to contain solvent,
2. Extractor tube fitted with a siphoning system, and
3. Water condenser.

The coarsely powdered drug is filled in an appropriate thimble leaving a margin of at least 1cm from the top. A round piece of filter paper is placed over the drug. The packed thimble is then placed inside the extractor tube. The required amount of solvent is put inside the round bottom flask. Over it the extractor tube containing filled thimble is fitted and then the water condenser is attached to it. Water is circulated through the condenser. The whole apparatus is put over a heating mantle.

The volume solvent required is less, about 2.5 – 3 ml per g of drug.

Difference between Maceration and Percolation

Maceration	Percolation
The drug is crushed to coarse powders.	The drug is crushed to coarse powders.
The drug is immersed (macerated) in about 75% of total volume of the extract for 2 – 7 days.	The drug is soaked(macerated) with sufficient solvent for some time to dissolve the soluble constituents.
Frequent agitation is necessary during maceration.	No agitation is required during percolation, the solvent moves through the column of drug.
Solvent used for maceration may be cold or warm.	Usually done with cold solvent.
Maceration makes the solvent saturated, unless it is displaced further extraction is difficult.	The macerated drug is packed in suitable column and solvent is poured to keep the solvent level just above upper surface of the drug column.
This may be simple or multiple type.	This may be simple, interrupted and continuous type.
This requires more time up to 7 days.	This requires less time compared to maceration.

Mostly the extracts are manufactured by the method of percolation and the percolates are concentrated either by distillation under reduced pressure or by evaporating at low temperature, so that during concentration the drugs are not exposed to high heat. Depending on the state of the concentrates the extracts are classified into three categories;

- Semi-liquid or fluid extract of syrupy consistency,
- Plastic mass, also known as pilular or solid extract, and
- Dry powder known as powdered extract.

The pilular extract may be converted into powdered extract for definite purpose, but each has its own pharmaceutical advantages.

Fluid extract is a liquid preparation of vegetable drugs and contains alcohol as a solvent which serves the preservative function also. Sometimes on storage fluid extract deposits sediment. In such cases it is either to be filtered or decanted to separate the clear supernatant liquid and the extract after filtration or decantation should conform to the specific standards.

Dilution of extracts:

The extracts particularly powdered extracts are sometimes necessary to be diluted to adjust the prescribed standards.

Type of extract	Diluents, commonly used
Pilular extract	Liquid glucose, malt extract, glycerin, etc.
Powdered extract	Dried starch, lactose, sucrose, powdered glycyrrhiza, Magnesium oxide, magnesium carbonate, calcium phosphate, etc.

To obtain a colour similar to that of natural extract, the diluent used to be coloured with chlorophyll or caramel.

Formulations:

Product: Senna Liquid Extract, BPC

Standard for product:

Weight per ml at 20°C: 1.02 – 1.09 g,

Alcohol content : 22 – 25%v/v,

Total solids : 17 – 25%w/v.

Use: Laxative

Lot size: 50 ml

Manufacturing Formula:

Senna Fruits, crushed	50 g
Coriander oil	0.3 ml
Alcohol (90%)	12.5 ml
Purified water	q.s

Manufacturing Method:

- Take the weighed quantity of senna fruits, crushed to coarse powder, in a 500 ml beaker,
- Add 250 ml of chloroform water, macerate for 8 hours,
- Decant the clear liquid, and strain, reserve the extract in a 500 ml beaker, cover it,
- Repeat the process twice with 100 ml of the chloroform water for each maceration,
- Lightly press the marc, strain the expressed liquid, mix it with the previously decanted liquid,
- Heat the liquid in a covered vessel for 3 minutes at 80°C, allow to stand for 24 hours, and filter,

- Evaporate the filtrate to 37.5 ml under reduced pressure at a temperature below 60°C,
- Add coriander oil dissolved in alcohol, if necessary, add sufficient purified water to make up the volume to 50 ml,
- Allow to stand for 24 hours, filter through muslin cloth,
- Carry out the tests, fill in suitable glass bottle, seal with a pilfer proof cap and label.

Product: Datura Liquid Extract

Standard for product: Total alkaloids; 2.25 – 2.75%w/v calculated as Hyoscyamine. Alcohol content; 28 – 44%v/v.

It contains 0.25%w/v of the alkaloids calculated as hyoscyamine.

Use: Parasympatholytic

Lot size: 50 ml

Manufacturing Formula:

Datura herbs, moderately coarse powder 50 g

Alcohol (45%)   q.s

Manufacturing Method:

- Take a 250 ml percolator (alternatively separating funnel), plug the valve with a layer of cotton, close the valve and transfer the datura herbs,
- Add 40 ml of alcohol (45%) to the herb, cover the percolator tightly and allow it stand for 24 hrs,
- Allow percolation to continue, collect and reverse the percolate. Continue percolation till the percolate shows the presence of alkaloid,
- Reserve about 43 ml of initial percolate. Keep rest of the percolate separately. After completion of extraction distil the percolate under vacuum at a temperature not exceeding 60°C. Remove the soft residue from the distilling flask and add in the reserved percolate, mix thoroughly,
- Determine the content of alkaloid and of alcohol, adjust the strength of the alcohol by adding required amount of alcohol (95%), if necessary,
- Set aside for not less than 24 hrs, filter through a cloth, if necessary,
- Fill in a clean, dry bottle, seal and label properly.

Product : Glycyrrhiza Extract (Aqueous)

This is a black, pilular mass having a characteristic odour and sweet taste.

Use: used in Aromatic Cascara Sagrada Fluid Extract

Lot size: 50 ml

Manufacturing Formula:

Glycyrrhiza roots or rhizomes, dried and powdered (40 mesh)   50 g

Purified water   q.s

Dilute Ammonia solution   q.s

Manufacturing Method:

- Taker the glycyrrhiza powder into a 100 ml beaker, add sufficient boiling water to macerate the powder, cover the beaker and allow to stand for 2 hrs,
- Transfer the macerate completely into a suitable percolator, plugged with a thin layer of cotton, rinse the beaker with little boiling water and add to the percolator,
- Continue percolation with boiling water until the glycyrrhiza is completely exhausted,
- To the percolate add sufficient dil. Ammonia till the mixture gives a distinct ammoniacal odour,
- Boil the liquid under and reduce the volume to 75 ml, filter through a cloth filter/bag filter,
- Evaporate the liquid until a soft mass is obtained. Cool to room temperature,
- Pack in a suitable wide mouth clean and dry container, seal and label properly.

Product: Glycyrrhiza Fluid Extract

Brown to dark brown colour liquid with characteristic odour and sweet in taste. It contains the extract of glycyrrhiza in hydro alcohol.

Standard for product: Alcohol content 20 – 24%v/v.

Use: Sweetening and bitter taste masking, mild expectorant

Lot size: 50 ml

Manufacturing Formula:

Glycyrrhiza roots or rhizomes,dried and powdered(40 mesh)   50 g

Alcohol(97%)   12.5 ml

Purified water   q.s

Dilute Ammonia solution   q.s

Manufacturing Method:

- Taker the glycyrrhiza powder into a 100 ml beaker, add sufficient boiling water to macerate the powder, cover the beaker and allow to stand for 2 hrs,

- Transfer the macerate completely into a suitable percolator, plugged with a thin layer of cotton, rinse the beaker with little boiling water and add to the percolator,

- Continue percolation with boiling water at a rate of 1-3 ml per minute until the glycyrrhiza is completely exhausted,

- To the percolate add sufficient dil. Ammonia till the mixture gives a distinct ammoniacal odour,

- Boil the liquid under and reduce the volume to 37.5 ml, Cool to room temperature,

- Add 12.5 ml of alcohol (97%) to the extract, mix thoroughly. Adjust the volume, if necessary, with purified water,

- Determine the alcohol content, fill in a clean, dry bottle, seal and label properly.

Tinctures

These are manufactured either by maceration or percolation. Either from vegetable drugs or from chemical substances, the alcoholic or hydro alcoholic solutions are prepared. The drug content of different tinctures may not be identical but, must be within the limits of established standards. The tinctures of potent drugs usually have the drug content of 10%. The potency is normally adjusted after completion of the test for drug content (assay). There are five methods for preparing a tincture or an extract; maceration, digestion, decoction, infusion and percolation.

Tinctures may be intended for oral administration and for external application depending on the active ingredient. Examples of both types are presented.

Formulations:

Product: Benzoin Tincture, BPC

Standard for product: Alcohol content: 81 – 85 %v/v

Weight per ml at 20°C: 0.845 – 0.860g

It contains extract of Benzoin in Alcohol (90%v/v).

Use: Topical protectant, expectorant, provides comfort by steam inhalation in acute laryngitis

Lot size: 100 ml

Manufacturing Formula:

Benzoin, crushed	10 g
Alcohol (90%)	q.s

Manufacturing Method:

- Take weighed quantity of benzoin in a 100 ml stopper measuring cylinder, add 80 ml of alcohol (90%), stopper the cylinder, shake frequently for one hour,
- Filter through cotton wool, pass sufficient alcohol (90%) to make 50ml, mix thoroughly,
- Determine the weight per ml at 20°C and alcohol content,
- Fill the product in a clean dry bottle, seal and label properly.

Product: Tincture of Capsicum, U.S.P.

Standard for product:

Content of capsaicin: not less than	0.025%w/v
Alcohol content :	83 – 88 %v/v

It contains extract of Capsicum in Alcohol (60%v/v).

Use: Carminative, appetizer, stomachic

Lot size: 100 ml

Manufacturing Formula:

Capsicum, moderately coarse powder	5 g
Alcohol (60%)	q.s

Manufacturing Method:

- Take weighed quantity of capsicum in a 100 ml stopper measuring cylinder, add 80 ml of alcohol (60%), stopper the cylinder, shake frequently for one hour,
- Filter through cotton wool, pass sufficient alcohol (60%) to make 50 ml, mix thoroughly,
- Determine the weight per ml at 20°C and alcohol content,
- Fill the product in a clean dry bottle, seal and label properly.

Product: Cardamom Tincture, Aromatic. BPC

It contains extract of Cardamom in Alcohol (90%v/v).

Standard for product:

Alcohol content	84 – 87 %v/v
Weight per ml at 20°C:	0.825 – 0.845g

Use: Flavouring vehicle

Lot size: 100 ml

Manufacturing Formula:

Cardamom seeds, freshly removed from fruits and immediately bruished:	6.85 g
Strong Ginger Tincture	6.25 ml
Caraway oil	1.04 ml
Cinnamon oil	1.04 ml
Clove oil	1.04 ml
Alcohol (90%)	q.s

Manufacturing method:

- Take weighed quantity of bruished cardamom seeds in a 250 ml stopper conical flask, add 75 ml of alcohol (90%), stopper the flask, macerate for 7 days with occasional shaking,
- Strain and press the marc into a 100 ml measuring cylinder, wash the marc with 3x5ml of alcohol (90%), add the strong ginger tincture, caraway oil, cinnamon oil and clove oil accurately drawn through pipette, make up the volume with alcohol (90%) and mix thoroughly,
- If required, filter through cotton wool,
- Determine the weight per ml at 20°C and alcohol content,
- Fill the product in a clean dry bottle, seal and label properly.

Product: Catchue Tincture, BPC

It contains extract of Catchue in Alcohol (45%v/v).

Standard of product:

Total solids: 12 – 17%w/v

Alcohol content: 36 – 40 %v/v

Weight per ml at 20°C: 0.990 – 1.010 g

Use: Astringent, cough and diarrhoeia

Lot size: 100 ml

Manufacturing Formula:

Catchue, crushed	20 g
Cinnamon, bruished	5 g
Alcohol (45%)	q.s

Manufacturing Method:

- Take weighed quantity of catchue, previously crushed and cinnamon, previously bruised, in a 100 ml stopper conical flask, add 75 ml of alcohol (45%), stopper the flask, macerate for 5 days with occasional shaking,
- Strain and press the marc into a 100 ml measuring cylinder, wash the marc with 2 × 5 ml of alcohol (45%), make up the volume with alcohol (45%) and mix thoroughly,
- Determine the weight per ml at 20°C and alcohol content,
- Fill the product in a clean dry bottle, seal and label properly.

Product: Belladonna Tincture USP

Standard for product:

> Alkaloid content: 0.027 – 0.033%w/v calculated as hyoscyamine.
>
> Alcohol content: 65 – 70%

Use: Parasympatholytics

Lot size: 100 ml

Manufacturing Formula:

> Belladonna leaf, moderately coarse powder: 10 g
>
> Alcohol (70%)   q.s

Manufacturing Method:

- Take weighed quantity of Belladonna leaf, moderately coarse powder in a 100 ml stopper conical flask, add 10 ml or sufficient alcohol(70%) to damp the powders evenly and distinctly, stopper the flask, allow to stand for 15 minutes,
- Transfer the mass into a suitable percolator, pack firmly, add 15 ml or sufficient alcohol(70%) to saturate the drug, cover the percolator, allow to stand till the solvent start dripping, close the lower orifice and allow to stand for 3 days,
- Percolate slowly and reserve the extract. Add 15 ml of fresh alcohol (70%) to the percolator, close the valve and cover the percolator, allow it to stand for 1 day,
- Percolate till the percolate respond to the test for alkaloids,
- Close the valve, add the extract to the reserved extract. Add15 ml of fresh alcohol(70%) to the percolator,
- Percolate completely, add the extract to bulk reserved extract,
- Make up the volume with alcohol (70%), mix thoroughly,
- Determine the drug (alkaloids) content and alcohol content,
- Fill the product in a clean dry bottle, seal and label properly.

Product: Tincture of Chiretta

It contains extract of Chiretta in Alcohol (60%v/v).

Standard for product: Alcohol content: 57 – 60%v/v.

Use: Bitter tonic

Lot size: 100 ml

Manufacturing Formula:

    Chiretta, 40 mesh coarse powder   10 g

    Alcohol(60%)   q.s

Manufacturing Method:

- Take weighed quantity of chiretta powder in a 100 ml stopper measuring cylinder, add 50 ml of alcohol(60%), stopper the cylinder, shake frequently for 4 hours,

- Transfer the mass into a percolator, add 15 ml of alcohol (60%), allow to percolate about 7-8 ml, close the valve, add the percolate to the percolator, cover the percolator, keep it for 3 days,

- Percolate and reserve the extract. Add 15 ml of fresh alcohol (60%) to the percolator, close the valve and cover the percolator, allow it to stand for 2 days,

- Percolate, Close the valve, add the extract to the reserved extract. Add15 ml of fresh alcohol (60%) to the percolator, cover the percolator and keep it for 24 hrs,

- Percolate completely, add the extract to bulk reserved extract,

- Make up the volume with alcohol (60%), mix thoroughly,

- Determine the weight per ml at 20°C and alcohol content,

- Fill the product in a clean dry bottle, seal and label properly.

Aromatic Waters

Aromatic waters are clear, saturated solution of volatile oils or other aromatic or volatile substances in water. They are also called as *medicated waters*. The odour and taste of the aromatic water is similar to the drug or substance from which it is prepared. There should not be any empyreumatic (smoke-like) and any other foreign odour in these preparations.

Some of these preparations have a mild therapeutic action, but they are mostly used for their flavouring properties in vehicles of the oral preparations of the medicaments. In case of an official preparation, the substances from which aromatic water is to be prepared should be of pharmacopeal quality, while in case of non-official preparations to get the best quality of flavour. The substance to be used should be of best quality. There are mainly two methods for manufacturing aromatic waters – distillation and solution.

The former method is an old and traditional one, but it is slow and expensive. Care should be taken to protect the drug from direct heat and instead of direct heat, steam should be used for distillation.

The most common problem in using aromatic waters in pharmaceutical preparations is *salting out* action of certain very soluble inorganic salt on the solubility of organic constituents of the volatile oils. In contact with an inorganic salt, the dissolved volatile oils separate out from the solution producing a cloudiness in the preparation. Hence, aromatic waters should be evaluated in terms of salting out effect before use in the preparations.

Aromatic waters should be stored in light-resistant, air-tight containers; since, these are susceptible to deterioration on storage. Volatilization, decomposition or growth of mould are the common reasons for deterioration of aromatic water.

General methods for Preparation of Aromatic waters

1. ***Dilution of concentrated water***:

   Dilute the concentrated water with 39 times its volume of water. Aromatic water prepared in this manner contains a small proportion, usually about 1.5%v/v of alcohol (90%).

2. ***Solution***:
   (a) Shake the essential oil with 500 times its volume of water, shake at intervals of 15 mins, repeatedly; allow to stand for 12 hrs and filter.
   (b) Triturate the oil with a sufficient quantity of talc or kieselguhr or pulped filter paper, add gradually 500 times its volume of water with stirring and filter.

3. ***Distillation***:

   Distil the drug or essential oil with the water until the specified volume of distillate has been collected; shake the distillate thoroughly and allow to stand for not less than 12 hrs; remove any excess of oil.

   When an aromatic water is prescribed, the distilled preparation not being specified, the aromatic water made by any of the methods described above may be dispensed.

   Aromatic waters B.P. are not prepared by distillation.

Formulations:

Product: Concentrated Anise Water

Standard for product:

>   Alcohol content: 51 – 55%v/v
>   Weight per ml at 20°C: 0.917 – 0.925g

Composition:

It contains Anise oil 2%v/v in hydro alcoholic base.

Use: Flavouring agent

Lot size: 100 ml

Manufacturing Formula:

>   Anise oil   2 ml
>   Alcohol(90%v/v)   60 ml
>   Purified water   q.s

Manufacturing Method:

- Measure 60 ml of alcohol (90%) and transfer into a 250ml conical flask,
- Add drop wise 2 ml of Anise oil drawn through a 2ml pipette with shaking,
- Add about 38 ml of purified water slowly with constant shaking,
- Transfer the solution into a measuring cylinder and make up the volume with purified water,
- If the solution is not clear, add 10g of purified talc and shake occasionally for 3 hrs,
- Filter through cotton wool, recycle the first filtrate until a clear filtrate is obtained,
- Fill the solution in a clean, dried bottle, seal and label properly,
- Determine the alcohol content and weight per ml at 20°C.

Product: Concentrated Caraway Water

Standard for product:

>   Alcohol content: 51 – 55%v/v
>   Weight per ml at 20°C   0.917 – 0.925g

Composition:

It contains Caraway oil 2%v/v in hydro-alcohol base.

Use: Flavouring agent

Lot size: 100 ml

Manufacturing Formula:

Caraway oil	2 ml
Alcohol(90%v/v)	60 ml
Purified water	q.s

Manufacturing Method:

- Measure 60 ml of alcohol (90%) and transfer into a 250ml conical flask,
- Add drop wise 2 ml of Caraway oil drawn through a 2ml pipette with shaking,
- Add about 38 ml of purified water slowly with constant shaking,
- Transfer the solution into a measuring cylinder and make up the volume with purified water,
- If the solution is not clear, add 10g of purified talc and shake occasionally for 3 hrs,
- Filter through cotton wool, recycle the first filtrate until a clear filtrate is obtained,
- Fill the solution in a clean, dried bottle, seal and label properly,
- Determine the alcohol content and weight per ml at $20^{\circ}C$.

Product: Concentrated Chloroform Water

Standard for product:

Alcohol content:	$51 - 55\%v/v$
Weight per ml at $20^{\circ}C$:	$0.953 - 0.969g$

Composition:

It contains Chloroform 10%v/v in hydro alcohol base.

Use: Flavouring agent.

Lot size: 100 ml

Manufacturing Formula:

Chloroform	10 ml
Alcohol(90%v/v)	60 ml
Purified water	q s

Manufacturing Method:

- Measure 60 ml of alcohol (90%) and transfer into a 250 ml conical flask,
- Add drop wise 10 ml of Chloroform drawn through a 10ml pipette with shaking,
- Add about 38 ml of purified water slowly with constant shaking,

- Transfer the solution into a measuring cylinder and make up the volume with purified water,
- Fill the solution in a clean, dried bottle, seal and label properly,
- Determine the alcohol content and weight per ml at 20 °C.

Product: Chloroform Water

Composition:

It contains Chloroform 0.25%v/v in purified water.

Use: Preservative and co-solvent

Lot size: 100 ml

Manufacturing Formula:

      Chloroform   0.25 ml

      Purified water   q.s

Manufacturing Method:

- Measure 95 ml of purified water and transfer into a 250ml stopper conical flask,
- Add drop wise 0.25 ml of Chloroform drawn through a 1ml pipette, stopper and shake till the solution is effected,
- Transfer the solution into a measuring cylinder and make up the volume with purified water, mix thoroughly,
- Fill the solution in a clean, dried bottle, seal and label properly.

Note:

The use of Chloroform in any pharmaceutical preparation is now banned.

Product: Concentrated Spearmint Water

Standard for product:

      Alcohol content: 52 – 56 %v/v

      Weight per ml at 20°C 0.912 – 0.920 g

Composition

It contains Spearmint oil 2%v/v in hydro alcohol base.

Use: Flavouring agent

Lot size: 100 ml

Manufacturing Formula:

Spearmint oil	2 ml
Alcohol(90%v/v)	60 ml
Purified water	q.s

Manufacturing Method:

- Measure 60 ml of alcohol (90%) and transfer into a 250 ml conical flask,

- Add drop wise 2 ml of Spearmint oil drawn through a 2 ml pipette with shaking,

- Add about 38 ml of purified water slowly with constant shaking,

- Transfer the solution into a measuring cylinder and make up the volume with purified water,

- If the solution is not clear, filter it through cotton wool, recycle the first filtrate till a clear solution is effected,

- Fill the solution in a clean, dried bottle, seal and label properly,

- Determine the alcohol content and weight per ml at 20 °C.

Infusions

Infusions are dilute solutions. These contain the readily soluble constituents of crude drugs. Formerly, these were freshly prepared by macerating the drug for a short period in cold or hot, boiling water and used. Presently, infusions are commonly prepared by diluting one volume of concentrated infusion to ten volumes with water. Sometimes, the dilution may be 1:7. Concentrated infusions have been omitted from B.P. and B.P.C.

These are susceptible to growth of fungous and bacterial growth. Thus, once prepared an infusion should be used within twelve hours of its preparation.

Preparation of Infusions: Concentrated infusions are usually prepared on a small scale by the method of maceration unless otherwise mentioned in an individual monograph. The same preparation when manufactured in larger quantities, the same method should be appropriately scaled up. In certain cases infusions may be prepared by any suitable method used for preparation of liquid extract.

Formulations:

Product: Orange Peel Infusion, Concentrated

Standard for product:

Alcohol content, 18 – 23%v/v Total solids, 10 – 15%w/v;

Weight per ml at 20 °C, 1.01 – 1.04 g.

Use: Flavouring agent.

Lot size: 50 ml

Manufacturing Formula:

Dried, Bitter-orange Peel, small pieces	25 g
Alcohol (25%)	67.5 ml

Manufacturing Method:

- Take weighed quantity of dried bitter-orange peel in a 100 ml clean stopper conical flask, add 50 ml of diluted alcohol (25%), stopper the flask,
- Allow to macerate for 48 hours with occasional swirling,
- Press out the liquid and transfer the extract into another 100 ml clean, dry, stopper cylinder,
- Take the marc into the conical flask, add 17.5 ml of alcohol (25%) to the marc and stopper the flask, allow to macerate for 24 hours with occasional swirling,
- Press out the liquid, add the extract to the first extract, stopper the flask and allow the mixed extract for fourteen days,
- Filter the solution through muslin cloth, carry out the tests, fill the product in an amber colour bottle, seal with a pilfer proof cap and label.

Note:

Orange peel infusion is prepared by diluting one volume of this product to ten volumes with purified water.

Product: Senegra Infusion, Concentrated

Standard for product:

Alcohol content, 19 – 23%v/v, Total solids, 10 – 13%w/v

Weight per ml at 20°C, 1.01 – 1.03g.

Use: Diaphoretics and expectorant

Lot size: 50 ml

Manufacturing Formula:

Senegra, coarse powder	25 g
Dilute Ammonia solution	q s
Alcohol (25%)	q s to make 50 ml

Manufacturing Method:

- Extract the senegra with alcohol by percolation using suitable percolator,
- Reserve the 37.5 ml of the percolate,

- Continue extraction until further 50 ml has been collected, evaporate to a syrupy consistence,
- Dissolve the residue in the reserved extract, add diluted ammonia solution gradually until the preparation is faintly alkaline, add sufficient alcohol to make up the volume,
- Allow to stand for 14 days in a stopper cylinder, filter through muslin cloth, carry out the tests, fill the preparation in an amber colour bottle, seal with a pilfer proof cap and label.

Note:

Orange peel infusion is prepared by diluting one volume of this product to ten volumes with purified water.

Suspensions

Suspension can be defined as a coarse dispersion system in which insoluble solid particles (drug) are dispersed (dispersed phase) in a dispersion medium (usually an aqueous or in some cases, organic or oily liquids). Suspension can be used as oral dosage form, applied topically on to the skin or mucous membrane surfaces, or given parenterally by injection.

Depending on the particle size of the dispersed solids it may be classified as,

Size range of the dispersed particles	*Type of dispersion*
1.0 nm – 0.5 µm	Colloidal dispersion
0.5 µm – 10 µm	Fine dispersion
10 µm – 50 µm	Coarse dispersion

It is desired that in any suspension the solid particles should remain uniformly dispersed throughout the dispersion, so that, a correct dose can be dispensed. Since coarse dispersions contain particles of relatively larger size range, sedimentation of particles is also faster. However, it is essential that the suspension, if sedimented, it must be redispersible with minimum agitation and should be easily pourable. Thus, it is customary to mention in the label, "shake well before use". These suspensions are called *ready-to –use.*

There are certain drugs whose suspensions are prepared only before use by adding a suitable vehicle, *reconstituted suspension*. Because of stability and other reasons these formulations are prepared and marketed as dry powders. There are certain problems in formulating and stabilizing suspension dosage forms, even then these are prepared because,

- some drugs are not stable in solution state, but stable in suspension,
- to some patients like infants and elderly it is convenient to swallow,
- like other liquid dosage forms, it provides the opportunity to adjust the dose as and when required,
- suspension dosage form has good patient's acceptability for its elegance, taste and flavour.

For prolonged therapy parenteral suspension are best. When an aqueous or oleaginous suspension of a drug is injected subcutaneously or intramuscularly, at the site of injection a depot or reservoir of drug is formed which slowly release the drug. The rate of release of the drug depends on intrinsic aqueous solubility of the drug and the type of vehicle of the suspension. Most common example is Procaine Penicillin G injection.

Types of suspension: Suspensions can be classified sinto various types based on its particle size, density and suspension character of the dispersed particle, route of administration, etc.

Criterion	Type of suspension
Size of dispersed particles	colloidal suspension and coarse suspension
Density of dispersed particles	suspension with diffusible solids and suspension with indiffusible solids
Dispersion character	flocculated suspension and deflocculated suspension
Route of administration	suspension for internal use and suspension for external use

Advantages of suspensions:

- An insoluble drug can be formulated as a liquid dosage form with improved organoleptic properties.
- Patient compliance, in terms of palatability, is better.
- Easy to administer to the patients who cannot swallow tablets or capsules.
- Increased surface area of the dispersed drug particles provide better therapeutic action, e.g. antacid.
- Bioavailability of drugs is expected to be better than other solid dosage forms (tablets, capsules), since it contains fine particles of drug, no need of disintegration.
- Compared to solutions the suspension can preserve the drug better, as the drug remains mostly in solid state; hence, the stability of the drug is better than in solution.
- It can be designed conveniently for slow and sustained release of drug.

Limitations of suspensions

- Water soluble drugs are not suitable for making suspensions.
- Reduction of particle size makes the drug thermodynamically unstable and hence, invites some problems in formulation.
- Although the drugs mostly remain insoluble in suspensions, a fraction which gets dissolve in the solvent can lead to physical instability of the preparation.
- There is chance of adsorption of preservative and colour present in the suspension by the fine solid particles; thus, the concentration of preservative needs to be increased, this is not desirable.
- The rate of absorption of drug from suspension is slower than that from a solution.
- The uniformity of dose depends on the redispersibility of the sedimented drug.

Formulation Consideration

Suspension, usually, contains dispersed phase and a dispersion medium. The solids may be hydrophilic or hydrophobic. Solids which are wetted with water without any surfactant, are called hydrophilic. Hydrophilic solids can absorb moisture at a relative humidity less than 70%. The hydrophobic solids have higher interfacial tension and cannot be easily wetted by water without using a suitable surfactant. These can be wetted by oils or semipolar liquids and thus, these are also called lipophilic.

The drug substance(s) being used for suspension should be microcrystalline powders of uniform or at least of narrow size range (preferably below 10 µm) and there should be no impurities adhered on the surface of the particles.

The stability of a suspension formulation depends on various factors. Some key points required to develop a stable suspension are listed below.

- Powders to be wetted completely for at least 10 hrs with minimum amount of suspending vehicle without agitation.
- Selection of the suspending and wetting agent should be proper in terms of their grade and concentration. No extra material should be included in the formula.
- The suspending agent should be dispersed or dissolved in the vehicle and sufficient time to be allowed for complete hydration.
- The mass of wetted particles is to be added slowly to the dispersion medium with low stirring.

- Weak monovalent acids, bases, salts or any electrolyte should be used for adjustment of pH and/or tonicity. No strong acid, base or electrolyte should be used which can change the particle charge abruptly.

- After complete preparation, the suspension should be milled or homogenized.

- The preparation should be stored carefully and protected from any microbial contamination.

A well formulated oral suspension may contain the following types of additives according to the requirement:

- wetting agent

- viscosity imparting agent (suspending agent)

- buffer and/or stabilizing agent

- preservatives

- sweetening agent

- colour

- flavouring agent

The parenteral suspension does not contain any sweetening, colouring and flavouring agent, while suspension for external use does not contain any sweetening agent.

Additives used in pharmaceutical suspensions are presented in the Table 4.7 and Table 4.8 below

TABLE 4.7

Lists of surfactants commonly used as wetting agents

Type & Name	HLB value	Remarks
Anionic		
Sodium Lauryl Sulphate	40	Foaming agent, bitter in taste
Sodium Docusate	24	- do -
Non-ionic		
Polysorbate 80	15	Most commonly used, bitter in taste
Polysorbate 65	10.5	Bitter in taste
Polysorbate 60	14.9	- do -
Polysorbate 40	15.6	Toxicity is less, bitter in taste
Polysorbate 20	16.7	Bitter in taste
Octoxynol 9	12.2	- do -
Nonoxynol 10	13.2	- do -
Polyoxamer 188	29	Foaming agent
Poloxamer 235	16	Toxicity is less, taste is good

TABLE 4.8

List of Suspending agents commonly used in suspensions

Type & Name	Effective at pH	Incompatibilities
Cellulose		
Carboxymethyl cellulose sodium Methyl cellulose, microcrystalline Cellulose.	3 – 10	Higher concentration of salts, tannins, Cationic surfactants.
Hydroxyethylcellulose	2 – 10	Insoluble in alcohol above 10%
Hydroxypropylcellulose	2 – 10	- do -
Hydroxypropylmethylcellulose	2 – 10	- do -
Gums		
Guar gum	3 – 9	Alcohol, borax, glycerine above 10%, Calcium and aluminium ions.
Gum acacia	3 – 9	Insoluble in alcohol above 10%
Pectin	2 – 9	Zinc oxide, alcohol above 10%
Sodium alginate	4 – 10	Calcium ions, alcohol above 10%
Tragacanth	3 – 9	Bismuth salt, alcohol above 40%
Xanthan gum	4 – 10	Borax, cationic surfactants
Agar	4 – 10	Alcohol, borax, glycerin above 10%, Calcium and aluminium ions.
Carrageenan	4 – 10	Alcohol, borax, glycerin above 10%, Calcium and magnesium ions.
Clays		
Bentonite (Colloidal aluminium silicate)	3 – 10	Viscosity is increased by polyvalent cations and calcium ions.
Attapulgite (colloidal magnesium aluminium silicate)	3 – 10	Viscosity is increased by calcium ions.
Miscellaneous		
Polyethylene glycols(3350, 8000)	3 – 10	Phenols
Lecithin	5 – 8	Insoluble in water
Povidone (K30)	3 – 10	Oils and lecithin
Gelatin	5 – 8	Acids, bases and aldehydes.

Evaluation of Suspensions

The tests to be carried out for assessment of a suspension are given in the Table 4.9 below.

TABLE 4.9

The tests to be carried out for evaluation of a suspension

Test	Description
Appearance	Transfer the preparation slowly into a glass cylinder to avoid entrapment of air during pouring, keep it for some time, then observe the suspension for its – colour, odour, taste, uniformity of dispersion, entrapped air, if any.
Sedimentation Rate	Transfer the suspension in a measuring glass cylinder and note the initial height and falling heights of the interface (height of the dense dispersed phase below the supernatant liquid) with respect to time. Calculate the settling rate.
Sedimentation volume	If sedimentation occurs, note the volume of the sediment and that of the total preparation, calculate in terms of percent sedimented with time.
Redispersibility	After gentle agitation check the uniformity of the suspension.
Viscosity	Use a suitable, calibrated viscometer (preferably rotational) and measure the apparent viscosity at room temperature.
pH	Use a calibrated pH meter and measure the pH of the suspension.
Density or Weight/ml	Measure the density or weight/ml of the suspension at equilibrium condition and at specified temperature using a standard method. During pouring of the sample into the specific gravity bottle no air should be entrapped. RD bottle method can also be used.
Drug content uniformity	Carry out the test as per the method given in the Pharmacopoeaia.
Other Tests	Carry out the test as per the individual monograph.

Formulations:

Product: Antacid Suspension

Standard for drug: Dried Aluminium hydroxide gel should contain not less than 47.0% w/w and not more than 60.0%w/w of Al_2O_3.

Magnesium hydroxide should contain not less than 95%w/w and not more than 100.5%w/w of $Mg(OH)_2$.

Dimethicone should contain polydimethylsiloxane, $[-(CH_3)_2SiO-]_n$ within 90.0%w/w - 99.0%w/w and silicon dioxide, SiO_2, within 4.0 – 7.0%w/w.

Standard for product: Content of Aluminium hydroxide gel : 90%– 110%w/v of the stated amount, calculated as Al_2O_3.

Content of Magnesium hydroxide: 90% – 110%w/v of the stated amount, calculated as $Mg(OH)_2$,

Content of Dimethicone: 85% - 115%w/v of the stated amount.

Composition:

Each 5 ml contains

Dried Aluminium Hydroxide Gel	IP	250 mg
Magnesium Hydroxide	IP	250 mg
Dimethicone activated	IP	50 mg

Use: Antacid

Lot size: 25 ml

Manufacturing Formula:

Dried Aluminium Hydroxide Gel	IP	1.25 g
Magnesium Hydroxide	USP	1.25 g
Simethicone activated	IP	0.25 g
Sodium CMC	MV	0.125 g
Syrup	IP	18.5 g
Sorbitol Liquid(70%)	USP	1.25 g
Glycerin	IP	1.25 ml
Tween 80		2.5 mg
Methyl Paraben sodium	IP	0.05 g
Propyl Paraben sodium	IP	0.01 g
Sodium Benzoate	IP	0.125 g
Bronopol		2.5 mg
Colour (FCF)	FCF	0.5 mg
Peppermint oil		0.06 ml
Menthol		0.5 mg
Purified water	IP	q.s

Manufacturing Method:

- Take required quantity of syrup in a 25 ml clean beaker, heat on a boiling water bath, add weighed quantity of methyl paraben, propyl paraben, sodium benzoate, bronopol,
- Stir with a glass rod until dissolved,
- Add sodium CMC, stir with a glass rod until a mucilage is formed,
- Take aluminium hydroxide, magnesium hydroxide and sodium CMC in a clean mortar pestle, add simethicone and make a smooth paste,
- Transfer the contents of the beaker slowly with continuous trituration,

- Rinse the beaker with 4 ml of purified water and pour into the mortar,
- Add tween 80, glycerin, sorbitol liquid and colour, continue trituration,
- Add menthol and peppermint oil, triturate for at least 30 mins,
- Estimate the content of drugs,
- Transfer the suspension into a clean, dry bottle; seal with pilfer proof cap and label.

Product: Ibuprofen Suspension

Standard for drug: It should contain not less than 98.5% and not more than 101%w/w of $C_{13}H_{18}O_2$, calculated on dried basis.

Standard for product: It should contain not less than 90% and not more than 110%w/w of the stated amount of ibuprofen, calculated as $C_{13}H_{18}O_2$.

Composition:

     Each 5 ml contains

         Ibuprofen IP 100 mg

         In a coloured, flavoured base

Use: Analgesic

Lot size: 25 ml

Manufacturing Formula:

Ibuprofen	IP	0.50 g
Sorbitol liquid(70%)	USP	11.25 g
Sodium CMC, LV		0.75 g
Syrup	IP	6.8 ml
Sodium benzoate	IP	0.138 g
Methyl paraben sodium	IP	0.026 g
Propyl paraben sodium	IP	0.005 g
Tween 80		0.025 g
Citric Acid	IP	0.067 g
Colour (FCF)		0.5 mg
Flavour		0.16 ml
Purified water	IP	q.s

Manufacturing Method:

- Take 5 ml of purified water in a clean 25 ml beaker, add methyl paraben, propyl paraben, heat to dissolve, add sodium benzoate, stir with a glass rod to dissolve,
- Add sodium CMC, stir to make the mucilage,
- Add citric acid and dissolve,
- Take ibuprofen in a clean mortar pestle, triturate with tween 80,
- Add sorbitol solution and triturate,
- Transfer the contents from the beaker gradually with continuous trituration, add syrup,
- Rinse the beaker with 3 ml of purified water and add. Triturate the mixture for at least 30 mins,
- Carry out the tests as applicable, add colour and triturate well to mix properly,
- Add the flavour and mix,
- Fill the product in a clean, dry bottle, seal with a pilfer proof cap,
- Label properly.

Product: Ibuprofen and Paracetamol Suspension

Standard for drug: Ibuprofen: it should contain not less than 98.5% and not more than 101%w/w of $C_{13}H_{18}O_2$, calculated on dried basis.

Paracetamol: It should contain not less than 99% and not more than 101%w/w of $C_8H_9NO_2$, calculated on dried basis.

Standard for suspension: It should contain not less than 95% and not more than 105%w/w of the stated amount of ibuprofen, calculated as $C_{13}H_{18}O_2$ and not less than 90% and not more than 110%w/w of the stated amount of paracetamol, calculated as $C_8H_9NO_2$.

Composition:

Each 5 ml contains

Ibuprofen	IP	100 mg
Paracetamol	IP	125 mg

Use: Analgesic and antipyretic

Lot size: 25 ml

Manufacturing Formula:

Ibuprofen	IP	0.5 g
Paracetamol	IP	0.625 g

Aerosil powder		0.02 g
Sorbitol liquid (70%)	IP	11.25 g
Sodium CMC		0.075 g
Syrup	IP	6.8 ml
Sodium Benzoate	IP	0.138 g
Methyl paraben sodium	IP	0.026 g
Propyl paraben sodium	IP	0.005 g
Tween 80		0.025 g
Citric Acid	IP	0.067 g
Colour (FCF)		0.5 mg
Flavour		0.16 ml
Purified water	IP	q.s

Manufacturing Method:

- Take 5 ml of purified water in a clean 25 ml beaker, add methyl paraben, propyl paraben, heat to dissolve, add sodium benzoate, stir with a glass rod to dissolve,
- Add sodium CMC, stir to make the mucilage,
- Add citric acid and dissolve,
- Take ibuprofen and paracetamol in a clean mortar pestle, triturate with tween 80, add sorbitol solution and triturate,
- Transfer the contents from the beaker gradually with continuous trituration, add syrup,
- Rinse the beaker with 3 ml of purified water and add. Triturate the mixture for at least 30 minutes,
- Carry out the tests as applicable, add colour and triturate well to mix properly,
- Add the flavour and mix,
- Fill the product in a clean, dry bottle, seal with a pilfer proof cap,
- Label properly.

Product: Furazolidone, Pectin and Kaolin Suspension

Standard for drug: Furazolidone contains not less than 97% and not more than 103% of $C_8H_7N_3O_5$ on dried basis.

Standard for suspension: It should contain not less than 90% and not more than 110% of Furazolidone calculated as $C_8H_7N_3O_5$.

Composition:

    Each 5 ml contains

Furazolidone	33.3 mg
Pectin	75 mg
Kaolin	1.0 g

Use: Antidiarrhoeal

Lot size: 25 ml

Manufacturing Formula:

Furazolidone		0.183 g
Pectin		0.375 g
Kaolin, light		5.0 g
Sodium CMC, LV		0.025 g
Guar Gum	IP	0.025 g
Syrup	IP	9.5 ml
Sodium Benzoate	IP	0.125 g
Methyl paraben sodium	IP	0.05 g
Propyl paraben sodium	IP	0.01 g
Tween 80		0.025 g
Citric Acid	IP	0.067 g
Flavour		0.16 ml
Purified water	IP	q.s

Manufacturing Method:

- Take 10 ml of purified water in a 25 ml clean beaker, add methyl paraben, propyl paraben and heat to dissolve,
- Add sodium benzoate, sodium CMC, guar gum and pectin. Soak for 24 hrs. at room temperature,
- On the next day, take required quantity of furazolidone and kaolin in a clean mortar pestle, triturate with tween 80,
- Add the contents from the beaker gradually with constant trituration, add syrup and triturate properly,
- Rinse the beaker with 5 ml of purified water and to the mortar, triturate at least for 30 mins,
- Carry out the tests as applicable, add the flavour and mix well,
- Fill the product in a clean, dry bottle and seal with a pilfer proof cap,
- Label the product properly.

Product: Metronidazole Suspension

Standard for drug: It should contain not less than 98% and not more than 101%w/w of $C_{13}H_{13}N_3O_4$, calculated on dried basis.

Standard for product: It should contain not less than 90% and not more than 110%w/w of the stated amount of Metronidazole, calculated as $C_6H_9N_3O_3$.

Composition:

Each 5 ml contains

Metronidazole Benzoate	IP	
Equivalent to Metronidazole	IP	200 mg
In a flavoured palatable base.		
Colour: Tartrazine		

Use: Antiamoebic and antiprotozoal

Lot size: 25 ml

Manufacturing Formula:

Metronidazole benzoate	IP	1.0 g*
Guar Gum	IP	0.125 g
Sorbitol liquid (70%)	USP	1.25 g
Liquid Glucose		0.625 g
Polysorbate 80		25 mg
Methyl Paraben sodium	IP	25 mg
Propyl paraben sodium	IP	5 mg
Syrup	IP	11.5 ml
Colour	FCF	1.0 mg
Flavour		3 .0 mg
Purified water	IP	q.s

*Calculate the amount on the basis of assay value of the supplied drug.

Manufacturing Method:

- Take 10 ml of purified water in a 25 ml clean beaker, add required quantity of methyl paraben, propyl paraben, place over a boiling water bath, stir to dissolve,
- Remove from heat,
- Add guar gum and mix well to make a mucilage, add syrup, sorbitol liquid and mix thoroughly,

- Take required quantity of metronidazole benzoate into a clean mortar pestle, triturate with polysorbate 80, add liquid glucose with continuous trituration. Once a smooth paste is made, add gradually the contents from the beaker, continue to triturate,

- Add colour and triturate, rinse the beaker with 4 ml of hot purified water and pour into the mortar,

- Continue trituration for at least 30 mins., add flavour and triturate to mix thoroughly,

- Carry out the tests as applicable, fill in a clean, dry bottle and seal with a pilfer proof cap,

- Label properly.

Mixtures

A mixture is a liquid medicinal preparation for internal use, of which a single dose or several doses are contained in a single bottle. These contain one or more medicaments either dissolved or suspended in a suitable vehicle. Usually the vehicle is aqueous, sometimes it may be a non-aqueous also. Some preparations cannot be stored for long time and hence, these should be freshly prepared. Thus, all suspensions may be called mixture, but all mixtures are not suspensions.

The medicament may be,

1. Soluble substance, e.g. sodium chloride, ammonium bicarbonate, potassium iodide, etc.

2. Diffusible (substances which easily redisperse uniformly on shaking, e.g. magnesium carbonate (light or heavy), quinine sulphate, rhubarb, light kaolin, etc.

3. Indiffusible (do not redisperse easily and need a suitable dispersing or suspending agent), e.g. acetyl salicylic acid, barbitone, jalap resin, quinine salicylate, sulphadimidine, etc.

4. Precipitate forming liquids, e.g. tincture of benzoin, tincture of tolu, tincture of myrrh, etc.

5. Slightly soluble liquids, e.g. creosote, paraldehyde, etc.

The most common dispersing agent used are compound tragacanth powder, tragacanth mucilage, sodium carboxymethylcellulose, etc.

The medicament is finely powdered and triturated and mixed with the suspending agent, if required, followed by the addition of vehicle to form a smooth paste, finally the volume is made up with vehicle.

In case the preparation is to be freshly prepared and used, it is not necessary to use additional substances. But, care should be taken while water is used for dispensing. Since, water is a good source of micro-organism, at least potable water is to be used for the preparations which need not to be preserved for long time. Otherwise purified water should be used. A proper instruction should be given to the dispenser or user in this regard.

Dilution of mixture is sometimes permitted in the individual monograph. If a dose prescribed or ordered is less than 5 ml (one tea-spoonful), a mixture can be diluted with the vehicle either which has been used in the preparation or as directed in the individual monograph, so that a measureable volume is obtained for the patient's convenience.

If known, advice should be given on the stability of a diluted mixture and if not known or not given in the individual monograph, it is to be assumed that the diluted mixture is less stable than the original preparation and diluted preparation should not be stored for more than two weeks.

Labelling: Other than the general informations, the label of a mixture should contain the following informations.

For a mixture other than one directed in the individual monograph to be freshly or recently prepared:

- the name and concentration of the active ingredient in a mixture,
- the direction for storage.

For a powder or granule mixture to be freshly prepared and issued –

- the name of the preparation in the form of powder or granules as specified in the individual monograph,
- the name and concentration of the active ingredient in the mixture when prepared as per the instruction of the manufacturer,
- direction for storage, and
- the date after which the preparation should not be used (the period should not be more than 2 weeks).
- the label must mention distinctly, SHAKE WELL BEFORE USE

Formulations:

Product: Succinylsulphathiazole Mixture, Paediatric.

Standard for drug: It should contain not less than 99% and not more than 101% of $C_{13}H_{13}N_3O_5S_2$ calculated on dried basis.

Standard for product: Content of Succinylsulphathiazole, 7.82 – 8.96%w/w, calculated as $C_{13}H_{13}N_3O_5S_2$.

Composition:

     Each 5 ml contains

        Succinylsulphathiazole   IP   500 mg

Use: Antibacterial

Lot size: 25 ml

Manufacturing Formula:

Succinylsulphathiazole, finely powdered	IP	2.5 g
Light Kaolin		1.5 g
Compound Tragacanth powder		0.25 g
Benzoic Acid	IP	0.25 g
Propylene glycol		15.0 ml
Amaranth red		25.0 mg
Soluble Essence of Raspberry		0.5 ml
Syrup	IP	5.0 ml
Purified water		q.s.

Manufacturing Method:

- Triturate the compound tragacanth powder, light kaolin and succinyl-sulphathiazole with syrup in a clean mortar pestle to make a smooth paste,

- Add benzoic acid to the paste and triturate with gradual addition of propylene glycol,

- Add amaranth and mix thoroughly,

- Add essence of raspberry and mix thoroughly,

- Transfer the mixture into a 25 ml measuring cylinder, rinse the mortar pestle with 3 ml of purified water and add to the bulk to make 25 ml,

- Stir the mixture well with a clean glass rod,

- Carry out the tests,

- Transfer the preparation into a clean, dry amber coloured bottle, seal with a pilfer proof cap,

- Label the preparation properly with a direction, SHAKE WELL BEFORE USE.

Product: Sulphadimidine Mixture, Paediatric.

Standard for drug: It should contain not less than 99% and not more than 101% of $C_{12}H_{14}N_4O_2S$ calculated on dried basis.

Standard for product: Content of Sulphadimidine, 8.48 – 9.56%w/w, calculated as $C_{12}H_{14}N_4O_2S$.

Composition:

      Each 5 ml contains

Sulphadimidine	IP	500 mg

Use: Antibacterial

Lot size: 25 ml

Manufacturing Formula:

Sulphadimidine, finely powdered	IP	2.5 g
Compound Tragacanth powder		1.0 g
Benzoic Acid	IP	0.25 g
Propylene glycol		15.0 ml
Amaranth red		25.0 mg
Soluble Essence of Raspberry		0.5 ml
Syrup	IP	5.0 ml
Purified water		q.s.

Manufacturing Method:

- Triturate the compound tragacanth powder and sulphadimidine with syrup in a clean mortar pestle to make a smooth paste,

- Add benzoic acid to the paste and triturate with gradual addition of propylene glycol,
- Add amaranth and mix thoroughly,
- Add essence of raspberry and mix thoroughly,
- Transfer the mixture into a 25 ml measuring cylinder, rinse the mortar pestle with 3 ml of purified water and add to the bulk to make 25 ml,
- Stir the mixture well with a clean glass rod,
- Carry out the tests,
- Transfer the preparation into a clean, dry amber coloured bottle, seal with a pilfer proof cap,
- Label the preparation properly with a direction, SHAKE WELL BEFORE USE.

Product: Sodium Salicylate Mixture, Strong.

Standard for drug: It contains not less than 99.5%w/w of sodium salicylate, calculated as $C_7H_5NaO_3$ on dried basis.

Standard for product: Content of sodium salicylate, 9.50 – 10.50%, calculated as $C_7H_5NaO_3$.

Composition:

Each 5 ml contains

Sodium Salicylate	IP	500 mg

Use: Analgesic.

Lot Size: 25 ml

Manufacturing Formula:

Sodium Salicylate		1.25 g
Sodium Metabisulphite		0.025 g
Concentrated Orange Peel Infusion		1.25 ml
Purified water	IP	q.s

Manufacturing Method:

- Dissolve sodium salicylate in 10 ml purified water,
- Dissolve sodium metabisulphite separately in 5 ml of purified water,
- Mix the two solutions in a 25 ml stopper cylinder,
- Add required amount of concentrated orange peel infusion and mix thoroughly,

- Make up the volume with purified water and mix well,
- Carry out the tests,
- Transfer the preparation into a clean bottle, seal the bottle with a pilfer proof cap,
- Label the bottle properly.

Note:

- *This preparation should be freshly prepared.*

Product: Sodium Bicarbonate Mixture, Paediatric.

Standard for drug: It contains not less than 99%w/w of sodium bicarbonate, calculated as $NaHCO_3$ on dried basis.

Standard for product: Content of sodium bicarbonate, 0.95 – 1.05%w/w calculated as $NaHCO_3$

Composition:

> Each 5 ml contains
>
> > sodium bicarbonate IP 50 mg

Use: Antacid

Lot Size: 25 ml

Manufacturing Formula:

Sodium Bicarbonate	IP	0.25 g
Concentrated Dill water	BPC	0.50 ml
Ginger Syrup	BPC	1.00 ml
Syrup	IP	9.25 ml
Purified water	IP	q s

Manufacturing Method:

- Dissolve sodium bicarbonate in 10 ml of purified water in a 25 ml stopper measuring cylinder,
- Add measured volume of syrup, ginger syrup and concentrated dill water, mix them thoroughly,
- Make up the volume with purified water and mix,
- Perform the tests,
- Transfer the preparation into a 25 ml amber bottle, seal with a pilfer proof cap,
- Label properly.

Note:

- *This preparation should be freshly prepared.*

Product: Sodium Chloride Mixture, Compound

Standard for drug: It contains not less than 99.5%w/w of sodium chloride, calculated as NaCl on dried basis.

Standard for product: Content of sodium bicarbonate, 4.75 – 5.25%w/w calculated as $NaHCO_3$, Content of sodium chloride, 1.90 – 2.10%w/w calculated as NaCl.

Composition:

Each 5 ml contains

Sodium Chloride	IP	100 mg
Sodium Bicarbonate	IP	250 mg

Use: Electrolyte replenisher

Lot Size: 25 ml

Manufacturing Formula:

Sodium Chloride	IP	500 mg
Sodium Bicarbonate	IP	1.25 g
Purified water	IP	q.s

Manufacturing Method:

- Dissolve sodium bicarbonate and sodium chloride in 20 ml of purified water in a 25 ml stopper measuring cylinder,
- Make up the volume with purified water and mix,
- Perform the tests,
- Transfer the preparation into a 25 ml amber bottle, seal with a pilfer proof cap,
- Label properly.

Note:

- *This preparation should be freshly prepared.*

Product: Ferrous Sulphate Mixture, Paediatric

Standard for drug: It contains not less than 99.5% and not more than 104.5%w/w of ferrous sulphate, calculated as $FeSO_4$, $7H_2O$.

Standard for product: Content of ferrous sulphate, 1.10 – 1.30%w/w calculated as $FeSO_4$, $7H_2O$.

Composition:

Each 5 ml contains

Ferrous sulphate   IP   60 mg.

Use: Haematinic

Lot Size: 25 ml

Manufacturing Formula:

Ferrous Sulphate	IP	300 mg
Ascorbic Acid	IP	25 mg
Orange syrup	BPC	2.5 ml
Purified water	IP	q.s

Manufacturing Method:

- Dissolve Ferrous sulphate and Ascorbic acid in 20 ml of purified water in a 25 ml stopper measuring cylinder,
- Add orange syrup and mix,
- Make up the volume with purified water and mix,
- Perform the tests,
- Transfer the preparation into a 25 ml amber bottle, seal with a pilfer proof cap,
- Label properly.

Emulsions

Emulsion is a dispersed system of two immiscible liquids in which one liquid is uniformly dispersed in another. The former liquid is called the dispersed phase or internal phase while the latter-dispersion medium or external phase.

The internal phase remains in the form of fine globules of colloidal dimensions. The size of the globules is very important for stability of emulsions. A third substance called emulsifying agent is added to the system to render the stability of the preparation.

Emulsions are used for oral, parenteral, topical administration including cosmetic purpose and also for diagnostic purposes. The emulsion may be of various types, - macroemulsion (conventional emulsion), microemulsion, multiple emulsion and gel emulsion.

Based on composition, emulsions are generally of two types – oil-in-water (o/w) and water-in-oil (w/o); but, there may be another two types – water-in-water (w/w) and oil-in-oil (o/o). W/w type contains aqueous solutions of immiscible/incompatible substances, like, polysaccharides, synthetic polymers, proteins, etc., while o/o type can be prepared from immiscible organic solvents stabilized by copolymers.

The therapeutic agents and other necessary additives are incorporated in this preparation by dissolving in either of the two phases. The preservatives commonly used in emulsions are chlorocresol, chlorobutanol, mercurals, benzoic acid, sorbic acid, p-hydroxybenzoic acids, etc. Since, the surface active agents (emulsifying agent) used in these preparations have a tendency to bind preservatives and thereby reduce the preservative action; so, the preservative should be carefully selected that can protect both the phases. Alkyl esters of p-hydroxybenzoic acids are found to be suitable for these preparations. For external use, choice of the type of emulsion depends on the nature of the drug substance being used, expected emollient effect, the condition of the skin surface, etc.

An emulsion can be diluted with the liquid that constitutes the external phase or is miscible with the external phase. In this process the viscosity of the emulsion will be reduced and in some cases the emulsion type may also be changed.

Classification of emulsions:

Based on different criteria emulsion can be classified into various types.

Criterion	Types of emulsion
Size of droplets/particles	Macroemulsion–Colloidal and Fine
	Microemulsion
Orientation of phase	Simple emulsion–water-in-oil (w/o) and oil-in-water (o/w)
	Multiple emulsion–water-in-oil-in-water (w/o/w) and oil-in-water-in-oil (o/w/o)
Physical state	Liquids
	Creams
Route of administration	Emulsions for internal use
	Emulsions for external use

Methods of identification of emulsion type

- Examining the miscibility of the continuous phase when diluted, either by shaking or by stirring, with oil or water should be taken for phase reversal (*Miscibility Test*).

- Measuring electrical conductance. Aqueous continuous phase will transmit electric current, while oily continuous phase will not transmit or will transmit less electric current (*Conductivity Test*).

- Examining fluorescence under microscope. Many oils fluoresce under ultra violet radiation (*Fluorescence Test*).

- If a drop of emulsion exposed to ultra violet radiation continuous fluorescence will be observed under microscope, if it is w/o type (*Colour Test*).

- The filter paper treated with cobalt chloride solution is dried. The dry paper when dipped into the emulsion. If the colour changes from blue to pink-red, the emulsion is oil-in-water type (*Cobalt paper Test*).

Emulsifying Agents

For pharmaceutical purposes the ideal emulsifying agent should be stable, inert, non-toxic, odourless, tasteless and colourless. At low concentration it should produce a stable emulsion.

Emulsifying agents can be broadly classified into three groups – synthetic, natural and finely divided solids.

Synthetic Emulsifying agents are of three types – anionic, cationic, non-ionic.

Anionic Emulsifying Agent

Soap is an example of this group. Soap is produced from long chain fatty acids, sulphated alcohol and sulphonates. On dissociation, the long chain anion renders the surface activity, while cation remains inactive. Soaps and similar anionic agents for their unpleasant taste and irritant act the intestinal mucosa, are not suitable for oral emulsion. With alkali soaps good o/w emulsion can be prepared but they are unstable at pH below 10 and are incompatible with acids, polyvalent inorganic and long-chain organic cations.

Calcium, magnesium, zinc and aluminium soaps are water insoluble and result w/o emulsions. Amine soaps produced from amine, e.g. triethanolamine, iso-propanolamine and fatty acids are less alkaline, stable and more resistant to Ca^{++} and to change of pH.

Cationic Emulsifying Agent

Quaternary ammonium compounds belong to this class of surface active agents. These have very good disinfectant and preservative actions and these are frequently used for this purpose. Simultaneously these can emulsify o/w emulsions also.

When this is used alone, a poor emulsifying activity is found. But, when used in combination with a fatty alcohol, excellent stability is attained. The classical example is cetrimide. It is a good disinfectant but poor surfactant, but in combination (1:9) with cetostearyl alcohol is an excellent surface active agent. Cetrimide cream BPC is a stable o/w cream which contains 50% of liquid paraffin, 44.5% of water and 5.5% of a mixture of cetrimide and cetostearyl alcohol (1:11).

These surfactants are quite stable within pH range from 3 to 7, these are compatible with other cationic compounds and with calcium and magnesium ions. But, very much incompatible with anionic surfactant and soap which even at minimum concentration can cause instability of the emulsion and can spoil the preservative action of the cationic surfactant. Because of their bactericidal activity no preservative is necessary if they are present in a formulation.

Non-ionic Emulsifying Agent

These surfactants have both hydrophobic and hydrophilic groups. Hydrophobic (lipophilic) group contains a long hydrocarbon chain which has very little affinity for water. A hydrophilic (lipophobic) group contains a functional group like carboxy, hydroxyl, amino, etc. which has affinity for water.

Such a surface active agent when added to an emulsion the molecules of the surfactant are adsorbed at the oil-water interface, the lipophilic groups direct towards oil phase and the hydrophilic groups direct towards water phase resulting formation of a film at the o/w interface. Depending on the dominating groups the surfactant may be either hydrophilic, suitable for o/w emulsion or lipophilic, suitable for w/o emulsion.

If the surfactant is a derivative of an alcohol and/or ethylene oxide, the hydrophilic groups will be dominating and the surfactant will be water soluble. If it is derived from a fatty acids of $C_{12} - C_{18}$ chain, the dominating character will be lipophilic and the surfactant will be water insoluble. However, by varying the number and type of group in the molecule the hydrophilic-lipophilic character can be modified. Esters of polyethylene or polyoxyethylene, oleic acid, lauric, palmitic or stearic acids, etc. belong to this class.

Selection of an Emulsifying Agent

- The selection of an emulsifying agent (emulgent) is based on the following factors, type of emulsion, w/o or o/w and the ultimate use, external or internal.
- ability to reduce the interfacial tension between the two immiscible liquids,
- physico-chemical stability of the emulsifying agent,
- compatibility with all ingredients of the formulation,
- inertness towards the organoleptic properties, like, colour, taste and odour should not be affected,
- ability to form coherent film around the globules of the dispersed phase,
- ability to prevent coalescence of the droplets of the dispersed phase,
- ability to produce and maintain the required viscosity of the preparation.

Comparison between suspension and emulsion

Suspension	Emulsion
Suspension is a dispersed system in which finely powdered solids (disperse phase) is dispersed in a liquid (dispersion medium).	Emulsion is a dispersed system in which one liquid remains dispersed (disperse phase) in the form of fine globules in an immiscible liquid (dispersion medium).
Suspension may be classified on the basis of size of the dispersed particles- colloidal dispersion having particle size ranging from 1nm - 1μm, and coarse dispersion having particle size larger than 1μm.	Emulsion contains dispersed globules with a size range from 0.1 to 100μm.
While preparing suspension a high shear is applied along with addition of a surface active agent to overcome the particle-particle attractive forces.	During emulsification the high shear is applied break the liquid (disperse phase) into fine globules with addition of a surface active agent for dispersion of the globules.
Suspensions are thermodynamically unstable due to excess surface free energy of the dispersed particles.	Emulsions are also thermodynamically unstable due to excess surface free energy of the dispersed globules.
Usually suspensions are oil-in-water(o/w) dispersion.	Emulsions may be of both types, oil-in-water (o/w) and water-in-oil (w/o).
Suspension requires a third substance called suspending agent for suspending the particles.	For emulsification, it also requires another substance called emulsifying agent.
These are viscous liquid preparations with adequate pourability.	Emulsions are also viscous preparations with adequate pourability.
In suspension the distribution of dispersed particles may be fairly uniform.	In emulsions the distribution of dispersed globules are uniform.
Suspensions suffer from aggregation, sedimentation and caking.	Emulsions suffer from creaming, cracking and breaking.

Formulations:

Product: Benzyl Benzoate Application

It contains Benzyl Benzoate 25%w/v

Standard for drug: It contains not less than 99% and not more than 100.5%w/w of $C_{14}H_{12}O_2$.

Standard for product: It contains not less than 22.5% and not more than 27.5%w/w of benzyl benzoate, $C_{14}H_{12}O_2$.

Use: Anti-parasitic (scabicide) for external application

Lot size: 50 ml

Manufacturing Formula:

Benzyl Benzoate	12.5 g
Emulsifying wax	1.2 g
Purified water	q s

Manufacturing Method:

(a) *Preparation of Emulsifying Wax, 10 g.*

Cetostearyl alcohol	9 g
Sodium Lauryl sulphate	1 g
Purified water	0.4 ml

Take the cetostearyl alcohol in a 50 ml beaker and heat to about $80°C$, add sodium lauryl sulphate, stir with a glass rod to mix thoroughly. Add purified water, heat to $115°C$. Continue heating at $115°C$ with vigorous stirring till frothing cesses and the product becomes translucent. Filter the product while hot through a clean cloth, cool, pack in a suitable container.

(b) *Preparation of benzyl Benzoate Emulsion*

- Take the emulsifying wax in a 100 ml beaker, heat to melt, add sodium lauryl sulphate to the molten wax, mix with a glass rod. Place the molten mass at $45°C \pm 2°C$ over water bath/ hot plate.
- Take 35 ml of purified water in a 50 ml beaker, heat to $45°C$.
- Attach a high speed stirrer to the beaker containing molten wax mixture. Add warm water very slowly (preferably as a slow stream) with constant high speed stirring, continue stirring for 2 hrs.
- Stop stirring and make up the volume with warm water, then continue stirring for another 1 hr with high speed.
- Remove the hot plate from water bath and stir until the emulsion attains room temperature.
- Determine the content of benzyl benzoate.
- Fill the emulsion in a clean, dry bottle, seal and label properly.

Product: Liquid Paraffin and Magnesium Hydroxide Emulsion

Standard for drug: Magnesium Hydroxide contains not less than 95% and not more than 100.5% of $Mg(OH)_2$.

Standard for product: It should contain 4.9 – 6.7 %w/w of Magnesium hydroxide calculated as $Mg(OH)_2$ and 19.7 – 24 %w/w of Liquid Paraffin.

Composition:

It contains

Magnesium hydroxide	6.2%
Liquid paraffin	27%

Use: Antacid and osmotic laxative

Lot size: 50 ml

Manufacturing Formula:

Liquid paraffin	IP	12.5 ml
Magnesium hydroxide mixture	BP	37.5 ml

Manufacturing Method:

- Transfer liquid paraffin into a 100 ml beaker marked at 50 ml, place it over a magnetic stirrer,
- Add magnesium hydroxide mixture gradually with constant stirring,
- Once emulsification is found to be complete, stop stirring. Remove stirrer,
- Transfer the product into a clean, dry bottle, seal and label properly.

Product: Cod-liver oil Emulsion

It contains Cod-liver oil 50%v/v.

Standards product: Vitamin A activity should not be less than 285 units/g

Use: Antixerophthalmic vitamin.

Lot size: 50 ml

Manufacturing Formula:

Cod-liver oil	25 ml
Acacia powder	6.25 g
Tragacanth powder	0.35 g
Volatile Bitter Almond oil	0.005 g
Chloroform	0.1 ml
Saccharin sodium	0.0025 g
Purified water	q.s

Manufacturing Method:

- Triturate the cod-liver oil with the acacia powder and tragacanth in a mortar pestle, add 20 ml of purified water, continue trituration until a creamy emulsion is formed,

- Add saccharin sodium solution (prepared separately in 2 ml of water), add volatile bitter almond oil dissolved in chloroform, continue trituration,

- Transfer the emulsion into a 50 ml measuring cylinder, make up the volume with purified water, transfer it again into the mortar pestle and triturate. Once emulsification is complete, fill the product in a clean, dry bottle, seal and label properly.

Product: Liquid Paraffin and Phenolphthalein Emulsion

(Compound Liquid Paraffin Emulsion)

Standard: It should contain 44 – 49 %w/w of Liquid Paraffin, and 0.28 – 0.35 %w/w of Phenolphthalein.

Composition:

It contains

Liquid paraffin	50%v/v
Phenolphthalein	0.34%w/v

Use: Laxative

Lot size: 50 ml

Manufacturing Formula:

Phenolphthalein	0.1715 g
Liquid paraffin	25 ml
Methyl cellulose20	1.0 g
Chloroform emulsion	2.5 ml
Vanillin	0.025 g
Saccharine sodium	0.0025 g
Benzoic acid solution	1.0 ml
Purified water	19.5 ml

Manufacturing Method:

- Take 17.5 ml of boiling purified water in a 100 ml beaker marked at 25 ml and 50 ml, place it over a magnetic stirrer, sprinkle methyl cellulose over it and stir, allow to stand for 2 hrs with constant stirring,

- Alternatively, mix the methylcellulose with 6 ml of boiling purified water, when the powder is thoroughly hydrated add sufficient purified water in the form of ice to make 17.5 ml continue stirring till a homogeneous mucilage is formed,

- Add chloroform emulsion, followed by benzoic solution, vanillin and saccharin sodium dissolved in purified water separately. Continue stirring. Make up the volume to 25 ml,

- Add gradually liquid paraffin to this aqueous phase with constant stirring, continue stirring till emulsification is completed,

- Pass the emulsion through a homogeniser,

- Fill the product in a clean, dry bottle, seal and label properly.

Product: Emulsion of Peppermint

It contains Peppermint oil 10%v/v.

Use: Carminative, flavoured vehicle

Lot size: 50 ml

Manufacturing Formula:

Peppermint oil	5 ml
Quillaia liquid extract	0.125 ml
Purified water	45 ml

Manufacturing Method:

- Take quillaia liquid extract in a 100 ml beaker marked at 50 ml, place it   over a magnetic stirrer, add peppermint oil with constant stirring,

- Add purified water gradually with constant stirring, continue stirring till emulsification is complete. Stop stirring, make up the volume with purified water and continue stirring,

- Transfer the product into a clean, dry bottle, seal and label properly.

Microemulsions are mixtures of oil and water stabilized by surfactant (amphiphile). These are optically isotropic, thermodynamically stable liquid systems. The average diameter of droplet in a microemulsion may vary from 10mµ to 50 mµ. Type of emulsion o/w or w/o, formed greatly depends on the oil and surfactant used for the preparation. Microemulsion (o/w) of many oils including volatile oils, vitamin A, D, and E oils, can be prepared by using suitable hydrophilic surfactants. For this purpose surfactants having HLB values within the range from 15 to 18 are most commonly used. These preparations are not exactly solutions but, dispersions. Usually such oral preparations contain polysorbate 60 and polysorbate 80. The principal advantages of a microemulsion are,

1. compared to any solid dosage form, such preparation can deliver the drug more rapidly and efficiently when administered orally,

2. better drug diffusion through skin from a microemulsion when applied transdermally,

3. microemulsion can be greatly used for developing artificial red blood cells and drug targeting for treatment of cancer.

Multiple emulsion is an emulsion of emulsion. In this emulsion system the drops of the dispersed phase contain smaller droplets having the same composition as the external phase. Accordingly the multiple emulsion may be of two types,- w/o/w and o/w/o. Thus, an emulsion of a particular type, o/w or w/o is inverted to o/w/o or w/o/w respectively, such inverted emulsion suffers from inherent instability unless a proper surfactant is used during preparation of each type. For example, to produce a w/o emulsion, a suitable lipophilic surfactant of low HLB value is to be used. For further emulsification of w/o emulsion into w/o/w, a hydrophilic surfactant of higher HLB value becomes necessary and using low shear the stability of the final emulsion can be optimized reasonably. Preparation of w/o/w type of multiple emulsion can be facilitated by using a microporous glass membrane with narrow pore size. Water being the external phase and the viscosity being lower, such preparation can be easily injected. As the oil phase lies between two aqueous layers it can control the drug release like a membrane and this type (w/o/w) of multiple emulsion can be used to prepare a sustained-release dosage form. Similarly, the aqueous layer of o/w/o type of emulsion can be used as liquid membrane to separate hydrocarbons.

Gel emulsions are water rich w/o emulsions. These contain much of water and minimum amount of a non-ionic surfactant. This gives a gel-like appearance, the transparency of the preparation depends on the composition and temperature maintained during preparation. As the amount of dispersed phase is very high, close packing of liquid droplets are not observed, the droplets turns into polyhedral shape and occupy the available space. Under this situation the internal structure of a gel emulsion may seem to be a multiple emulsion. Gel emulsions have the applications in pharmaceutical, cosmetic, food, chemical engineering.

Solution used in Body Cavity

Gargles

These are solution preparations intended for use as a prophylactic or in the treatment of throat infection. These are used either as is or after dilution with water. They may contain antiseptics, antibiotics with or without an anaesthetic. The preparation is taken in mouth and held in throat, then air from the lung is forced through the solution (gargle). After this the gargle is spitted or expectorated from the mouth. However, very few preparations are swallowed after gargling. The repeated process brings the medicaments of the gargle into intimate contact with the membranous lining of the throat where mild sore is present and a relief to the throat-sore is achieved.

The gargle does not make any protective covering on the throat membrane, hence, no oily substance with or without any suspending agent, or no drug with mucilaginous nature should be used in these preparations.

Gargle is packed in white fluted bottle and its label should be such that it can be easily distinguished from a preparation intended for internal administration, except those are advised to swallowed after gargling. For example, during treatment of oral fungal infection, half of the dose of nystatin solution is taken in each side of the mouth, swished around as long as possible, then gargled and finally swallowed.

If the preparation contains any light sensitive material a coloured bottle should be used.

Formulations:

Product: Phenol Gargle

Standard for phenol: It contains not less than 99.0%w/w of phenol, calculated as C_6H_6O.

Standard for product: Content of Phenol: 0.84 – 1.13%w/v calculated as C_6H_6O.

Composition:

It contains Phenol Glycerin BPC 5%v/v in water.

Colour used, Amaranth.

Use: Bactericidal gargle

Lot size: 20 ml

Manufacturing Formula:

Phenol Glycerin BPC	1.0 ml
Amaranth solution, 1.0%	0.2 ml
Purified water IP	q.s

Manufacturing Method:

Preparation of Phenol Glycerin

Phenol	1.6 g
Glycerin	8.4 g

Transfer accurately weighed amount of phenol into a 25ml clean, dry beaker, add glycerin and stir to dissolve, if required heat the mixture until phenol is completely dissolved.

Note:

- *Handle phenol carefully, it is very caustic and whitens the skin. Use spatula and gloves.*

Preparation of phenol gargle:

- Take volumetrically 1.0 ml of phenol glycerin in a 25 ml measuring cylinder,
- Add 0.2 ml of amaranth solution to it, mix,
- Make up the volume with purified water, stopper and shake,
- Filter the solution through cotton wool, fill the solution in a clean, amber bottle, seal and label properly,
- Carry out the test.

Note:

- *The label must mention, NOT TO BE SWALLOWED.*

Product: Potassium Chlorate and Phenol Gargle

Standard for potassium chlorate: It should be of reagent grade or pharmaceutical grade as per IP.

for Liquefied phenol: It contains not less than 88.0%w/w of phenol, calculated as C_6H_6O.

Standard for product: Content of Phenol, 1.10 – 1.40%w/v, calculated as C_6H_6O.

Content of potassium chlorate, 2.85 – 3.15%w/v, calculated as $KClO_3$

Composition:

It contains   Phenol IP 1.25%w/v

Potassium chlorate IP 3.0%w/v

Liquefied Phenol IP 1.25%w/v in purified water,

Colour used: Amaranth

Use: Antiseptic (Bactericidal) and mild astringent gargle

Lot size: 20 ml

Manufacturing Formula:

Liquefied Phenol	IP	0.3 ml
Potassium chlorate	IP	0.6 g
Amaranth solution, 1.0%		0.2 ml
Purified water IP	q.s	

Manufacturing Method:

- Take weighed quantity of potassium chlorate in a clean 25 ml stopper cylinder, add about 10 ml of purified water, shake until dissolve,

- Add measured volume of liquefied phenol, mix thoroughly,

- Add measured volume of amaranth solution and make up the volume with purified water, stopper the cylinder and shake,

- Filter the solution through cotton wool and fill in a colour bottle, seal with a pilfer proof cap,

- Carry out the tests and label properly.

Note:

- *The label must mention,* NOT TO BE SWALLOWED.

Mouthwashes

These are aqueous solutions, sometimes concentrated solutions, commonly used for cleansing and deodorizing the buccal cavity. The solution is swished in the oral cavity and then thrown out.

Mouthwashes are formulated and used for:

1. Therapeutic purposes,

2. Diagnostic purposes and

3. Cosmetic use.

The therapeutic mouthwashes are used for the treatment of plaque, gingivitis, dental carries and stomatitis. For example, a mixture of antihistaminic, hydrocortisone, nystatin and tetracycline is used for stomatitis which is a painful side effect of cancer chemotherapy. Pilocarpine is used for dry mouth (xerostoma). Chlorhexidine gluconate is used for plaque. The mouthwash can also be used for diagnostic purpose. Oral cancer or lesions can be diagnosed by using toludine blue mouthwash.

The cosmetic mouthwash contains antimicrobial drugs with or without a flavour and is used to reduce the bad breath.

Besides active constituents a mouthwash contain other excipients like alcohol, surface active agents, humectant, colouring agents and flavouring agents.

- Alcohol is used in the range from 10% to 20%. At this concentration it can act as a cosolvent, preservative, solubiliser and enhancer of flavours and taste masking agent for the unpleasant taste of the drug.

- Glycerin or sorbitol are used as humectant to increase the viscosity, sweetness of the mouthwash. It can improve the mouth feel or body to the preparation and preservation of the product.
- A suitable surface active agent, non-ionic, anionic or cationic is used in the concentration of 0.1% - 0.5% to solubilise the flavour, to remove the debris from the preparation through foaming action.

Containers: Mouthwashes are usually packed in white fluted bottles.

Labelling: Along with necessary information a direction should be given whether the preparation is to be diluted before use and the proportion of dilution. The label must clearly and distinguishably mention that the preparation is not intended for internal administration.

Formulations:

Product: Sodium Chloride Mouth-wash, Compound

Standard for sodium chloride: It should contain not less than 99% and not more than 100.5%w/w of NaCl on dried basis.

Standard for sodium bicarbonate: It should contain not less than 99% and not more than 101%w/w of $NaHCO_3$.

Standard for product: Content of Sodium Chloride; 1.42 – 1.58%w/v calculated as NaCl.

Content of Sodium Bicarbonate; 0.95 – 1.05%w/v calculated as $NaHCO_3$.

Composition:

It contains

Sodium Chloride IP	1.5%
Sodium Bicarbonate IP	1.0%
Quillaia Extract	0.025%

In flavoured aqueous base.

Use: Cleansing of mouth.

Lot size: 20 ml

Manufacturing Formula:

Sodium Chloride	IP	0.3 g
Sodium Bicarbonate	IP	0.2 g
Peppermint oil, 0.4% solution in alcohol		0.5 ml
Quillaia Liquid Extract, 0.5%w/v		0.1 ml
Purified water	IP	q.s

Manufacturing Method:

- Take 1 ml of peppermint oil solution in a clean test tube add 0.2 ml of quillaia extract and mix,
- Dissolve sodium chloride and sodium bicarbonate in purified water, freshly boiled and cooled, into a clean 25 ml measuring cylinder,
- Add 0.6 ml of peppermint oil and quillaia mixture into bulk solution and mix thoroughly, make up the volume with purified water and mix,
- Carry out the tests, if necessary, filter through cotton wool,
- Fill the solution into a fluted bottle and seal with a cap,
- Label the preparation properly.

Note:

- *This preparation should be diluted with equal volume of warm water before use.*

Product: Zinc Sulphate and Zinc Chloride Mouthwash

Standard for zinc sulphate: It should contain not less than 99% and not more than 104%w/w of $ZnSO_4$, $7H_2O$.

Standard for zinc chloride: It should contain not less than 95% and not more than 100.5%w/w of $ZnCl_2$.

Standard for product:

Content of Zinc; 0.89 – 0.98%w/v calculated as Zn.

Composition:

It contains

Zinc Sulphate	IP	2.0%
Zinc Chloride	IP	1.0%

Use: Prevention of sour and bitter taste in the mouth

Lot size: 20 ml

Manufacturing Formula:

Zinc Sulphate	IP	0.4 g
Zinc Chloride	IP	0.2 g
Tartrazine solution, 1.0%		0.2 ml
Dil. Hydrochloric Acid		0.2 ml
Purified water	IP	q.s.

Manufacturing Method:

- Take weighed quantity of Zinc Sulphate and Zinc Chloride in a 25 ml stopper measuring cylinder, dissolve in purified water,
- Add measured volume of dilute hydrochloric acid, mix thoroughly,
- Add tartrazine solution and make up the volume,
- Determine the content of zinc,
- Filter the solution through cotton wool, if necessary, and fill in white fluted bottle, seal with a cap and label.

Note:

- *This preparation should be diluted to 20 times with warm water before use.*

Enemas

There are certain solutions or suspensions intended for rectal or vaginal administration. These may be aqueous or oily solutions or suspensions and are used either for their local effects or for systemic absorption of the medicament. These are called *enemas*. The enemas may be classified according to their use into two categories,

1. Retention enemas, and
2. Evacuation enemas.

Retention enemas are solutions intended for rectal administration for local effects, for example, hydrocortisone enema, or for systemic absorption, e.g. aminophylline enema. If aminophylline is administered orally the unwanted gastro-intestinal problems occur, which can be avoided through rectal administration in the form of its enema. Within half an hour from rectal administration the drug can reach to its effective concentration in the blood. Inflammation of ulcerative colitis is sometimes treated with retention enema of corticosteroids. Example of therapeutic enemas are, chloral hydrate, paraldehyde (sedative); barium sulphate enema for X-ray examination of the lower bowel, etc.

Evacuation enemas are commonly used to evacuate the bowel. Enemas of definite volume are commercially available. For example, solutions of sodium phosphate and sodium biphosphate, light mineral oil, etc. The mechanism of action of this type of enema may be either stimulation of peristalsis or lubrication of impacted faeces. Stimulation of peristalsis is done either by larger volume, from 500 ml to 1 Lt or due to osmotic retention of water in the bowel. The later type is of lesser volume, usually 100 ml. 5% solution of soft soap, turpentine enema, are of this type. Olive oil, arachis oil enemas are lubricating enemas.

Large volume enemas should be administered after warming to body temperature. Small volume (100 ml) enemas available in disposable sealed polythene bags fitted with a rectal nozzle are convenient for self administration. The user needs to insert the nozzle and squeeze the bag. When oral or nasal feeding are not possible, the nutrients can also be administered rectally.

Containers: Enemas should be supplied in coloured fluted glass bottles or in single use plastic packs fitted with a rectal nozzle.

Formulations:

Product: Paraldehyde Enema

It contains Paraldehyde 0.1%v/v in sodium chloride solution.

Use: Sedative

Lot size: 500 ml

Manufacturing Formula:

Paraldehyde	USP	50 ml
Sodium chloride	IP	40 g
Purified water, freshly boiled and cooled	IP q.s	500 ml

Manufacturing Method:

- Take sodium chloride in a 500 ml clean beaker,
- Add about 400 ml of purified water and stir to dissolve sodium chloride,
- Transfer the solution into a 500 ml clean measuring cylinder, add measured volume of paraldehyde and stir to dissolve,
- Make up the volume with purified water, mix thoroughly,
- Fill the solution in a suitable bottle, seal and label properly.

Note:

- *It must be freshly prepared.*

Dose:

- 5 ml per kg of body weight, maximum of 300 ml for rectal administration.

Product: Sodium phosphate Enema

Standard for product: Content of sodium acid phosphate: 15.2–16.8%w/v calculated as $NaH_2PO_4, 2H_2O$.

Content of sodium phosphate: 5.6 – 6.4%w/v calculated as $Na_2HPO_4, 12H_2O$.

Use: Evacuation of bowel

Lot size: 100 ml

Manufacturing Formula:

Sodium Acid Phosphate	IP	16 g
Sodium Phosphate	IP	6 g
Purified water, freshly boiled and cooled,	IP q.s	100 ml

Manufacturing Method:

- Take 90 ml of freshly boiled and cooled purified water in a clean 250 ml beaker,
- Add weighed quantities of sodium acid phosphate and sodium phosphate, stir to dissolve,
- Transfer the solution into a clean 100 ml measuring cylinder, make up the volume with purified water, carry out the tests,
- Filter the solution through 0.2 μ membrane filter under aseptic environment,
- Fill in suitable sterile bottle and seal with sterile rubber stopper and aluminium cap,
- If necessary keep the bottle in boiling water for 50 mins or sterilise at a temperature 116°C for 45 minutes, Label the bottle properly.

Note:

- *If not sterilised or filtered through membrane filter, a suitable preservative can be used.*

Spirits

These are alcoholic or hydroalcoholic solutions. These may contain medicinal substances or flavouring agents, usually of volatile in nature. Aromatic Spirit of Ammonia is prepared by a process of distillation but most other spirits are prepared by the process of simple solution. Concentration of alcohol in spirits are quite high, generally 60% and more. The volatile substances are soluble in alcohol, their solubility in water is not sufficient to make their aqueous solutions. Hence, depending on the solubility of a particular volatile substance in water and alcohol, the ratio of alcohol-water is determined as the solvent. The spirits usually contain more amount of volatile substances than a corresponding aromatic water. These preparations when diluted with water, the volatile constituents separate out from the solution in colloidal form and the solution becomes turbid or opalescent or milky depending on the amount of separated solutes. This process of separation is called salting out. Thus, when a spirit is used in another preparation as a flavouring agent, it should be carefully mixed to avoid salting out.

Spirits may be used as medicinal preparation for the therapeutic value of the aromatic constituents present.

Spirits may be used for

1. preparing oral formulations,
2. external application, and
3. inhalation.

During oral administration these diluted with water to minimize the pungency of the alcohol.

Spirits should be stored in tightly closed containers and at cool place.

Formulations

Product : Spirit of Camphor

Standard for product:

Weight/ml at $20^{\circ}C$: 0.835 – 0.843 g

Alcohol content : 79 – 82% v/v

Camphor content : 9.2 – 10.4% w/v as $C_{10}H_{14}O$

Composition:

Each 100 ml contains:

Camphor	10g
Alcohol (90%v/v)	q s

Use: Flavoured vehicle

Lot Size: 50 ml

Manufacturing Formula:

Camphor	5 g
Alcohol (90%v/v)	q s

Manufacturing Method:

*   Weigh accurately 5 g of camphor, transfer it into a stopper 100 ml conical flask.
*   Add about 40 ml of diluted alcohol (70%), stopper and shake thoroughly till camphor is completely dissolved.
*   Transfer the solution into a 50 ml measuring cylinder and make up the volume with diluted alcohol.
*   Transfer the product into a dry well-closed container, stopper tightly and label properly.

Product: Spirit of Anise

Standard for product:

Alcohol content, 78 – 82%v/v,

Weight per ml at 20°C, 0.830 – 0.840 g

Each 100 ml contains:

Anise oil   10 ml

Alcohol (90%v/v) q.s

Use: Flavouring agent

Lot size: 50 ml

Manufacturing Formula:

Anise oil   5 ml

Alcohol (90%v/v)   q.s

Manufacturing Method:

- Take 45ml of alcohol (90%) in a 100ml stopper conical flask,
- Pipette out 5 ml of anise oil and add to alcohol gradually with swirling,
- Mix thoroughly. If the solution is not clear, add 25 g of purified talc and shake for 15 minutes,
- Filter through Whatman filter paper No.1. Recycle the first 10 ml filtrate or until a clear filtrate is obtained,
- Transfer the clear filtrate into a well-closed container and label it properly.

Product : Spirit of Peppermint

Standard for product:

Alcohol content,   78 – 82% v/v,

Weight per ml at 20°C,   0.83 – 0.84 g

Each 100ml contains

Peppermint oil   10 ml

Alcohol (90%v/v) q.s

Use: Flavouring agent

Lot size: 50 ml

Manufacturing Formula:

Peppermint oil   5 ml

Alcohol (90%v/v) qs

Manufacturing Method:

- Take 45ml of alcohol (90%) in a 100ml stopper conical flask,
- Pipette out 5 ml of cinnamon oil and add to alcohol gradually with swirling,
- Mix thoroughly. If the solution is not clear, add 25 g of purified talc and shake for 15 minutes,
- Filter through Whatman filter paper No.1. Recycle the first 10ml filtrate or until a clear filtrate is obtained,
- Transfer the clear filtrate into a well-closed container and label it properly.

Product : Lemon Spirit

Standard for product:

Alcohol content, 84 – 87% v/v,

Weight per ml at 20°C, 0.814 – 0.823 g

Content of Aldehydes, 3.45 – 4.60% w/v, calculated as $C_{10}H_{16}O_5$.

Each 100 ml contains:

Terpeneless Lemon oil	10 ml
Alcohol (95%v/v)	q.s

Use: Flavouring agent

Lot size: 50 ml

Manufacturing Formula:

Lemon oil (Terpeneless)	5 ml
Alcohol (95%v/v)	q.s

Manufacturing Method:

- Take 45ml of alcohol (95%) in a 100ml stopper conical flask,
- Pipette out 5.0 ml of lemon oil and add to alcohol gradually with swirling,
- Mix thoroughly and make up the volume with alcohol (95%v/v). If the solution is not clear, add 25 g of purified talc and shake for 15 minutes,
- Filter through Whatman filter paper No.1. Recycle the first 10ml filtrate or until a clear filtrate is obtained,
- Transfer the clear filtrate into a well-closed container and label it properly.

Product: Surgical Spirit

Standard for product:

       Methyl salicylate - 90 – 110%v/v of the stated amount.

       Diethyl phthalate - 90 – 110%v/v of the stated amount.

Each 100 ml contains

Castor oil:	2.5 ml
Methyl salicylate:	0.5 ml
Ethyl phthalate:	2.0 ml
Industrial methylated spirit q.s	

Composition:

    It contains

Castor oil:	1.25 ml
Methyl salicylate:	0.25 ml
Diethyl phthalate:	1.0 ml
Industrial methylated spirit q s	

Use: Antiseptic

For external use only

Lot size: 50 ml

Manufacturing Method:

(a) *Preparation of industrial methylated spirit*:

    It contains Wood naphtha – 5% in Alcohol(90%v/v)

    Method: For 50 ml take 2.5 g wood naphtha accurately weighed in a 50 ml volumetric flask, add 40 ml of alcohol IP(90%v/v), stopper and shake until dissolve. Make up the volume with alcohol 90%v/v and shake again.

(b) *Preparation of surgical spirit*:

- Measure accurately 0.25 ml of methyl salicylate using a 1ml graduated pipette and transfer into a 50 ml clean stopper conical flask previously dried.
- Separately measure 1 ml of ethyl phthalate and transfer into the conical flask.
- Add about 40 ml of industrial methylated spirit and until dissolve.
- Using another 2ml graduated pipette transfer 1.25 ml of castor oil into the flask and shake.

- Once the solution is made, transfer the solution into a clean, dried measuring cylinder and make up the volume with methylated industrial spirit.

- Transfer solution into a well-closed container, stopper tightly, shake and label properly.

Liquid Preparations for External use

The solutions intended for external use, particularly the antiseptic solutions are susceptible to be contaminated with resistant microorganisms. Hence, precautions should be taken as mentioned below.

- Water to be used for making the solution should be freshly distilled or freshly boiled.

- The container to be used to store water should be properly cleaned, if necessary, should be sterile.

- The closures of cork or containing cork liners should not be used.

- Once the container is opened, it is better not to use the content after one week.

- Non sterile solution of antiseptic should not be applied over broken skin or to eyes or be introduced into the body cavity.

Formulations:

Product: Strong Iodine Solution

Standard for drug: It should contain not less than 99.5% and not more than 100.5%w/w of I.

Standard for product:

    Content of Iodine: 9.5 – 10.5% w/v,

    Potassium iodide: 5.7 – 6.3% w/v

    Alcohol: 74 – 79% v/v

Composition:

    It contains:

Iodine IP	10%
Potassium iodide IP	6%
In hydro alcohol base.	

Use: Antiseptic and Source of iodine, For external use only

Lot size: 50 ml

Manufacturing Formula:

Iodine IP	5 g
Potassium iodide IP	3 g
Purified water	5 ml
Alcohol (90%)	q s

Manufacturing Method:

- Take weighed quantity of potassium iodide in a 50 ml stopper cylinder, add weighed quantity of iodine, stopper and mix these as far as possible,
- Add measured volume of purified water to the cylinder, stopper and shake occasionally till iodine is dissolved,
- Add alcohol (90%) to make up the volume, stopper the cylinder ad shake thoroughly,
- Transfer the solution into a clean, dry, amber coloured bottle, seal and label properly,
- Determine the iodine content and alcohol content.

Product: Weak Iodine Solution (Tincture of Iodine)

Standard for drug: It should contain not less than 99.5% and not more than 100.5% w/w of I.

Standard for product:

Content of Iodine: 1.8 – 2.2% w/v,

Potassium iodide: 2.1 – 2.6% w/v

Alcohol: 48.4 – 49.5 %v/v

Composition:

It contains:

Iodine IP	2%
Potassium iodide IP	2.5%

In hydro alcoholic base.

Use: Local antiseptic

For external use only

Lot size: 50 ml

Manufacturing Formula:

Iodine	IP	1 g
Potassium iodide	IP	1.25g

| Alcohol | IP | 25 ml |
| Purified water | IP | 25 ml |

Manufacturing Method:

- Take weighed quantity of potassium iodide in a 50 ml stopper cylinder, add weighed quantity of iodine, stopper and mix these as far as possible,
- Add 40 ml of alcohol (50%), stopper the cylinder and shake frequently till complete solution is effected, make up the volume with alcohol (50%), stopper and shake thoroughly,
- Transfer the solution into a clean, dry, amber coloured bottle, seal and label properly,
- Determine the iodine content and alcohol content.

Product: Borax-Glycerin Solution

Standard for borax: It contains an amount of sodium borate, $Na_2B_4O_7$ equivalent to not less than 99% and not more than 105% of $Na_2B_4O_7,10H_2O$.

Standard for glycerin: It contains not less than 95%w/v of $C_3H_8O_3$.

Composition:

It contains

Borax IP 1.2% w/w in glycerin.

Use: Throat ulcer

Lot size: 50 ml

Manufacturing Formula:

| Borax | IP | 6 g |
| Glycerin | IP | 44 g |

Manufacturing Method:

- Take the glycerin by weight in a 100 ml beaker, heat it, add borax and stir with a glass rod. Continue heating with occasional stirring until the borax is completely dissolved,
- Filter the solution through a clean cloth of 100 mesh, allow it to cool,
- Make up the volume with little glycerin, if necessary,
- Determine the content of borax,
- Fill in a clean, dried bottle, seal and label properly.

Product: Alcoholic Chlorhexidine Solution

Standard for drug: Chlorhexidine Gluconate Solution contains not less than 19.0%w/v and not more than 21.0%w/v of $C_{22}H_{30}Cl_2N_{10},2C_6H_{12}O_7$.

Standard for product: It contains 0.45–0.55%w/v of Chlorhexidine Gluconate, calculated as $C_{22}H_{30}Cl_2N_{10}, 2C_6H_{12}O_7$.

It contains Chlorhexidine solution BPC 2.5%v/v in hydro alcoholic base.

Use: Antiseptic for external use

Lot size: 50 ml

Manufacturing Formula:

Chlorhexidine Gluconate solution,(20%) BPC	1.25 ml
Alcohol (95%v/v), IP	35 ml
Purified water, freshly boiled and cooled q.s	

Manufacturing Method:

- Take the alcohol in a 50 ml measuring cylinder, add chlorhexidine gluconate solution, mix,
- Add purified water gradually to make up the volume, stopper and mix well,
- Fill the solution in a clean, dry bottle, seal and label properly,

Note:

- *Alcohol(95%) can be replaced by industrial methylated spirit, if the law permits. However, isopropyl alcohol can be used in place of alcohol.*
- *The shelf-life of the preparation containing alcohol or methylated spirit is one year, while the shelf-life is three years if isopropyl alcohol is used.*

Product: Chloroxylenol Solution

Standard for chloroxylenol: It should contain not less than 98% and not more than 103%w/w of C_8H_9ClO.

Standard for product: Content of chloroxylenol: 4.5–5.5%w/v calculated as, C_8H_9ClO.

Alcohol content: 16 – 20%v/v

Composition:

It contains:

Chloroxylenol 5 %w/v

In hydro alcoholic soap base.

Use: Antiseptic for external use.

Lot size: 50 ml

Manufacturing Formula:

Chloroxylenol		2.5 g
Potassium hydroxide	IP	0.68 g
Oleic acid	USP	0.38 ml
Castor oil	IP	3.15 g
Terpineol		5.0 ml
Alcohol (95%v/v)	IP	10.0 ml
Purified water	IP q.s	50.0 ml

Manufacturing Method:

- Weigh accurately potassium hydroxide and transfer into a clean 100 ml beaker, add 0.75 ml of purified water and dissolve the alkali,
- Mix separately castor oil and 3.15 ml of alcohol, add this solution to alkali solution and mix, cover the beaker, keep it for one hour or until a mixture of one drop of this solution and 19 drops of purified water is found to be clear (test for complete saponification),
- Add oleic acid and mix,
- Mix separately chloroxylenol with 6.85 ml of alcohol, add terpineol to this solution, mix, pour this solution to the soap solution in a thin stream with constant stirring,
- Add sufficient purified water with stirring and make up the volume,
- Carry out the tests,
- Fill the solution in a clean bottle and seal with a pilfer proof cap and label.

Collodions

These are liquid preparations containing pyroxylin dissolved in a mixture of solvents commonly ether and alcohol. These are intended for application over the skin. Either a glass applicator or camel's hair brush is used to apply. Since these contain volatile solvent, the solvent quickly evaporates and leaves an occlusive protective film of pyroxylin on the skin. These may or may not contain any medicament. When a medicated collodion is applied, the medicated film adheres to the skin firmly. Hence, before application the skin should be made dry properly.

Pyroxylin is a soluble gun cotton, collodion cotton (nitrated cellulose) prepared from the reaction between defatted cotton and a mixture of nitric acid and sulphuric acid. Its main constituent is cellulose tetranitrate. It looks like cotton wool but is harsh to touch. Commercially it is available as moistened with diluted alcohol or industrial methylated spirit. As it is highly inflammable, it is stored in well-closed container in a loose, soft pack, away from light and in cool place. It is dried before use.

Pyroxylin is slowly soluble in 25 parts of a mixture of alcohol and ether(1:3), in acetone and glacial acetic acid. For preparing the solution pyroxylin is shaken with the solvent in a well-closed, light-resistant container and kept for few days in a cool place to allow the impurities to settle completely. The supernatant clear solution is finally decanted.

There are two types of official collodions- Flexible Collodion BP and salicylic Acid Collodion BPC.

Flexible collodion: It contains 3% of castor oil and 2% of camphor. Castor oil makes the collodion flexible and camphor makes it waterproof. Thus, the use of collodion over the skin becomes comfortable. Sometimes, this is used as a coating over bandages or stitched incisions for waterproof protection from external stress.

Salicylic acid collodion: It is the flexible collodion containing 10-12% of salicylic acid. Because of keratoytic activity of salicylic acid, it is mainly used to remove corns from the toes. However, during use of salicylic acid collodion for corn removal care should be taken that only one drop is put directly on the corn at a time. Once this is dried the second drop can be put. It should not touch the adjacent normal skin. Since salicylic acid irritates the normal skin. The container should be tightly closed after use, as the solvent present in the collodion is very volatile.

The label should clearly mention the following information, *For external use only, Store in a cool place, Highly inflammable, keep away from flame.*

Formulations:

Product: Flexible Collodion

Standard for product: Content of Alcohol: 21 – 25%v/v.

Composition:

> Each g contains
>> Camphor   IP   20 mg
>> In alcoholic solution of flexible collodion.

Use: Protective

Lot size: 20 ml

Manufacturing Formula:

Camphor	IP	0.4 g
Castor oil	IP	0.6 g
Flexible collodion		19.0 g

Manufacturing Method:

Take all the ingredients, accurately weighed in a 50 ml clean, dry bottle, cap the bottle tightly,

Shake the bottle occasionally till camphor is dissolved, keep it for 7 days, observe for sedimentation, if any, filter after 7 days through G_4 sintered glass crucible,

Determine the alcohol content,

Fill the preparation in a clean, dry, coloured bottle and seal with a pilfer proof cap, Label properly.

Product: Salicylic Acid Collodion

Standard for product: Content of salicylic acid: 9.5 – 11.5%w/v calculated as $C_7H_6O_3$.

Composition:

> Each ml contains
>
>> Salicylic acid 100 mg
>>
>> in flexible collodion.

Use: Keratolytic

Lot size: 20 ml

Manufacturing Formula:

Salicylic acid	IP		2.0 g
Flexible collodion	USP	q.s	20.0 ml

Manufacturing Method:

- Take required quantity of salicylic acid in a 25 ml measuring stopper cylinder, add 18 ml of flexible collodion, stopper the cylinder tightly,
- Shake occasionally till salicylic acid is completely dissolved, make up the volume with flexible collodion,
- Keep the solution for 7 days for settling, if any,
- Filter the solution through G_4 sintered glass crucible, fill the filtrate in a coloured bottle, seal with a pilfer proof cap and label properly.

Liniments

These are either solutions or emulsions of medicinal substances which are applied by rubbing on the skin. Two types of solvents are commonly used to prepare liniments, one is alcoholic and the other is oleaginous. For example, Soap Liniment BPC contains alcohol while, Methyl Salicylate Liniment BPC or Camphor Liniment BP contains oil. The medicinal substances which have analgesic, counterirritant, rubefacient action or which need to penetrate the skin, are prepared in the form of liniment using alcohol or hydroalcohol as vehicle. Because, alcohol helps the medicament to penetrate the skin. The pain from fibrositis, sciatica and similar problems can be masked by alcohol based liniments by producing warmth sensation on the affected area of the skin. If the liniment is used for massage, oil based preparation is suitable. The oil based liniments are less irritating than alcohol based liniments. They also have better spreadability. Thus, during formulation of a liniment, selection of a proper vehicle is important. The selection of vehicle is based on two criteria- the type of action desired and the solubility of the medicament. Liniment should not be applied to broken or bruised skin, as it may increase the irritation.

For preparation of oleaginous liniments either fixed oils, e.g. sesame oil, peanut oil, cotton seed oil, almond oil, arachis oil, etc. or a mixture of fixed oils and volatile oils, e.g. turpentine oil, wintergreen oil, etc. can be used.

The label of liniments must mention the statements, *For external use only, Not to be applied to wounds or broken skin.* If the liniment contains alcohol, that should also mention *Inflammable* with a note, *Keep away from flame.* The liniment which is an emulsion or contains some insoluble substances, if any, should bear the label with a statement, *Shake well before use.*

The liniments should be packed in tightly closed containers, like coloured, fluted bottles; and should be stored in a cool place.

Containers: Liniments should be filled in coloured fluted bottles.

Labelling: The label should clearly mention, For external use only

Formulations:

Product: Methyl Salicylate Liniment

It contains Methyl Salicylate 25%v/v in arachis oil.

Standard for product:

        Content of Methyl Salicylate: 23 – 26.5%v/v.

        Weight/ml at 20 °C : 0.973 g - 0.989 g

Use: Pharmaceutical aid

Lot size: 20 ml

Manufacturing Formula:

Methyl Salicylate		5.0 ml
Arachis oil	q.s	20.0 ml

Manufacturing Method:

- Take the measured volume of methyl salicylate in a clean, dry measuring cylinder,
- Add arachis oil sufficiently to make up the volume,
- Mix thoroughly, carry out the tests and transfer the solution into an amber coloured bottle, seal with a pilfer proof cap,
- Label properly.

Product: Soap Liniment

It contains Camphor 4% in hydroalcoholic flavoured base.

Standard for product:

Content of Oleic acid: not less than 3.8%w/v.

Weight/ml at 20°C : 0.880 g – 0.900 g

pH : 7.4 – 8.0

Use: Local antipruritic

Lot size: 20 ml

Manufacturing Formula:

Camphor			0.8 g
Oleic Acid			0.8 g
Rosemary Oil			0.3 ml
Potassium hydroxide solution, 5% w/v			2.80 ml
Alcohol, 95%	IP		13.3 ml
Purified water, freshly boiled and cooled,	IP	q.s	20.0 ml

Manufacturing Method:

- Transfer the measured volume of oleic acid into a clean, dry 25 ml beaker, add 7 ml of alcohol and stir with a glass rod to dissolve oleic acid,
- Add measured volume of potassium hydroxide solution with stirring,
- Dissolve weighed quantity of camphor separately in 3 ml of alcohol in a 10 ml beaker and add measured quantity of rosemary oil to this, mix well,
- Add this solution to the bulk and mix well,
- Add sufficient purified water with stirring to make up the volume,
- Transfer the preparation into a clean, dry, amber bottle, seal tightly with a pilfer proof cap, keep it for 7 days, filter through a G_4 sintered glass cruisible under vacuum,

- Carry out the tests,
- Fill finally into a clean, dry, amber coloured bottle, seal with a pilfer proof cap and label properly.

Product: White liniment

Standard for product:

Content of volatile oil : 24.5 – 27.5%v/w,

Refractive index of the oily distillate at 20°C : 1.465 – 1.477

Use: Counterirritant and rebefacient

Lot size: 20 ml

Manufacturing Formula:

Ammonium chloride	0.25 g
Dilute Ammonia solution, 37.5%v/v	0.9 ml
Oleic acid	1.7 ml
Turpentine oil	5.0 ml
Purified water, freshly boiled and cooled,	12.5 ml

Manufacturing Method:

- Take measured volume of oleic acid into a clean, dry 50 ml stopper measuring cylinder, add measured volume of turpentine oil and mix,
- Add dilute ammonia solution and mix,
- Add 7.6 ml (0.9+1.7+5.0 = 7.6, accurately measured) of warm (40-45°C) purified water and shake, carefully to avoid spouting,
- Dissolve ammonium chloride separately in 10 ml of purified water in a 25 ml clean beaker and add to the bulk solution, mix well,
- Rinse the beaker with purified water and add to the bulk solution, make up the volume and shake well,
- Carry out the tests and fill the preparation into a clean, dry, amber coloured bottle, seal with a pilfer proof cap and label properly.

Lotion

Lotions are liquid preparations intended for application over the skin. Lotions should be taken on lint or other soft absorbent material and applied without any friction. Most of the lotions are solutions and their main ingredients are simple salts, e.g., copper and zinc sulphates, lead subacetate, etc,. which are water soluble. For preparing salicylic acid lotion alcohol is used as solvent. Medicaments which can treat the skin conditions or can treat local infection are primarily selected for lotions. For example, copper and zinc sulphate lotion is used for its astringent action, salicylic lotion for treating dandruff, mixture of salicylic acid and mercuric chloride for treating follicular infection. Salicylic acid is also used for its anti-fungal, keratolytic and bacteriostatic activity. If alcohol is present in a preparation, it accelerates the rate of drying of the lotion and provides a sensation of cooling effect on the skin. When glycerin is incorporated in a preparation, it protects the skin from drying and renders the skin moist for a considerable time. If the alcohol content is high in a lotion, castor oil should be used to counteract the defatting action of alcohol.

Since lotions may contain highly inflammable solvents like acetone, alcohol, caution should be mentioned in the label for their proper storage and the label should mention clearly. *For external use only* and SHAKE WELL BEFORE USE.

Formulations:

Product: Copper and Zinc sulphate Lotion

Each 100 ml contains:

Copper sulphate IP	914 mg
Zinc sulphate IP	137 mg
Camphor water	q.s

Standard for product:

Copper sulphate: 0.86 – 0.97%w/v calculated as $CuSO_4$, $5H_2O$

Zinc sulphate: 1.30 – 1.47%w/v calculated as $ZnSO_4$, $7H_2O$

Use: Astringent

Lot size: 50 ml

Manufacturing Formula:

Copper sulphate	457 mg
Zinc sulphate IP	68.5 mg
Camphor water	q.s

Manufacturing Method:

- Take 50 mg of camphor accurately weighed in a 100 ml stopper conical flask, add 50 ml of purified water, stopper tightly and until dissolved,

- Take 457 mg of copper sulphate and 68.5 mg of zinc sulphate accurately weighed in a separate 100 ml conical flask, add about 45 ml of camphor water, stopper tightly and shake well till a clear solution is effected,
- Transfer the solution into a measuring cylinder, make up the volume with camphor water, mix thoroughly,
- Transfer into a well-closed container and label it properly.

Product: Calamine Lotion

Standard for calamine: It should contain not less than 98% and not more than 100.5% of ZnO, calculated on dried basis.

Standard for product: Content of Zinc oxide: 14.4 – 17.6%w/v calculated as ZnO.

Each 100 ml contains:

Calamine	8 g
Zinc oxide	8 g
In flavoured vehicle	

Use: Topical protectant

Lot size: 50 ml

Manufacturing Formula:

Calamine	4 g
Zinc oxide	4 g
Bentonite	0.625 g
Glycerin IP	1 ml
Calcium Hydroxide Solution	36.5 ml
Purified water	q.s

Manufacturing Method:

Preparation of calcium hydroxide solution:

- Take 100 ml of purified water in a stopper conical flask, cool it. Transfer 0.3 g of calcium hydroxide into the flask and shake occasionally for 1 hr., allow to settle, decant about 60 ml of supernatant liquid carefully,
- Take 25 ml of hot purified water in a 100 ml beaker, sprinkle 0.625 g of bentonite in portions, allowing each portion to become thoroughly wetted without stirring. Allow it to stand for overnight, then mix thoroughly with a glass rod until a uniform mucilage is obtained,
- Add 12.5 ml of calcium hydroxide solution to the bentonite mucilage and mix thoroughly,

- Triturate 4 g of calamine and 4 g of zinc oxide with 1 ml of glycerin in a mortar pestle, add about 5 ml of bentonite mucilage in portions, triturate properly after each addition until a smooth uniform paste is obtained,

- Transfer the paste into a 100 ml beaker marked at 50 ml, attach to a suitable electric stirrer, continue stirring, rinse the mortar pestle with the bentonite mucilage in portions to effect complete transfer of calamine paste. Continue stirring for 1 hour. Stop stirring and uplift the stirrer,

- Make up the volume with calcium hydroxide solution, continue stirring for at least 2 hrs,

- Determine the content of zinc oxide, fill in suitable bottle, seal properly and label.

Product: Oily Calamine Lotion

Standard for calamine: It should contain not less than 98% and not more than 100.5% of ZnO, calculated on dried basis.

Standard for product: Content of Zinc - 2.52 – 3.35 5 w/v calculated as Zn.

Composition:

      Each 100 ml contains:

            Calamine 5 g

            In a oily flavoured base.

Use: Topical protectant

Lot size: 50 ml

Manufacturing Formula:

Calamine	2.5 g
Wool fat	0.5 g
Oleic acid	0.25 ml
Arachis oil	25 ml
Calcium hydroxide solution	q.s

Manufacturing Method:

- Take weighed quantity of wool fat, oleic acid and arachis oil in a 50 ml beaker; heat to melt and stir with a glass rod,

- Take the calamine in a mortar pestle, add the molten mass and triturate properly to make a uniform smooth slurry,

- Transfer the slurry into a 100 ml beaker marked at 50 ml, attach the beaker with a suitable electric stirrer; continue stirring, rinse the mortar pestle with 4 ml of calcium hydroxide solution for 4 to 5 times, add to the slurry and continue stirring for 2 hrs,

- Stop stirring, make up the volume with calcium hydroxide solution and continue stirring for further 2 hrs,

- Fill in the clean and dried bottle, seal and label properly.

Calcium hydroxide solution is to be prepared as per the method described under calamine lotion.

Product: Phenolated Calamine Lotion

Standard for calamine: It should contain not less than 98% and not more than 100.5% of ZnO, calculated on dried basis.

Standard for product: Content of Zinc oxide: 14.4 – 17.6% w/v calculated as ZnO.

Composition:

Each 100 ml contains:

Calamine	8 g
Zinc oxide	8 g
Liquefied Phenol	1 ml

Use: Antiseptic and protectant

Lot size: 50 ml

Manufacturing Formula:

Calamine	4 g
Zinc oxide	4 g
Glycerin	1 ml
Avicel	1 g
Sodium carboxymethyl cellulose	1 g
Liquefied Phenol	0.5 ml
Calcium hydroxide solution q s	50 ml

Manufacturing Method:

- Prepare the mucilage of sodium carboxymethyl cellulose with 25 ml of calcium hydroxide solution in a 100 ml beaker, add avicel and mix thoroughly with a glass rod,

- Take the calamine and zinc oxide in a mortar pestle, ad glycerin and triturate properly to make a smooth, uniform paste. Add sodium CMC mucilage in portions, continue trituration,

- Transfer the slurry into a 100 ml beaker marked at 50 ml, attach with a suitable electric stirrer, continue stirring, rinse the mortar pestle with 4 ml of calcium hydroxide solution for 4 to 5 times, add to the slurry and continue stirring for 2 hrs,

- Stop stirring, make up the volume with calcium hydroxide solution and continue stirring for further 2 hrs,

- Determine the content of zinc oxide,

- Fill in the clean and dried bottle, seal and label properly,

*Calcium hydroxide solution is to be prepared as per the method described under calamine lotion.

- Dissolve 6.855 g of ferric ammonium citrate, accurately weighed, in 40 ml of chloroform water in a 50 ml stopper cylinder,

- Make up the volume with chloroform water,

- Determine the content of ferric ammonium citrate and calculate in terms of Fe,

- Fill in a clean bottle, seal and label properly.

Magmas

According to USP magmas are suspensions of poorly soluble drugs in a water medium and are distinguished from gels mainly in that the suspended particles are larger. Thus they tend to separate on standing and require a label directing that they be shaken well before each use.

Among various types of gels, most of the inorganic hydrogels and magmas are two phase system. For example, bentonite magma and aluminium hydroxide gel. Some of the magmas and inorganic hydrogels can be prepared by precipitating the dispersed phase. This results reduction of size of the dispersed particles and the particle become more fines. Due to such precipitation the subdivided particles acquire a gelatinous character. Such gelatinous precipitate are also obtained when solutions of some inorganic salts react to form microcrystalline precipitates that have greater degree of affinity towards water. These microcrystalline precipitated particles attract water molecules strongly and become gelatinous particles. These gelatinous particles further combine and form gelatinous precipitate. For example, solution of aluminium phosphate when mixed with solution of sodium hydroxide aluminium phosphate reacts with sodium hydroxide and forms insoluble gelatinous precipitate of aluminium hydroxide, called aluminium hydroxide gel.

Some of the magmas are prepared by dispersing the inorganic substance in the solvent, usually water.

When such material is dispersed, the solid particles become hydrated due to their strong affinity towards water and form a gelatinous mass. For example, bentonite, a naturally occuring aluminium silicate, insoluble in water. When dispersed in water at a concentration of about 4-5%, it swells to about 12 times of its volume and form a gelatinous mass called bentonite magma.

Such inorganic magmas or gels are pH sensitive. For example, pH of the bentonite magma normally remains within 9.5-10.5. Bentonite is also used as suspending agent. If the pH is less than 7, it loses its suspendability.

Both magmas and gels can remain almost uniform for fairly sufficient time due to the strong attraction between disperse phase and dispersion medium. The dispersed phase settles very slightly. After a long standing a little supernatant layer of the dispersion medium can be seen over the dispersed phase. However, on shaking the preparation is uniformly dispersed.

When the magma is kept undisturbed for sufficient time, it sets to a gel which on agitation turns into a sol. This property is called thixotropy and the process can be repeated indefinitely.

Some official magmas are Dihydroxy aluminium Aminoacetate Magma, USP, Bentonite Magma, NF.

Because of this orally administered drugs can be satisfactorily dispensed through their magmas or gel preparations.

Milk of Magnesia

Magnesium hydroxide is an inorganic compound with the chemical formula $Mg(OH)_2$. As a suspension in water, it is often called **milk of magnesia** because of its milk-like appearance.

The term *milk of magnesia* was first used for a white-coloured, aqueous, mildly alkaline suspension of magnesium hydroxide formulated at about 8%w/v by Charles Henry Phillips in (1880) and sold under the brand name *Phillips' Milk of Magnesia* for medicinal usage.

When dilute solution of sodium hydroxide is added to dilute solution of magnesium sulphate in a thin stream, sodium hydroxide reacts with magnesium sulphate and a fine, flocculating, gelatinous precipitate of insoluble magnesium hydroxide is formed.

$$2NaOH + MgSO_4 \rightarrow Mg(OH)_2\downarrow + Na_2SO_4$$

Sodium sulphate is removed by repeated washing of the precipitate with purified water. Finally the requisite amount of purified water added to prepared desired volume of the preparation. This preparation is industrially prepared by direct hydration of magnesium oxide. The method is more economical.

$$MgO + H_2O \rightarrow Mg(OH)_2$$

The milk of magnesia is an opaque, white, viscous preparation which when kept undisturbed varying proportions of water separate. Hence, it should be shaken before use. Since, the suspension is alkaline, pH is about 10, a reaction between the glass and magma may take place, and the product may acquire a bitter taste. By adding 0.1% citric acid the product can be stabilized. Addition of suitable flavour, maximum up to 0.05%, the palatability of the product can be improved.

The optimum storage temperature is within 35°C in a tightly closed glass container. At freezing temperature the fine dispersed particles coalesce and at higher temperature the gel structure is affected

Glycerites

A glycerite is a fluid extract of an herb or other medicinal substance made with glycerin.

According to King's American Dispensatory (1898) a glycerite is Glycerita.—Glycerites. This class of preparations is generally understood as solutions of medicinal substances in glycerin, although in certain instances the various Pharmacopoeias deviate to an extent. The term Glycerita as here applied to fluid glycerines, or solutions of agents in glycerin, is preferable to the ordinary names, "glyceroles," "glycerates," or "glycemates," etc., and includes all fluid preparations of the kind referred to, whether for internal administration or local application. Many solutions of glycerin or glycerin and water, are apt upon standing to develop microscopic cryptogams, unless a certain proportion of alcohol is added to the solutions. On this account, it is better to prepare many members of this class of solutions in small quantity at a time, and only as they are wanted.

Glycerites are frequently used as a substitute for alcohol in tinctures, as a solvent that will create a therapeutic herbal extraction. Glycerine is less extractive and is approximately 30% less able to be absorbed by the body due to processing in the liver. Fluid extract manufacturers often extract herbs in hot water before adding glycerin to make glycerites to increase extraction.

Glycerin will not extract the same constituents from plants that alcohol will. From "Herbal Preparations and Natural Therapies" by Debra St. Claire:

- glycerin will extract the following-sugars, enzymes (dilute), glucosides, bitter compounds, saponins (dilute), and tannins

- absolute alcohol will extract the following-alkaloids (some), glycosides, volatile oils, waxes, resins, fats, some tannins, balsam, sugars, and vitamins.

Formulations:

Product: Starch Glycerite

Composition:

It contains

Starch 10%

Benzoic acid 2%

Glycerine 70% in purified water.

Use: Topical vehicle and protectant

Lot size: 10 ml

Manufacturing Formula:

Starch	1.0 g
Benzoic acid	0.2 g
Glycerine	7.0 g
Purified water	q.s

Manufacturing Method:

- Weigh accurately starch and benzoic acid, transfer into a 100 ml clean conical flask, add 3 ml of purified water, mix well,
- Add required volume of glycerin and mix thoroughly, stopper the flask with a rubber stopper,
- Heat the mixture in a hot oil bath at 140°C with occasional shaking, continue heating until the mixture becomes translucent,
- Cool the preparation and pack in a wide mouth bottle, seal with a pilfer proof cap and label.

Paints

These are liquid preparations for application to the skin or mucous surfaces. These may be aqueous or alcoholic solutions and sometimes, are prepared with a collodion basis. Usually these contain the medicament like antiseptic, astringent, caustic or analgesic properties. Resinous substances like benzoin, prepared storax, or tolu balsam in ethereal solution are used as bases of medicated varnishes.

Containers: These are normally dispensed in coloured fluted bottles to distinguish them from the preparations intended for internal use. The bottles should be fitted with glass stoppers or other suitable closures.

Labelling: The label should mention distinctly, For external use only, besides all other relevant information.

Storage: These are to be packed in airtight containers and stored in a cool place.

Formulations:

Product: Coal Tar Paint

Standard for product: weight per ml at 20°C, 0.850 – 0.870 g.

Use: Local anti-eczematic

Lot size: 25 ml

Manufacturing Formula:

Coal tar   2.5 g

Acetone and

Benzene (nitration grade) of equal volumes to make   25 ml.

Manufacturing Method:

- Prepare 28 ml of a mixture of acetone and benzene (nitration grade) at a ratio of 1:1.

- Dissolve weighed quantity of coal tar in the solvent mixture and make up the volume.

- Determine the weight/ml at 20°C and filter through G_4 sintered glass crucible, fill in suitable bottle and seal immediately with a pilfer proof cap. Label properly.

Note:

- *The label should state 'This preparation is inflammable'.*

- *Keep away from a naked flame.*

Product: Crystal Violet Paint

Standard for product: Light absorption, dilute 5 ml to 250 ml with water, dilute 5 ml of this solution to 250 ml water and measure the extinction of a 1-cm layer at the maximum at about 585 nm; the extinction should not be less than 0.32.

Use: Antiseptic and disinfectant

Lot size: 25 ml

Manufacturing Formula:

Crystal violet   0.125 g
Purified water   q.s

Manufacturing Method:

- Dissolve weighed quantity of crystal violet in purified water sufficient to make 25 ml,
- Filter the solution through a clean, wet cloth,
- Fill in a suitable bottle, seal with a pilfer proof cap and label properly.

Product: Brilliant Green and Crystal Violet paint

Standard for product:

Weight per ml at 20°C, 0.930 – 0.950 g;

Alcohol content, 42 – 48%v/v.

Use : Antiseptic

Lot size: 50 ml

Manufacturing Formula:

Brilliant green	0.25 g
Crystal violet	0.25 g
Alcohol (90%)	25.0 ml
Purified water q.s	

Manufacturing Method:

- Dissolve weighed quantity of brilliant green and crystal violet in measured volume of alcohol, add sufficient purified water to make 50 ml,
- Determine the weight per ml and alcohol content,
- Filter the solution through a clean, wet cloth, fill in a clean and dry bottle, seal with a pilfer proof cap,
- Label correctly.

Exercises

Short Questions

1. (a) Define elixir and linctuses.
   (b) Why the simple syrup does not contain any preservative?
   (c) Name the additives used in oral liquids.
   (d) Why are sodium sulphite, sodium metabisulphite used in liquid preparations?
   (e) Name the flavours suitable for masking bitter taste in a liquid preparation.

(f) What are the flavours commonly used to mask sour taste in a liquid preparation?

(g) Name five flavours commonly used in oral liquids.

(h) Name five colours used in oral liquids.

(i) Name four preservatives used in oral liquids.

(j) What are the tests to be performed during mixing step of liquid manufacturing?

(k) Name the tests to be performed during extraction.

(l) Name the tests to be performed during filtration.

(m) What is invert syrup?

(n) What is surface dilution?

(o) What is the maximum time beyond which a diluted syrup or elixir cannot be used?

(p) What is organised drug?

(q) For maceration whether organised or unorganised drugs are suitable?

(r) What are the ideal characteristics of a solvent for extraction?

(s) What is simple maceration/

(t) What is fresh infusion?

(u) What is digestion?

(v) What are common problems in suspension?

(w) Name various types of emulsifying agents.

(x) Name the suspending agents commonly used in suspension.

(y) Name the commonly used surface active agents.

(z) Name the tests to be performed during formulation of a suspension.

2. What are different methods of preparing simple syrup?

3. Write down the various steps of manufacturing a solution preparation.

4. What information should be provided in a label for an oral liquid? Present a label.

5. Describe the general method of manufacturing of a suspension.

6. Discuss the common problems and their solutions associated with suspension preparation.

7. Write down the general methods of preparation of an aromatic water.

8. Write down the additives with example and function commonly used in suspension formulation.

9. Distinguish between suspension and emulsion.

10. Describe the general method of manufacturing of an emulsion.

11. Describe the general method of preparing tinctures.

12. Short notes on;
    (a) Enemas,
    (b) Gargles,
    (c) Mouthwashes,
    (d) Liniments,
    (e) Spirits,
    (f) Paints,
    (g) Collodions,
    (h) Elixirs,
    (i) Linctuses,
    (j) Mixtures,
    (k) Lotions,
    (l) Wetting agents,
    (m) Suspending agents,

5 Sterile Preparations

Parenteral Preparations (Injectables)

Other than Blood Products and Immunological Products

These are sterile preparations intended for administration into the body by injection, infusion or implantation. There are five main types of parenteral preparations - Injections, Powders for Injection, Intravenous Infusion, Concentrated Solutions for Injection and Implants.

Parenteral preparations may be of small volume parenteral (SVP) and large volume parenteral (LVP).

The manufacturing method of these preparations should be designed in such a way that the final product is completely free from foreign particles, pyrogen or bacterial endotoxins, and any micro-organism. The product should remain sterile during its shelf-life.

Parenteral preparations that are solutions or suspensions require vehicle in which the medicaments are either dissolved or suspended. Most common vehicle is Water for Injection. Any other suitable vehicle can be used which is safe in the volume of injection, inert with respect to therapeutic efficacy and the tests of the active ingredient.

Sometimes these preparations contain certain compatible additives like buffers, stabilisers and antimicrobial preservatives to enhance the stability of the product during its shelf-life. The additives should not interfere with the therapeutic action of the drug and with any test carried out on the product. *But no colouring agent and flavor should be present in a parenteral preparation.*

Aqueous Parenteral preparations intended for subcutaneous, intradermal, intramuscular administration or large volume parenterals, if possible, should be made isotonic with blood by addition of sodium chloride or any other suitable substances. The preparations intended for intraocular, intravenous injection or any product that may gain access into cerebrospinal fluid should not contain any buffering agent.

Parenteral preparations packed in mu dose container, regardless the method of sterilisation, may contain suitable antimicrobial agent (preservative) in appropriate concentration, unless otherwise directed in the individual monograph, or unless the drug itself is bacteriostatic.

When the volume to be injected as a single dose exceeds 15 ml, the preparation should not contain any preservative unless otherwise justified; or when the preparation is intended for administration by the intraocular, intracardiac or intracisternal routes or other route resulting access to the cerebrospinal fluid.

Where preservatives should not be used

(a) Injection containing an ingredient which itself has anti-bacterial activity,

(b) Single dose intravenous injection, where dose is more than 15 ml,

(c) Injection used as intracardiac, intrathecal, intra-arterial, intracisternal and peridural,

(d) Injection prepared by heating with bactericide.

Where the drug is susceptible to oxidative degradation a suitable antioxidant may be added and/or the air in the container may be displaced by nitrogen or any suitable inert gas.

To make the product sterile there are different methods of sterilisation. The method selected for sterilisation of a particular product should be investigated for its effect on the product and before practice the procedure needs to be validated also. The absolute definition of sterility is *complete absence of viable micro-organism*, but in practice the term sterility is defined in terms of probability and sterility of a final product is achievable only through GMP. However, the different methods of sterilisation are steam sterilisation (moist heat sterilisation), dry heat sterilisation, sterilisation by filtration, gas sterilisation and sterilisation by ionic radiation.

General Standards for Injections (solution, emulsion or suspension) other than stated in the monograph.

Particulate matter: the solutions should be clear and free from any visible particle when examined on visual inspection by unaided eye under suitable conditions of visibility.

Injection with a nominal content of 100 ml or more should comply with the limit test for particulate matter.

Uniformity of content: Should comply with the test for uniformity of content.

Extractable volume: Should comply with the test for Extractable volume.

Sterility: Injections should comply with the test for sterility.

Pyrogens: Unless otherwise mentioned in the individual monograph, when the volume of a single dose is 10 ml or more, the preparation should comply with the test for pyrogens/ the test for bacterial endotoxins.

Standards for Injections (Powders)

In addition to the standards stated in individual monograph these products should comply with the following general standards.

Uniformity of content: Should comply with the test for uniformity of content.

Uniformity of weight: Take 20 filled containers from a pooled sample. Remove the labels wrapped over the containers. Transfer the content from each container as much as possible into a weighing bottle which is clean, dry and weighed. Weigh the individual contents after each transfer. Make the average. Not more than 2 of the individual weights deviate from the average weight by more than 10% and none should deviate by more than 20%.

For powders for injection which have been tested for uniformity of content need not to be tested for this test.

Sterility: Powders for Injection shall comply with test for sterility.

Intravenous Infusions

These are sterile aqueous solutions or emulsions (o/w type), free from pyrogens or bacterial endotoxins, foreign particle visible to the naked eye, intended for intravenous administration. These are isotonic to the blood and do not contain any anti-microbial preservative. Their nominal content is 100 ml or more.

Particulate matter: Should comply with the limit test for particulate matter.

Sterility: Should comply with the test for sterility.

Pyrogens: Where the test for bacterial endotoxins is not prescribed, the preparation should comply with the test for pyrogens.

Concentrated Solutions for Injection

These are sterile solutions intended for administration either by injection or intravenous infusion only after dilution with a suitable liquid.

Standards: After dilution it should comply the standards for either Injections or Intravenous Infusion depending on its nominal volume and use.

Implants

These are sterile solid preparations of size suitable for implantation into the body tissues for release of the drug over an extended period of time. These are usually packed individually in sterile containers.

General Standards

Sterility: Should comply with the test for sterility.

Formulation Considerations

During formulation development work for these preparations the following important factors are needed to be considered.

- the suggested route of administration,
- the volume of injection,
- the solvent to be used to dissolve or disperse the drug (s),
- stability criteria of the proposed preparation, (whether a stabiliser is required or not),
- pH of the product,
- osmotic pressure of the solution,
- specific gravity/wt. per ml of the product, particularly when intended for spinal anaesthesia,
- selection of preservative system, if required,
- method of sterilisation,
- physical stability of a suspension or emulsion for accurate withdrawal of dose,
- working environment, method of manufacture and finally biopharmaceutical aspects.

Additives used in sterile preparations: The list of additives commonly used is presented in the Table 5.1 below.

TABLE 5.1

Common additives used in sterile preparations

Category	Name of the substance	Usual concentration	
Preservative	Benzalkonium chloride solution	0.02%	
	Chlorhexidine acetate	0.01%	w/v
	Benzyl alcohol	0.5 – 10%	
	Benzethonium chloride	0.01%	
	Butylparaben	0.015%	
	Methylparaben	0.01 – 0.2%	
	Propylparaben	0.005 – 0.035%	
	Chlorocresol	0.1%	
	Chlorbutol	0.25 – 0.5%	
	Metacresol	0.10 – 0.3%	
	Phenol	0.06 – 0.5%	
	Phenyl mercuric acetate	0.001%	
	Phenylmercuric nitrate	0.001%	
	Thiomersal	0.001 – 0.02%	

Table 5.1 contd....

Category	Name of the substance	Usual concentration
Buffer	Sodium acetate	0.8%w/v
	Sodium citrate	4.0%
	Sodium benzoate and benzoic acid	5.0%
	Sodium phosphate, monobasic	1.7%
	Sodium phosphate,dibasic	0.71%
	Sodium bicarbonate	0.005%
	Sodium carbonate	0.06%
	Sodium tartrate	1.2%
	Potassium phosphate	0.1%
	Acetic acid	0.22%
	Adipic acid	1.0%
	Citric acid	0.5%
	Lactic acid	0.1%
	Maleic acid	1.6%
	Tartaric acid	0.65%
Stabiliser	Creatinine	0.5 – 0.8%
	Glycine	1.5 – 2.25%
	Niacinamide	1.25 – 2.5%
	Sodium caprylate	0.4%
	Sodium saccharine	0.03%
	Sodium acetyl tryptophanate	0.53%
Antioxidant	Ascorbic acid	0.02 – 0.1%
(Reducing agent)	Sodium bisulphite	0.1 – 0.15%
	Sodium metabisulphite	0.1 – 0.15%
	Sodium formaldehyde sulphoxylate	0.1 – 0.15%
	Thiourea	0.005%
(Blocking agents)	Tocopherols	0.05 – 0.075%
	Ascorbic acid esters	0.01 – 0.015%
	Butylated hydroxy toluene	0.005 – 0.02%
Synergist	Ascorbic acid	0.01 – 0.05%
	Citric acid	0.005 – 0.01%
	Citraconic acid	0.03 – 0.45%
	Phosphoric acid	0.005 – 0.01%
	Tartaric acid	0.01 – 0.02%
Chelating agent	Disodium edentate	0.01 – 0.075%
	Disodium calcium edentate	0.04%
Solubiliser	Dimethyl actamide	0.01%
Wetting agent	Dioctyl sodium sulphosuccinate	0.0150%

Table 5.1 *contd....*

Category	Name of the substance	Usual concentration
Emulsifiers	Ethyl alcohol	0.6 – 49%
	Ethylacetate	0.1%
	Glycerin	14.6 – 25%
	Eggyolk	1.2%
	Lecithin	0.5 – 2.3%
	Polyethylene glycol 40 castor oil	7 – 11.5%
	Polyethylene glycol 300	0.01 – 50%
	Polyethylene glycol	0.2 – 50%
	Polysorbate 20	0.01%
	Polysorbate 40	0.05%
	Polysorbate 80	0.04 – 4.0%
	Povidone	0.2 – 1.0%
	Sodium desoxycholate	0.21%
	Sorbitan monopalmitate	0.05%
	Theophylline	5.0%
Suspending agent	Gelatin	2%
	Methylcellulose	0.03 – 1.05%
	Pectin	0.2%
	Polyethylene glycol 4000	2.7 – 3.0%
	Sodium carboxymethylcellulose	0.05 – 0.75%
	Sorbitol solution	50%
Tonicity	Glycerin	1.6 – 2.25%
Adjusting agent	Lactose	0.14 – 5.0%
	Mannitol	0.4 – 2.5%
	Dextrose	3.75 – 5.0%
	Sodium chloride	quantity required
	Sodium sulphate	1.15%
	Sorbitol	2.0%
Local	Procaine hydrochloride	1%
Anaesthetics	Benzyl alcohol	5%

List of non-aqueous solvents is given below in the Table 5.2

TABLE 5.2

List of non-aqueous solvents commonly used in sterile preparations

Water miscible	Water immiscible
Dioxolanes	Fixed oils
Dimethyl acetamide	Ethyl oleate
N-(β-hydroxyethyl)-lactamide	Isopropyl myristate
Butylene glycol	Benzyl benzoate
Polyethylene glycol 400-600	
Polyethylene glycol	
Glycerin	
Ethyl alcohol	

Different steps involved in the manufacture of small volume parenterals (SVPs), large volume parenterals (LVPs) and powder injections (PIs).

Sl. No.	Manufacturing steps	Type of preparation		
		SVP	LVP	PI
1.	Washing and sterilisation of containers and closures	Y	Y	Y
2.	Preparation of pyrogen free distilled water	Y	Y	N
3.	Preparation of solution	Y	Y	N
4.	Filtration of solution	Y	Y	N
5.	Filling and sealing	Y	Y	Y
6.	Terminal sterilisation of product	Y	Y	Y
7.	Inspection	Y	Y	Y
8.	Labelling and packing	Y	Y	Y

General Method

1. **Washing of containers and closures:**

   (a) **Ampoules (1-10 ml capacity):** Wash successively with soft feed water filtered through G_4 sintered disc/0.8 μ membrane filter, then with compressed air filtered through Norgan Air Filter, rinse with pyrogen free distilled water filtered through G_4 sintered disc/0.8 μ membrane filter, finally with compressed air filtered through Norgan Air Filter,

   (b) **Ampoules (above 10 ml capacity) and vials:** Soak the ampoules and vials in hot detergent (Teepol/Homacel) solution 0.5% for 4-8 hrs.,
   - Wash with soft feed water, soak in 0.5% hydrochloric acid solution for 2 hrs.,
   - Wash with filtered soft feed water,
   - Wash the ampoules with filtered compressed air,
   - Wash the ampoules/vials with pyrogen free distilled water, and
   - Finally with filtered compressed air.
   - Check the pH of the final washing, it should be 6-7.

   (c) **Closures:** Soak the rubber closures in 0.5-1% solution of detergent (Teepol/Homacel), boil for 30 mins.
   - Wash with soft feed water till complete removal of detergent,
   - Soak the closures in hot 0.5% hydrochloric acid contained in suitable stainless steel container for 2 hrs,

- Wash with soft feed water till complete removal of acid,
- Soak the closures in hot, 0.5% solution of sodium bicarbonate for 2 hrs,
- Wash with soft feed water till complete removal of alkalinity,
- Finally wash with pyrogen free filtered distilled water till the pH of the washing is 6.5.

2. **Sterilisation of containers and closures:** Sterilise the washed containers in a dry heat steriliser at $200 - 250°C$ for $2 - 4$ hrs.

   Sterilise the washed closures in a steam steriliser (Autoclave) at $116 °C$ (i.e., under 10 lbs/sq.inch pressure) for 30 min.

   Note: If the product contains a preservative, soak the washed rubber closures in the solution of the preservative at its double concentration for 24 hrs, then wash the closures till the washing is free from preservative. Then sterilise the closures.

3. **Distilled water:** Purified water is prepared either by deionization or distillation. This water cannot be used in parenteral preparations as the solvent.

   Water for injection is the water purified by distillation and used as a solvent only in parenteral preparations   which are to be sterilised after preparation.

   Sterile water for injection is the water for injection which is sterilised and suitably packed. It is pyrogen free and may contain a bacteriostatic agent when packed in containers of 30 ml or smaller. This water needs to comply with the test for pyrogen as per IP.

Standards

Test	Purified water	Water for injection	Sterile water for injection
Description	clear, colourless, and odourless	clear, colourless, and odourless	Clear, courless and odourless or it may contain. the odour of the bacteriostatic agent, if present.
Chloride	-	-	Not more than 0.5 mcg/ml.
Sulphate	-	-	-
Ammonia	Not more than 0.3mcg/ml	Not more than 0.3 mcg/ml	-
Calcium	-	-	-
Heavy metals	-	-	-
Oxidisable Substances	pink colour should not disappear completely.	Pink colour should not disappear completely.	NA, if contains preservative.

Table contd....

Test	Purified water	Water for injection	Sterile water for injection
Total solids	Not more than10mcg/ml	Not more than 10 mcg/ml	Not more than 40 mcg/ml, If package is 30ml or less. Not more than 30 mcg/ml, If package is 30ml – 100 ml. Not more than 20 mcg/ml, if package is more than 100 ml
Sterility	-	-	should be sterile
Pyrogen	-	should be pyrogen free	should be pyrogen free

4. **Environment:** Before starting of the manufacturing operation, check the environment of the manufacturing area for,

   (i)   Microbial count test,

   (ii)   Positive air pressure,

   (iii) Cleanliness of the equipments to be used,

   (iv)   Complete analysis of water for injection to be used,

   (v)   Clothing uniforms of the working personnel for sterility.

5. **Preparation of solution:**

   - Accurately weigh required quantity of each ingredient as per the,
   - Manufacturing Formula,
   - Transfer into clean suitable container and add required quantity of water for injection or the specified solvent and stir till dissolved,
   - Make up the volume with the solvent and mix well,
   - Carry out the tests like assay, pH, etc on a sample of the solution prepared as per the In-process control tests for injection.

6. **Filtration of solution:**

   - Filter the solution through Whatmann filter paper No.1 or G_4 sintered glass,
   - If the filtrate is not clear, use charcoal (not more than 0.4% w/v) for Decolourisation,
   - Filter the filtrate again through a membrane filter of porosity 0.2 μ under Aseptic condition,
   - Collect the filtrate in a suitable pre-sterilised container.

Note: If charcoal is used, ensure that it is free from pyrogen and other impurities that may affect the quality of the product.

7. **Filling and sealing:**
   - Fill the solution into desired pre-sterilised pack container like ampoules,
   - Vials or bottles, if necessary flash with inert gas like nitrogen,
   - The filling should be done under laminar air flow,
   - Seal the containers by fusion (if ampoules) or with appropriate closures,
   - (Pre-sterilised) and with the clean aluminium cap (if vials or bottles),
   - Carry out the test for *clarity* and *extractable volume* on filled packed,
   - Containers randomly.

   Note: In case of ampoules seal immediately after filling and, if necessary after filling replace the air in the ampoules by flashing with an inert gas, e.g. nitrogen before sealing.

8. **Sterilisation:** Absolute sterility of individual product of a lot cannot be guaranteed without loss of each and every unit, which is not practically possible. hence, the sterility of a lot/batch is a probability and can be assured by compliance of an established procedure according to GMP.

   The effectiveness of sterilisation process is established by validation and certification of the process. The basis of validation and certification are;
   - Capacity of the sterilising equipment within the required parameters,
   - Ability of the control system to record the operational parameters of the Sterilising equipment,
   - Reproducibility of the sterilising efficacy of the equipment and process,
   - Monitoring system during routine operation and re-qualification of the equipment, if necessary,
   - Documentation system of the complete operation and validation protocols,
   - Selection of the method of sterilisation should consider the following aspects,
   - The effect of the method on the product and package or container,
   - In case of terminal sterilisation, the aspect of physical, where relevant,
   - chemical conditions inside the sterilising chamber,
   - Detection of location(s) inside the sterilising chamber where the effect of sterilising agent is/are minimum (coolest points in an autoclave),
   - Loading arrangement of each type and size of containers with respect to cooler parts in an autoclave,

- Ensuring whether all loads receive consistently the specified,
- Exposure/treatment.

Methods of Sterilisation

Moist Heat Sterilisation

The process utilizes saturated steam as heating material or sterilising agent and an autoclave or a pressure cooker as the equipment. The materials sterilised by this method are aqueous preparations packed in containers and surgical materials. The seal containers are exposed to saturated steam for a definite period of time. The maintenance of an effective combination of time and temperature ensure sterility.

Combination of temperature and time normally used are as follows:

Holding Temperature ($^{\circ}$C)	Holding Time (min.)
115 – 118	30
121 – 124	15
126 – 129	10
134 – 138	3

The holding time and temperature can be changed if the process can ensure sterility within the established tolerance when operated routinely. The F_o concept can be used for establishing the sterilisation cycle parameters.

The F_o value of a saturated steam sterilisation process is the lethality expressed in terms of the equivalent time in minutes at a temperature of 121°C delivered by that process to the product in its final containers with reference to microorganisms possessing a Z-value (the change in temperature required to alter the D-value by a factor of 10) of 10. In general for aqueous preparations a microbiologically validated steam sterilisation process that delivers, in total (i.e., including the heating up and cooling down phases of the cycle), an F_o value of not less than 8 to every container in the load is considered satisfactory.

For the heat sensitive products and in certain cases, where a process which produces, in total, F_o less than 8 is necessary, attention must be taken to ensure that an adequate assurance of sterility is consistently achieved. Microbiological validation of the process is not only necessary. It is necessary to demonstrate, through routine practice, that the microbiological parameters are also within the established tolerances to achieve a theoretical level of not more than one living microorganism per 10^6 containers in the final product.

During sterilisation of surgical items in an autoclave the steam should neither be superheated nor contain more than 5% of entrained moisture. Moreover, the air inside the autoclave, both jacket and chamber, should be replaced by the steam. Most dressings can conveniently be sterilised at 134-138 °C for 3 min.

Dry Heat Sterilisation

The products suitable for this process are heat-stable, non-aqueous products and powders.

Holding temperature and holding time in this process are usually as follows;

Holding Temperature (°C)	Holding Time (min.)
180	30
170	60
160	120

The preparations to be sterilised by this method is distributed in the final containers which are then either finally sealed or temporarily closed and exposed to an established set of holding time and temperature. The containers which have been temporarily closed are to be finally sealed under aseptic conditions to maintain sterility.

The process is usually carried out in a sterilising oven designed especially for the purpose. The oven should also be attached to the devices for sensing, monitoring and controlling the critical parameters.

The validation of this process can be done in a manner similar to that for the steam sterilisation. When the containers, to be used for filling intravenous solution, are sterilised by this method, there should be no particulate matter inside the oven.

For heat-stable articles the microbial survival probability of 10^{-12} can be achieved using this method.

Sterilisation by Filtration

Liquids or solutions of heat-sensitive materials are sterilised by this method. This method is a physical process. The microorganisms are removed from the preparation by adsorption on a filter medium of nominal pore size of 0.2 μm. The filter medium should,

- Produce a filtrate completely free from microorganisms, spores and particulate matter from the solution.
- Not change the composition of the solution (i.e., should be perfectly inert).
- Not shed any fibre during filtration.

The process is completed in two steps:

Pre-filtration and membrane filtration: Pre-filtration removes all visible particles as well as particles below the visible range. Since the asbestos filters may have a tendency to shed fibres, filters made of nitro-cellulose are preferred. The solution is forced through such filters with either negative or positive pressure and filled into sterile containers. Excessive positive pressures and leakage of air in negative pressure equipment should be avoided, since any leakage of air have the risk of contamination. If the filtration process is too prolonged, the filter should be changed occasionally, since colonies of micro-organisms may become well enough established in the filter pores to contaminate the filtrate. The entire process must be carried out under aseptic and particle free environment only.

The integrity of the filtration system should be checked before and after use by carrying out tests like bubble point, pressure hold or diffusion rate, etc., appropriate to the type of filter used and the stage at which the test is carried out.

This process of sterilisation should be validated with respect to the microbial load in the filtering solution.

Gas Sterilisation

The solids, e.g. Sodium Penicillin G which are not heat stable, are sterilised by this method. The sterilising agent is a gas, ethylene oxide alone or mixed with some other inert gas. Ethylene oxide is toxic and when mixed with air is explosive also. Hence, this process is to be used for those materials which are not inflammable and are compatible with this gas. The sterilising efficiency of ethylene oxide depends on

- The concentration of the gas,
- Duration of exposure,
- Temperature,
- Humidity and
- Nature of the material to be sterilised (load).

Suitable biological indicator should be distributed throughout the load to assess the sterilising efficacy in each cycle. At the end of each process sufficient time should be allowed for dispersal of residual gas and other volatile residues. The amount of residual ethylene oxide, ethylene glycol and ethylene chlorhydrin are to be determined by a suitable method like gas chromatography.

The most important limitation of this method is the extent of penetration of the gas inside the load. Thus, the design and arrangement of the load become a factor for sterilisation efficiency of the gas. The depth of the load should such that the gas can easily penetrate to the bottom most layer and there is least resistance to the dispersal of the gas after completion of exposure.

Sterilisation by Ionizing Radiations

In this method the sterilising agent is the ionizing radiation in the form of gamma radiation from a suitable radio-isotope, *e.g.* Cobalt-60, Cesium-137 or of electrons energised by a suitable accelerator. The drug substances, dosage forms and medical devices can be sterilised in the final containers or packages by exposing the articles to the radiation for definite period of time.

In both the cases the degree of sterility depends on

- The dose of the radiation,

- Number of exposures, and

- Nature of the articles (load).

The effective and tolerable sterilising dose of gamma radiation is about 25 kGy (2.5 Mrads). This causes minimum damage to the material.

Microbiological monitoring is necessary if the dose is reduced. Validation of the sterilising efficacy of the process, particularly at lower exposure level, needs:

- to measure the resistance of the microbial population in the product to the magnitude (number and/or degree) of the radiation,

- loading pattern, and

- radiation dose absorbed by the material.

Validated dosimetry method can be used to measure the radiation dose absorbed by the material being irradiated. This may involve the determination of induced changes in the optical properties of plastics. Clean plastics or plastics containing radiation sensitive dyes whose colour intensity changes with the amount of radiation energy absorbed.

Biological Indicators: According to I.P. the biological indicators are characterised and standardised preparations of specific microorganism with known stability, high resistance to one or more sterilisation processes.

The biological indicators are used as a tool to:

1. Qualify the physical operation of a steriliser,
2. validate and a sterilisation process with respect to the materials for sterilisation and process,
3. monitor the operation routinely.

Factors that influence the selection of a biological indicator are:

1. Stability of the non-pathogenic strain,
2. Resistance of the strain to sterilisation process,
3. Reproducibility of the recovered strain after cultivation under standardised conditions.

Recommended Biological Indicators with respect to process is given in the Table 5.3 below.

TABLE 5.3

Biological indicators with respect to sterilisation processes

Sterilisation Process	Biological Indicator
Moist Heat Sterilisation	NCTC 10007 (spores of Bacillus stearothermophilus) or NCTC 8594 (spores of Clostridium sporogenes)
Dry Heat Sterilisation	NCIMB 8058 (spores of Bacillus subtilis var. niger)
Radiation sterilisation	NCTC 10327 (spores of Bacillus pumilus)
Ethylene oxide sterilisation	NCTC 10073 (spores of Bacillus subtilis var. niger)

9. Inspection:

- On the following day of sterilisation inspect visually each filled container against black and white background whether there is any visible particulate matter inside.

- Carefully invert the container without creating any turbulence in the solution movement, place under the visual inspection table and see carefully, the white particle will be visible over black back ground and black particle will be visible over white background.

- Discard the container having any visible particle.

Note: *Particulate matter means any extraneous, mobile, undissolved substance unintentionally present in injection. But not the gas bubbles.*

10. **Labelling and packing:** The containers used for packing injectables should also be sterile and they should be inert, sufficiently transparent and non-diffusible. These may be glass ampoules, vials, bottles or plastic bottles or bags. The container may be for single dose or multiple doses.

Vials and bottles need closures to ensure a reliable seal which can prevent the access of micro-organisms and other contaminants and can allow the puncture with minimum shedding of particles during withdrawals of contents either in portions or in whole without being removed. These may be made of rubber or plastic material which is compatible with the injectable preparation. Like the container as it remains directly in contact with the preparation, a closure should be thoroughly cleaned and sterilised before use. When the preparation contains any ingredient, e.g. preservatives, or any other additive which can be absorbed by the closure, the closures should be heated with the solution of such ingredient(s) for sufficient time before being used. The concentration of those ingredients should be double of the actual and volume should be sufficient to immerse the closures completely.

While labelling the containers, the size of the label should be such that it leaves a space of full length sufficient for inspection of the content visually. Besides this the label shall provide following information.

- The name of the product,
- Composition along with strength in terms of percentage concentration or in dose-volume,
- Name and concentration of preservative and stabilising agent, if present,
- Storage conditions of the product.

For the parenteral preparation which needs to be constituted or diluted before use, the label should state in addition to the above information

- Composition/name of the recommended diluent, the amount of the diluent necessary to make specific concentration of the drug and final volume of the solution or suspension to be prepared,
- Storage conditions for the diluted preparation, and period within which the constituted/diluted preparation is to be used under the recommended storage conditions.

Adjustment of isotonicity/iso-osmocity of sterile preparations

The parenteral and ophthalmic preparations should be iso-osmotic or isotonic (as they may affect the blood cells) to blood and lachrymal secretions respectively.

The osmotic pressure of blood or lachrymal secretions is approximately 6.7 atm. Hence, a solution intended for parenteral or ophthalmic use should have osmotic pressure of 6.7 atm. A molar solution of a non-ionized solute (one gm mole in a litre) has osmotic pressure of 22.4 atm. So, 6.7/22.4 = 0.3 molar solution of a non-ionised solute will be iso-osmotic with blood or tears.

Example: The mol. wt. of Dextrose anhydrous = 180

A molar solution of dextrose means 180 g/lt.

So, 0.3 molar solution of dextrose means 0.3 × 180 = 54 g of dextrose/lt. i.e. 5.4 g in 100 ml or 5.4% w/v solution.

For calculating the amount of a non-ionised solute required for making an iso-osmotic solution the following formula is used,

$$\frac{M \times 0.3 \times 100}{1000} = w \text{ g of solute in 100 ml. where M is the molecular weight of the}$$

solute.

For ionisable solute the above formula is modified as,

$$\frac{M \times 0.3 \times 100}{1000N} = w \text{ g of solute in 100 ml.}$$

Where N is the nos. of ions produced on ionisation of one molecule of solute, and M is the mol. wt.

Example: At what concentration of NaCl will be iso-osmotic to blood?

Molecular weight (M) of NaCl = 58.5

On ionisation each molecule of NaCl produces Na^+ and Cl^- ions, i.e. N = 2

$$\frac{58.5 \times 0.3}{2 \times 10} = 0.88 \text{ g of sodium chloride in 100 ml, i.e. 0.9\%w/v solution.}$$

Process Control Tests for Injectables

The tests may vary with the type of parenteral preparations and however, the common tests to be carried out at different steps are mentioned below in the Table 5.4

TABLE 5.4

Process control tests with respect to manufacturing steps

Manufacturing step	Tests to be carried out
Preparation of solution	clarity, pH, content of active ingredients and preservatives, if any.
Filling of ampoules, vials	particulate matter, extractive volume.
Sterilisation (steam sterilisation)	checking and recording of steam pressure inside autoclave (chamber pressure), the temperature and sterilisation time.
Post sterilisation	Particulate matter, clarity, pH, extractable volume, uniformity of contents, sterility, pyrogen test/bacterial endotoxin.

General Method of Tests

1. **Colour and clarity of solution:** Take two clean and dry, flat bottom test tubes of diameter 15-25 mm, transfer suitable volume of the sample (preparation) into one test tube up to a depth of at least 4 cm. In other test tube take the volume of distilled water. Place the two test tubes vertically over a white tile or any white back ground, examine the two liquid columns from top in diffused light and compare the colour and clarity of   the sample with those of water. The test should comply with the *test for Description* mentioned in the individual monograph.

2. **pH:** Calibrate the pH meter using standard buffer solutions definite pH like 4.0, 7.0, 9.2. Wash the electrode with distilled water, then soak the electrode with tissue paper, pour the sample in a clean, dry beaker and check its pH.

3. **Content of active ingredient(s):** Proceed as per the method described in the individual monograph or as per the established method.

4. **Content of preservative:** Proceed as per the method described in the individual monograph or as per the established method.

5. **Particulate matter:** This test should be carried out in a room maintained with positive air pressure, the room should be supplied with filtered air and the test to be done under laminar air flow (horizontal) fitted with HEPA filter. The air flow rate should be maintained around 0.45±1 metre/second during testing.

The working place should be thoroughly cleaned. During the test properly cleaned glass ware, equipment and rubber or latex gloves are to be used.

Using a flat-ended forceps take one colour contrast grid membrane filter of 2.5 cm.

Diameter and porosity not more than 5μ, clean both the sides of the membrane with a jet of filtered water to remove the particles, if any, adhered to the membrane.

Place the membrane grid side up on the filter holder and install over the clean filtering funnel.

Open the container of the preparation (sample This is to protect the preparation being tested (sample) from extraneous particulate matter which may contaminate) carefully to avoid any extraneous contamination, transfer 25 ml of the sample into the filtering funnel and filter under vacuum. Wash the wall of the funnel not the membrane with a jet of filter water, rinse the membrane with filtered water remove the membrane using the flat-ended forceps and put it on a clean slide so that the grid side remains up. Partially cover and allow the filter to dry. Examine the membrane under a microscope and count the particles on the filter. Limit of particulate matter.

Particle size (in μm) equal to or larger than	Max. allowable nos. of particles/ml
50	50
25	5
50	Nil

6. **Extractable volume:** There are two methods. Method 1 applies to container having nominal volume (volume mentioned on the label) is not more than 5 ml. Method 2 applies to container where the nominal volume is more than 5 ml. Suspensions should be shaken before withdrawal of the contents, and oily preparations may be warmed, but cooled to 25 °C before the test. One syringe with a volume not more than twice the volume to be drawn and one clean, dry measuring cylinder having a capacity not more than 8 times of nominal volume of each container.

***Method* I:** Take 6 containers from randomly sampled pool, 5 for the test and one for rinsing the syringe. The syringe is fitted with a suitable needle. Open the container kept for rinsing purpose, draw a little amount and rinse the syringe, holding syringe upward discharge the content so as to expel any air. Withdraw as much as possible the content of one of the five containers, keeping the needle upward expel any from the syringe, note the volume and then transfer the content into the dry cylinder without emptying the needle. Repeat the process with rest four containers. Measure the total volume. The average content of the 5 containers should be within the stated limits.

***Method* II:** Carry out the same process on 3 containers. The average volume should be within the limits of the stated nominal volume.

Nominal volume	Limits of extractable volume
5ml or less	85-115% of nominal volume
More than 5 ml	85-115% of nominal volume

Multiple dose containers should contain sufficient excess amount to permit the stated number of withdrawals.

7a. Uniformity of content (Injection for solution, suspension or emulsion): Unless otherwise specified, single dose product, packed in single dose containing less than 10 mg or less than 10% of active ingredient shall comply with the following test. When more than one ingredient are present, each ingredient should be tested for compliance. Empty each container as completely as possible and determine the content (assay) of each ingredient. The test for uniformity of content should be carried out on a pooled sample of the preparation, not less than 10 containers sampled randomly.

The preparation complies with the test if the individual values thus obtained lie between 85-115% of the average value. If more than one individual value remains outside the limits, or if any one value remains outside the limit 75-125% of the average value, the preparation is declared as fail.

If one individual value is found outside the limit 85-115%; but inside the limit 75-125%; the test is to be repeated on a poled sample of 20 containers. If not more than 3 individual values out of 30 are outside the limit 85-115% and not more than one out of 30 is outside the limit 75-125% of the average value.

Note: *This test shall not be applied to suspension for injection containing multivitamins and trace elements.*

7b. Uniformity of content (powders for injection): Unless otherwise specified in the individual monograph, powders for injection containing less than 10 mg or less than 10% of active ingredient or that have a unit weight equal to or less than 50 mg shall comply with the test for uniformity of content described under Injections (solutions, suspension and emulsion). When more than one ingredient are present, each ingredient should be tested for compliance.

The test for uniformity of content should be carried out on a pooled sample of the preparation, not less than 10 containers sampled randomly.

8. **Sterility test:** The purpose of the test is to detect the presence of viable microorganism in the product and the test is designed in such a way that when the microorganism will be placed in a nutritive aqueous clear medium and kept at a favourable temperature, the organism will grow leading to formation of turbidity in the medium.

   Precaution is to be taken to avoid contamination of the product during the test; and the working environment (air, surface of the working area) should be maintained sterile.

   For which check tests on air and working surface should also be carried out at regular interval.

   This is also assumed that all the units of a batch/lot have been prepared in such a manner that the risk of contamination is same for each of the units and since, every unit of a lot cannot be tested, a minimum number of units depending on the lot size, have to be sampled and tested as shown in the Table 5.5 below.

Table 5.5

Batch size and minimum numbers of samples to be tested

Sl. No.	Batch size	Minimum nos. of units to be tested
I	*Injections*	10% or 4 whichever is more
	Less than 100 units	10
	100 – 500	2% or 20 whichever is less
	More than 500	
II	*Ophthalmic and other non-injectables*	5% or 2 whichever is more
	Less than 200	10
	More than 200	
III	*Bulk solids*	
	Lee than 4 containers	Each container
	4 – 50 containers	20% or 4 whichever is more
	More than 50 containers	2% or 10 whichever is more
IV	*Surgical Dressings*	
	Less than 100 packets	10% or 4 whichever is more
	100 – 500 packets	10
	More than 500	2% or 20 whichever is less

The probability of detecting viable microorganisms in the test for sterility depends on the number present in a given amount of the preparation being tested and on the species of microorganism present. Very low level of contamination cannot be detected on the basis of random sampling of a batch.

In fact, no sampling plan for applying the test to a specified proportion of discrete units selected from a batch is capable to ensure that all the untested units are in fact sterile.

Therefore, greater assurance of sterility can be achieved from reliable manufacturing process and compliance with Good Manufacturing Practices.

The test comprises the detection of aerobic and anaerobic bacteria and of fungi. There are two methods – Membrane Filtration (Method A) and Direct Inoculation (Method B).

Method A is preferred where the sample is (a) an oil, (b) an ointment that may be diluted to solution, (c) a non-bacteriostatic solid soluble in the culture medium, and (d) a soluble bacteriostatic/fungi static powder or liquid, (e) liquid product where each unit contains 100 ml or more.

Culture Media: The following media should be used for the sterility test.

Thioglycollate media: - pH 7.1 ± 0.2, to be sterilised before use.

Fluid Thioglycollate	**Alternate Thioglycollate medium**	
for clear food products	for turbid and viscid product, and for devices having tubes with small lumina.	
L-Cystine	0.5 g	0.5 g
Sodium chloride	2.5 g	2.5 g
Dextrose, monohydrate	5.5 g	5.5 g
Granular agar (moisture < 15%)	0.75 g	-
Yeast Extract (water soluble)	5.0 g	5.0 g
Pancreatic digest of casein	15.0 g	15.0 g
Sodium thioglycollate or	0.5 ml	0.5 ml
Thioglycollic acid	0.3 ml	0.3 ml
Resazurin (0.1% fresh solution)	1.0 ml	1.0 ml
Distilled water q.s	1000.0 ml	1000.0 ml

Soyabean-casein digest medium– pH 7.1 ± 0.2, to be sterilised before use.

Pancreatic digest of casein	17.0 g
Papaic digest of soyabean meal	3.0 g
Sodium chloride	5.0 g
Dibasic potassium phosphate (K_2HPO_4)	2.5 g
Dextrose, monohydrate	2.5 g
Distilled water q.s	1000.0 ml

Membrane Filtration Method (Method A)

- Use suitable membrane filtration unit fitted with membrane filter of diameter 47 mm and of pore size 0.45 μ. Sterilise the whole assembly before use. In case of an oil, use sterile dry membrane.

- Under specified environment filter the required quantity of sample or sample diluted with liquid (*e.g*: oils, oily solution, ointment, etc).

- If necessary, wash the membrane after filtration of the sample (*e.g.* antibacterial preparation) with suitable fluid, *e.g.* 0.1% sterile solution of peptic digest of animal tissue, adjusted to pH 6.9-7.3.

- After filtration take out the membrane, cut it in two halves. Immerse one half in 100 ml of soyabean casein digest medium and incubate at 20-25 °C for 7 days. Immerse the other half of the membrane in 100 ml of fluid thioglycollate medium and incubate at 30-35 °C for 7 days.

- During incubation period observe both the media at every 24 hours. If there is no sign of growth (turbidity, change of colour) during 7 days, the sample is said to pass the test for sterility.

- Quantity of samples to be used for injectable, ophthalmic and other non-injectable preparations are given in the Table 5.6 below.

TABLE 5.6

Quantity of sample to be used with respect to content in each container

Quantity in each container	Min. quantity to be used for each culture medium, unless otherwise mentioned.
Liquid Injectable	
Less than 1 ml	Total contents of a container
1 – 4 ml	half of the contents of a container
4 – 20 ml	2 ml
4 – 20 ml	10% of the contents of a container
100 ml or more	not less than half of the contents of a container

Table 5.6 *contd…*

Quantity in each container	Min. quantity to be used for each culture medium, unless otherwise mentioned.
Solid Injectables	
Less than 50 mg	Total content of a container
50 - 200 mg	50% of a container
200 mg or more	100 mg
Ophthalmic Solutions & other non-injectable liquid preparations.	
After mixing 10-100 ml	5-10 ml
Other preparations; solutions or dispersions in water or other suitable solvents.	
After mixing 1-10 g	0.5-1.0 g
Absorbent cotton	not less than 1 g of unit portion.

Direct Inoculation Method (Method B)

- When the quantity in a single container is insufficient to carry out the tests, the combined contents of two or more containers are to be used to inoculate the media.

- With a sterile pipette or syringe remove the adequate quantity of the sample and aseptically transfer to the culture medium.

- Mix the liquid with the medium but do not aerate excessively.

- Incubate the inoculate media for not less than 14 days, unless otherwise directed in the individual monograph, at 30°-35 °C in case of *fluid thioglycollate medium* and at 20°-25 °C in the case of *soyabean-casein medium.*

- If the sample makes the medium turbid on mixing so that the turbidity, if developed

- On incubation, cannot be detected on visual examination, transfer suitable portion of the medium between third and seventh day of the test to a fresh container and incubate for not less than 7 days and not less than 14 days after transfer.

- The amount of substance or preparation to be used for inoculation in the culture media varies according to the quantity in each container and is mentioned in the Table 5.7 below.

TABLE 5.7

Amount of substance or preparation to be used for inoculation

Type of product & Content of each container	Min. quantity of the product	Min. volume of culture medium (ml)
I Liquid injectables		
Less than 1 ml	Total contents of 1 container	15
1 - 5 ml	Half the content of a container	20
20 - 50 ml	5 ml	40
50 - 100 ml	10 ml	80
II Solids		
Less than 50 mg	Total content of a container	40
50 - 200 mg	50% of a container	80
200 mg or more	100 mg	80

Observation and Interpretation of Results:

Examine the incubated samples during and after incubation period for macroscopic evidence of growth of microbes. If no evidence of growth is found, the sample (product) tested passes the test for sterility.

If there is any evidence of microbial growth, reserve the container(s) showing growth and repeat the test as follows:

(a) If the growth is due to the presence of any microorganism, isolate and identify the organism(s).

(b) If the growth is not due to the sample, but found to be for other reason, the test is treated as **cancelled** and **repeat** with same number of samples as done earlier.

(c)   If no sign of growth is found in the repeat test, the sample (product) **passes** the test.

(d) If these are not readily distinguishable from those found in the reserved containers (control or blank) in the first test, the preparation being examined **fails** the test.

(e) If these are readily distinguishable from those found in the reserved containers (control or blank) in the first test, the preparation being examined should be **retested** with double the number of samples.

(f) If no sign of microbial growth is noticed in the repeat test, the preparation tested is declared as **passed**.

(g)   If there is growth in the second test the preparation is declared as **failed.**

9. Pyrogen test: Pyrogens are metabolic products of microorganisms. Chemically these are phospholipid attached to a polysaccharide carrier. They produce fever in human beings and animals. The main sources of pyrogens are equipments, fittings, water and materials. These can be destroyed either by heating at 250 °C for 45 min or by treating strong alkali (NaOH). Hence, proper cleaning of equipments, pipe lines and use of pyrogen free materials can only prevent the contamination.

The test is designed to measure the rise in body temperature of rabbits after intravenous injection of the preparation into the ear vein of the test rabbits.

Test Animals

1. Healthy, matured rabbits of either sex,
2. Weight of each rabbit should be not less than 1.5 kg maintained at least for one week,
3. The normal body temperature of each test rabbit should be within 38 °C-39.8 °C,
4. Rabbit once used for a test should be given a rest for at least 48 hrs, provided the sample tested earlier did not fail,
5. If the sample found to be pyrogenic, the rabbits used for that test should not be reused before 2 weeks and on those rabbits a **Sham test** is to be carried out 1-3 days before reuse,
6. The rabbits should be kept in a house away from disturbance or excitement,
7. The temperature of the rabbits' house and that of the test room should not differ by ± 3 °C.

Sham test: The test is done on the rabbits under following situations,

- Being used for the first time,
- Which were not used within last 2 weeks,
- The rabbits are to be conditioned for 1-3 days before the test. Record the temperature at least 90 minutes before the injection. Inject pyrogen-free normal saline solution warmed to about 38.5 °C at a dose of 10 ml per kg of body weight. Record the body temperature at interval of 1, 2 and 3 hours after the injection,
- Animal showing a temperature variation of 0.6 °C or more should be discarded.

Temperature Recording: Any device, *e.g.*, clinical thermometer, thermocouple or thermistor beads with standardised sensitivity of recording temperature is to be inserted into the rectum of the rabbits to a depth of not less than 7.5 cm and sufficient time should be allowed to reach the maximum, stable temperature.

Procedure

1. The test room should be free from noise, disturbance or excitement,
2. The difference between the initial body temperatures of any two rabbits (test animals) should not be more than 1°C,

3. Food is to be withhold with free access to water overnight and till the test is over, during the test no water should be given,

4. The syringes, needles and other glass wares are to be sterilised by heating at 250°C for at least 45 min,

5. The product (sample) is to be warmed to 37 °C,

6. Record the temperature, *control temperature*, of each rabbit prior to injection,

7. the sample is to be injected into the marginal ear vein of each of the three rabbits slowly over a period of not more than 4 minutes and at a dose of 10 ml per kg within 30 min. from the *control temperature* reading,

8. Record the temperature at 1, 2 and 3 hours after the injection.

Results and Interpretation

The preparation shall be considered to pass the test, if

(a) The sum of the responses (increase in temperature) of the three rabbits (group) is not more than 1.4 °C, and

(b) None of the individual responses is 0.6 °C or more.

When any of the above two conditions (a or b) is deviated, the test should be repeated with another 5 rabbits and the preparation shall pass the test, if

(a) The sum of 8 responses (including the previous responses of 3 rabbits) is not more than 3.7 °C, and

(b) Not more than 3 individual responses out of 8 responses (including the previous responses of 3 rabbits) are 0.6 °C or more.

Formulations:

Product: Dextrose Injection, I.P

Standard for drug: It contains not less than 99% and not more than 100.5% of Dextrose calculated as $C_6H_{12}O_6$, on dried basis.

Standard for product: Not less than 95% of the stated amount.

Strength: 10%w/v

Composition: It contains Dextrose I.P 10 g in sterile water for injection.

Packing: 540 ml bottle (USP Type III)

Use: Nutrient, fluid replenisher

Lot size: 1000 ml

Manufacturing Formula:

Dextrose	IP	100 g
Water for Injection	IP q.s	1000 ml

Manufacturing Method:

- Take properly cleaned and rinsed with water for injection 1000 ml beaker,
- Take 250 ml of freshly prepared pyrogen free water for injection, add 100 g of dextrose , dissolve, make up the volume with freshly prepared pyrogen free water for injection,
- Determine the content of dextrose and pH of the solution filter the solution through 0.2 μ membrane filter,
- Fill the solution in thoroughly cleaned bottle, rinsed with water for injection,
- Seal the bottle with washed rubber closure, finally seal with aluminium cap,
- Sterilise the filled bottle in an autoclave for 45 minutes under 15 lbs pressure,
- Check the contents of the bottle on the subsequent day for particulate matter,
- Carry out the test for pyrogen,
- Label the product.

Product: Isoniazid Injection

Standard for drug: It contains not less than 98.0% and not more than 101.0% of Isoniazid calculated as $C_6H_7N_3O$ on dried basis.

Standard for product: It contains not less than 95.0% and not more than 105.0% of Isoniazid calculated as $C_6H_7N_3O$.

Strength: 50 mg/2 ml

Composition: Each 2 ml contains

    Isoniazid I.P   50 mg

Packing: 2 ml in amber ampoule (USP Type I)

Use: Anti-tubercular

Lot size: 20 ml

Manufacturing Formula:

Isoniazid	I.P	0.5 g*
Hydrochloric acid, 0.1 N		q.s
Water for Injection	I.P	q.s

*calculate the quantity as per assay value.

Manufacturing Method:

- Take about 15 ml of hot (60°C) water for injection in a clean test tube,
- Add accurately weighed, required quantity of isoniazid and stir until dissolved,
- Allow the solution to cool, adjust the pH within 5.6 to 6.0 with either 0.1N HCl,
- Mix thoroughly and take a sample for assay,
- Based on the assay value calculate the quantity of isoniazid in remaining solution and make up the volume with water for injection,
- Filter the solution through 0.2 μ membrane filter, test for clarity,
- Fill the solution in 2 ml amber ampoules under nitrogen gas, seal the mouth of the ampoules by fusion,
- Sterilise the ampoules by autoclaving at 10 lbs per sq. inch for 45 min,
- Inspect the sterilised ampoules visually for particulate matter,
- Evaluate the product as per official monograph/test protocol,
- Label the ampoules properly.

Product: Sodium Bicarbonate Injection, 7.5% w/v, I.P

Standard for drug: It contains not less than 99% and not more than 101% w/w of sodium bicarbonate, calculated as $NaHCO_3$ on dried basis.

Standard for injection: It contains not less than 95% and not more than 105% of the stated amount

Strength: 75 mg/ml

Packing: 50 ml transparent ampoules

Composition:

Each ml contains

Sterile solution of Sodium Bicarbonate I.P 75 mg

Use: Systemic alkaliser.

Lot size: 250 ml

Manufacturing Formula:

Sodium Bicarbonate	I.P	375 mg.
Disodium Edetate	I.P	25 mg
Water for Injection	I.P	q.s

Manufacturing Method:

- Take 200 ml of hot (50 °C) water for injection in a clean 250 ml beaker fitted with a stirrer,

- Add weighed quantity of sodium bicarbonate gradually with continuous stirring,
- Add disodium edentate to the solution and stir to dissolve,
- Test for pH and assay, make up the volume with water for injection, mix thoroughly,
- Filter the solution through 0.45 μ membrane filter, fill the ampoules under CO_2 gas,
- Seal the filled ampoules and sterilise at 15l bs pressure for 40 – 45 min,
- On the next day check the ampoules for particulate matter and test completely as IP,
- Label the ampoules and pack suitably.

Note: *If necessary, the solution may be clarified with pyrogen free charcoal before membrane filtration.*

Product: Cyanocobalamine Injection

Standard for drug: It contains not less than 96% and not more than 102% of Cyanocobalamine, calculated as $C_{63}H_{88}Co\,N_{14}O_4P$ on dried basis.

Standard for injection: It contains not less than 95% and not more than 110% of Cyanocobalamine, calculated as $C_{63}H_{88}Co\,N_{14}O_4P$.

Strength: 1 mg/ml

Packing: 2 ml amber ampoules.

Composition:

Each ml contains

Cyanocobalamine IP	1 mg
Benzyl Alcohol IP	10 mg

Use: B-group vitamin; hemopoietic

Lot size: 20 ml

Manufacturing Formula:

Cyanocobalamine	I.P	25 mg*
Sodium Chloride	I.P	150 mg
Sodium Dihydrogen phosphate	I.P	6 mg
Benzyl Alcohol	I.P	200 mg
Water for Injection	I.P	q.s

*An overage of 25% assuming 100% assay value of the Cyanocobalamine being used.

Manufacturing Method:

- Dissolve weighed quantity of sodium chloride and sodium dihydrogen phosphate in 10 ml of warm freshly prepared water for injection, allow it to cool,
- Add weighed quantity of Cyanocobalamine in the solution and dissolve,
- Add required quantity of benzyl alcohol and mix thoroughly,
- Make up the volume with water for injection, mix well,
- Check the pH (4.75) and draw a sample for assay,
- Filter the solution through 0.2 μ membrane filter aseptically and fill in the ampoules under aseptic environment,
- Flush with nitrogen during filling and seal,
- Test the ampoules for particulate matters and other tests as per the monograph,
- Label the ampoules properly.

Note: *Since the product is sterilised by filtration, filling and sealing should be done strictly under aseptic environment, and the glass wares, filtration assembly must be sterile.*

Product: Chlorpheramine Maleate Injection

Standard for drug: It contains not less than 98% and not more than 101% w/w of Chlorpheramine Maleate, calculated as $C_{16}H_{19}ClN_2, C_4H_4O_4$ on dried basis.

Standard for injection: It contains not less than 90% and not more than 110% of Cyanocobalamine, calculated as $C_{16}H_{19}ClN_2, C_4H_4O_4$.

Strength: 10 mg/ml

Packing: 2 ml or 5 ml amber ampoules

Composition:

Each ml contains

Chlorpheramine Maleate, I.P	10 mg
Phenol I.P	1 mg

Use: Antihistaminic

Lot size: 50 ml

Manufacturing Formula:

Chlorpheramine Maleate,	I.P	500 mg
Phenol, I.P white crystals,	50 mg	
Water for Injection	I.P	q.s

Manufacturing Method:

- Dissolve chlorpheramine maleate, accurately weighed, in 35 ml of water for injection,

- Dissolve phenol separately in 10 ml of water for injection, add this solution to the bulk gradually with constant stirring, adjust the pH to 4.35,

- Make up the volume with water for injection, test for assay,

- Filter the solution through 0.45µ membrane filter,

- Fill in the 2 or 5 ml ampoules, seal and sterilise in an autoclave at 10 lbs pressure for 15 min,

- Inspect the ampoules visually for particulate matter,

- Label and pack properly.

Ophthalmics

Introduction

Preparations intended to be used topically to the eye for treatment of surface or intraocular disease called as ophthalmic products. Under normal condition the maximum volume of tear fluid can be retained in the human eye are:

- Before blinking 30 µl and after blinking 10 µl. normally, 7-8 µl.

- Thus, limited volume or amount of an ophthalmic preparation can be applied to eye.

- Only for flushing or bathing of eye large volume of ophthalmic preparations are necessary.

- If 20 drops make 1 ml, 1 drop amounts to be 50 µl, 50% of which an eye can accommodate and rest is drained out from the eye.

- Administration of more than one drop of a preparation to eye is unnecessary. An ophthalmic solution cannot stay on the eye surface for more than 1-2 minutes; the amount of drug absorbed would be less than 1% of the administered dose. Hence, the repeat administration is required to increase the absorption of drug.

- The ophthalmic preparations should be sterile, isotonic, properly buffered and adequately preserved.

- The viscosity enhances the retention period of the drug into the eye and hence, enhances the absorption of the drug. Special care should be taken to avoid contamination during manufacture and use of ophthalmics.

Eye Drops

These are sterile, aqueous or oily solutions or suspensions of one or more medicaments intended for instillation into the conjunctival sac. Unless in single-dose, aqueous eye drops contain a suitable preservative which is bactericide and fungicide. When medicament itself has adequate antimicrobial activity, no other antimicrobial preservative is used in the preparation.

These may contain suitable additives like buffers, stabilising agents, solubilising agents, and substances to adjust viscosity and tonicity of the preparation.

Eye drops prepared for use in surgical procedures should not contain any antimicrobial preservatives and should be packed in single dose container. Buffering or stabilising agent, if used in the preparation should be compatible with the drug and other ingredients present in the formulation. Any additive used should neither affect the therapeutic action of the drug nor cause any irritation after instillation of the product.

Most commonly used preservatives are phenylmercuric nitrate or acetate (0.002%), benzalkonium chloride (0.01%). The latter is not used in the preparation containing local anaesthetics.

Single-dose preparations contain about 0.5 ml in a sterile, flexible applicator pack enclosed in a sealed outer container.

Aqueous preparations are usually packed in multiple dose, usually not more than 10 ml in a container.

General Method of Preparation

The apparatus and the containers to be used in the preparation of eye-drops must be thoroughly cleaned before use. Unless otherwise mentioned in the individual monograph, eye-drops are prepared by the following method:

Method: The drug is dissolved in the aqueous vehicle containing a suitable preservative, and other excipients, if any.

Preparation of solution

- The solution is filtered through 0.45 μ or 0.8 μ membrane filter, (*filtration*)
- The filtered solution is then transferred to the final containers, (*filling*)
- The filled containers are sealed with rubber teats and aluminium caps (*sealing*)
- The filled and sealed containers are sterilised by any one of the three methods depending on the physic-chemical properties of the drug.

(a)   Heating in boiling water at 98°-100°C for 30-45 minutes,

(b)   Auto-claving at pre-determined pressure for definite period,

(c)   Filtering the solution through 0.2 μ sterilised membrane filter under complete sterile environment, (*sterilisation*),

- The sterilised products are evaluated physically, chemically and biologically to assess the quality (*quality control*),
- Labelled and suitably packed (*labelling and packing*).

Sterilisation: Eye drops are prepared by using methods designed to ensure their sterility and to avoid any contamination and growth of micro-organisms. Based on the physico-chemical properties of the drug and the product, a suitable method of sterilisation should be used for the manufacture of Eye Drops.

Containers: Eye Drops should be packed in containers made from the materials that do not cause any deterioration of the product due to

1. Diffusion into or across the material of the container,
2. By yielding any foreign substances to the content (leaching).

The container and package of a single dose preparation should ensure maintenance of the sterility of the contents and of the applicator up to the time of use.

For multiple doses the container should be fitted with an integral dropper or with a sterile screw cap of suitable material incorporating a dropper and plastic or rubber teat. Alternatively, such a sterilised cap assembly may be packed separately and provided for withdrawal of successive doses.

Eye drop in the form of solution shall be clear and free from any particle. It should comply with the test for clarity as per IP or any other Pharmacopoeia.

Eye drop in the form of suspension, if sedimented, the sediment should easily be dispersed uniformly after shaking so that a correct dose can be administered.

Some eye drops are supplied in dry form and need to be constituted in an appropriate sterile liquid before use.

Labelling

The label should mention

- The names and concentrations in percentages, or weight or volume per ml, of the active ingredients,
- The names and concentrations of any added antioxidant, stabilising agent or antimicrobial preservative,
- The conditions for storage of the product,

For multiple dose container the label should also state that

- Once the container is opened the content can only be used for one month,

- Care should be taken to avoid contamination during use,

- The preparation is not for injection.

General Standards

Uniformity of volume: Should comply with the test for content of packaged dosage forms.

Particle size: *This test is applicable only to the eye drop in the form of suspension.*

- Introduce a suitable volume of the suspension into a counting cell or onto a microscopic slide,

- Scan under the microscope an area corresponding to 10 µg of the solid phase,

- Scan at least 50 representative fields.

Limits:

1. Not more than 20 particles have a maximum dimension greater than 25 µm,

2. Not more than 10 particles have a maximum dimension greater than 50 µm and none has a maximum dimension greater than 100 µm.

Sterility: Both content and the dropper should comply with the test for sterility.

Remove the dropper aseptically and transfer into a tube containing suitable culture medium so that it is completely immersed. Incubate and carry out the test for sterility.

Formulations:

Product: Chloramphenicol Eye-drop

Standard for drug: It contains not less than 98% and not more than 102%w/v chloramphenicol, calculated as $C_{11}H_{12}Cl_2N_2O_5$ on dried basis.

Standard for product: Content of chloramphenicol; 0.45 – 0.55%w/v, it must meet all other standards for eye-drops as per the Pharmacopoeia.

Composition:

It contains

Chloramphenicol	IP	0.5%
Phenylmercuric nitrate	IP	0.002%

In a sterile buffered aqueous medium.

Use: Anti-bacterial

Lot size: 20 ml

Manufacturing Formula:

Chloramphenicol	IP	0.1 g
Phenylmercuric nitrate	IP	0.4 mg
Boric Acid	IP	0.3 g
Borax	IP	60.0 mg
Water for injection	IP	q.s

Manufacturing Method:

- Weigh accurately 50 mg of phenylmercuric nitrate and transfer into a clean 50 ml volumetric flask, pre-rinsed with water for injection, dissolve in water for injection, make up the volume with water for injection and mix thoroughly,

- Take weighed quantities of borax and boric acid into a clean 25 ml beaker, add about 15 ml of water for injection, stir with a glass rod, heat to 60°C to dissolve, add weighed amount of chloramphenicol, continue to heat at 60°C with stirring until a clear solution is obtained,

- Add 0.4 ml of phenylmercuric nitrate solution and mix, cool the solution to room temperature,

- Transfer the solution into a clean stopper measuring cylinder, make up the volume with water for injection, mix well,

- Determine the drug content,

- Filter the solution aseptically through 0.2 μ filter, fill the solution into pre-sterilised vials, seal immediately with pre-sterilised rubber closure and aluminium cap under aseptic environment,

- Carry out other tests as per the Pharmacopoeial monograph,

- Label properly.

Product: Sulphacetamide Eye-drop

Standard for drug: It contains not less than 99% and not more than 101%w/v of sulphacetamide sodium, calculated as $C_8H_9N_2NaO_3S$, on dried basis.

Standard for product: Content of Sulphacetamide sodium; 95%-105%w/v of the stated amount, calculated as $C_8H_9N_2NaO_3S, H_2O$.

It must meet all other standards for eye-drops as per the Pharmacopoeia.

Composition:

It contains sterile solution of

Sulphacetamide Sodium	IP	10.0%
Phenylmercuric nitrate	IP	0.002%
Sodium metabisulphite	IP	0.1%

Use: Antibacterial

Lot size: 20 ml

Manufacturing Formula:

Sulphacetamide Sodium	IP	2.0 g
Phenylmercuric nitrate	IP	0.4 mg
Sodium metabisulphite	IP	20.0 mg
Water for injection, freshly prepared IP		q.s

Manufacturing Method:

- Weigh accurately 50mg of phenylmercuric nitrate and transfer into a clean 50 ml volumetric flask, pre-rinsed with water for injection, dissolve in water for injection, make up the volume with water for injection and mix thoroughly,
- Take weighed quantity of Sulphacetamide Sodium into a clean 25 ml beaker, pre-rinsed with freshly prepared water for injection, add about 15 ml of water for injection, stir with a glass rod until a clear solution is obtained, add weighed amount of sodium meta-bisulphite and stir to dissolve, flush with nitrogen gas,
- Add 0.4 ml of phenylmercuric nitrate solution and mix,
- Transfer the solution into a clean stopper measuring cylinder, make up the volume with water for injection, mix well, flush with nitrogen gas,
- Determine the drug content,
- Filter the solution aseptically through 0.2 μ filter, fill the solution into pre-sterilised vials, flush with nitrogen gas and seal immediately with pre-sterilised rubber closure and aluminium cap under aseptic environment,
- Carry out other tests as per the monograph,
- Label properly.

Product: Pilocarpine Eye-drop

Standard for drug: It contains not less than 98.5% and not more than 101%w/v of pilocarpine nitrate, calculated as $C_{11}H_{16}N_2O_2$, HNO_3 on dried basis.

Standard for product: Content of Pilocarpine Nitrate; 90%-110%w/v of the stated amount, calculated as $C_{11}H_{16}N_2O_2$, HNO_3.

Composition:

It contains sterile solution of

Pilocarpine hydrochloride IP 5%w/v

Benzalkonium chloride   IP 0.02%v/v

Use: Cholinergic in glaucoma

Lot size: 20 ml

Manufacturing Formula:

Pilocarpine hydrochloride	IP	1.0 g
Benzalkonium chloride	IP	0.004 ml
Water for injection	IP	q.s

Manufacturing Method:

- Weigh accurately the required amount of pilocarpine hydrochloride and transfer into a clean 25 ml beaker, add 15 ml of freshly prepared water for injection and dissolve,
- Add 4 ml of 0.1%v/v solution of benzalkonium chloride in water for injection, mix thoroughly, make up the volume with water for injection, mix well,
- Carry out the test,
- Filter the solution aseptically through 0.2 μ filter, fill the solution into pre-sterilised vials, flush with nitrogen gas and seal immediately with pre-sterilised rubber closure and aluminium cap under aseptic environment,
- Carry out other tests as per the monograph,
- Label properly.

Product: Hypromellose Eye-drop, BPC

Standard for product: pH, 8.4 – 8.6

Composition:

It contains:

Hypromellose 4500		0.3% w/v
Benzalkonium Chloride Solution	IP	0.02% v/v
Sodium chloride	IP	0.45% w/v
Potassium chloride	IP	0.37% w/v

in sterile buffered solution.

Use: Artificial tears

Lot size: 20 ml

Manufacturing Formula:

Hypromellose 4500		0.06 g
Benzalkonium Chloride Solution	IP	0.004 ml
Sodium chloride	IP	0.09 g
Potassium chloride	IP	0.074 g
Boric Acid	IP	0.038 g
Borax	IP	0.038 g
Water for injection	IP	q.s

Manufacturing Method:

- Take 5 ml of hot (80°-90 °C) water for injection in a 25 ml clean beaker, add hypromellose, allow to be hydrated,
- Add 5 ml of cold water for injection in the form of ice, stir until homogenous solution is obtained,
- Take 7 ml of water for injection in another clean beaker, add weighed quantities of sodium chloride, potassium chloride, borax and boric acid, dissolve, add benzalkonium chloride solution mix,
- Mix the two solutions thoroughly and make up the volume with water for injection, mix thoroughly,
- Allow the solution to stand for overnight, decant and filter the supernatant liquid,
- Fill the solution in suitable container, seal with washed rubber closure and aluminium cap,
- Sterilise the filled containers in an autoclave at 10 lbs pressure for 30 minutes, redisperse the coagulated hypromellose by shaking on cooling,
- Label the preparation.

Product: Prednisolone Eye-drop

Standard drug: It contains not less than 96% and not more than 104%w/v of prednisolone, calculated as $C_{21}H_{28}O_5$ on dried basis.

Standard product: Content of Prednisolone sodium Phosphate IP 0.466 – 0.570%w/v pH, 7.0-8.5

Composition:

It contains

Prednisolone sodium phosphate	IP	0.5%

Benzalkonium Chloride solution	IP	0.02%v/v
Disodium Edetate	IP	0.01%w/v

In suitable buffered sterile aqueous medium

Use: Adrenocortical steroid

Lot size: 20 ml

Manufacturing Formula:

Prednisolone sodium phosphate	IP	0.1036 g
Benzalkonium Chloride solution	IP	0.004 ml
Disodium Edetate	IP	0.002 g
Sodium Acid Phosphate	IP	0.06 g
Sodium Chloride	IP	0.10 g
Sodium Hydroxide	IP	q.s
Water for injection	IP	q.s

Manufacturing Method:

- Take 10 ml of water for injection in a clean 25 ml beaker, dissolve sodium acid phosphate, prednisolone sodium phosphate, disodium edentate and sodium chloride,

- Add 4% solution of sodium hydroxide drop wise to adjust the pH of the solution to 8.0,

- Add 0.4 ml of diluted benzalkonium chloride solution (1 ml in 100 ml), make up the volume with water for injection, mix thoroughly, carry out the tests,

- Filter the solution through 0.2 μ membrane filter, fill in amber coloured vial, seal with rubber closure and aluminium cap,

- Sterilise the sealed vial by heating in boiling water for 30 minutes,

- Label properly.

Eye Lotions

Eye lotions are the solutions intended for washing or bathing the eyes. These may be of two types:

1. Sterile aqueous solutions which do not contain any added bactericide; these are used for first-aid or any purpose for a maximum period of 24 hrs.

2. Sterile aqueous solutions which contain added bactericide; these are used for intermittent domiciliary treatment or administration for up to 7 days.

Preparation of Eye Lotion

The apparatus and containers used for preparation of any eye lotion must be thoroughly cleaned before use. The drug is dissolved in water for injection

- The solution is filtered through appropriate filtering medium,
- The filtered solution is filled in suitable containers and sealed properly,
- The filled and sealed containers are sterilised by any of the established method, steaming in boiling water, autoclaving or filtration,

During dispensing of eye lotion, the user must be made aware how to use the preparation and how to avoid contamination of the preparation after opening the container.

For type (1) and type (2) preparations, the label should also state that

- Once the container is opened the content must be used within 24 hrs,
- Care should be taken to avoid contamination during use,
- The preparation is not for injection.

General Standards

Standards applicable to eye drops should be applicable to preparations of type (2).

Uniformity of volume: Should comply with the ***test for content of packaged dosage forms.***

Particle size: *This test is applicable only to the eye drop in the form of suspension.*

- Introduce a suitable volume of the suspension into a counting cell or onto a microscopic slide,
- Scan under the microscope an area corresponding to 10 μg of the solid phase.
- Scan at least 50 representative fields.

Limits:

1. Not more than 20 particles have a maximum dimension greater than 25 μm,
2. Not more than 10 particles have a maximum dimension greater than 50 μm and none has a maximum dimension greater than 100 μm.

Sterility: Both content and the dropper should comply with the test for sterility.

Remove the dropper aseptically and transfer into a tube containing suitable culture medium so that it is completely immersed. Incubate and carry out the test for sterility.

For preparations of type **(1)** – purity, clarity, pH, sterility, isotonicity and any others as mentioned in the monograph.

Containers and Closures

- Coloured fluted glass bottles are suitable for supply of eye lotions.
- The closures should be impermeable, must be covered with a readily breakable seal.
- No cork can be used as closure.
- The closures used must be stable at autoclaving temperature.

Formulations:

Product: Sodium Chloride Eye Lotion

Standard for product: Content of sodium chloride, 0.85-0.95%w/v calculated as NaCl.

It is a sterile solution of sodium chloride IP 0.9%.

Use: Washing or bathing of eyes

Lot size: 50 ml

Manufacturing Formula:

> Sodium chloride IP   0.45g
>
> Water for injection IP   q.s

Manufacturing Method:

- Weigh accurately the required quantity of sodium chloride, dissolve in sufficient volume of water for injection,
- Make up the volume with water for injection, determine the content of sodium chloride, pH,
- Filter the solution through a filter of 1.2 μ,
- Fill the solution in a fluted amber colour bottle, seal properly,
- Sterilize the filled and sealed bottle by autoclaving under 15 lbs pressure for a period of 45 minutes.

Note: All the apparatus and container used must be thoroughly cleaned.

Evaluation of Eye-drop, Eye-lotion, etc.,

Common tests to be employed for evaluation are:

1. Physical Tests
    1.1   Description - Colour, Clarity
    1.2   pH
    1.3   Uniformity of volume
    1.4   Particulate matters and Particle size

2. Chemical Tests
    2.1   Identification tests
    2.2   Assay
    2.3   Uniformity of contents

3. Biological Tests
    3.1   Microbiological assay, if applicable
    3.2   Sterility test

Eye Ointments

These are sterile, semi-solid preparations intended for application into the conjunctival sac or lid margin of the eye. Usually these contain antiseptics, anti-inflammatory, antimicrobial, mydriatic or miotic substances. These appear to be homogeneous and contain one or more medicaments dissolved or dispersed in a suitable basis. The bases which are usually non-aqueous, contain certain additives like stabilising agents, antimicrobial preservatives and antioxidants. The base used must be non-irritant to the conjunctiva and allow diffusion of the drug throughout the secretion of the eye. The base must be stable to retain the activity of the drug(s) throughout the shelf-life of the preparation.

Eye ointments are prepared in such a way that their sterility are ensured and no contaminant is introduced. While using eye ointment, care should be taken to avoid contamination.

Preparation of Eye Ointment

While preparing eye ointment the apparatus to be used should be properly clean and sterilised. Usually eye ointments are prepared by using the following basis.

Liquid paraffin   10 %w/w

Wool fat   10 %w/w

Yellow soft paraffin   80 %w/w

Heat all the three ingredients together, filter the hot mixture through a coarse filter paper in a hot funnel, sterilise the base by heating at 150°C for one hour. Allow to cool to room temperature before incorporating the sterile drug substance(s) and ensure that no contamination of microorganism takes place during cooling of base and incorporation of drug.

However, the above composition of the eye ointment base may be modified when the preparation is intended for use in tropical or subtropical climates. Hard paraffin may be included and amount of soft paraffin may be reduced to maintain desired viscosity of the ointment.

During preparation of an eye ointment any one of the following aseptic techniques is used.

Method **I:** The drug is readily soluble in water and its solution is stable

The solution is made with least amount of water and the solution is sterilised by either autoclaving or by filtration. The sterile solution is then gradually incorporated into sterile melted base with continuous stirring; continue stirring until the preparation becomes cold. Transfer the required amount of the preparation into suitable sterile final containers aseptically and the filled containers are immediately sealed so as to exclude micro-organisms.

Method **II:** The drug is not readily soluble in water or its solution is not stable

The drug is finely powdered and sterilised. It is mixed thoroughly with a portion of the melted sterile base. Then the rest amount of melted, sterile base is mixed gradually to make a homogeneous mixture. The ointment is filled into suitable sterile containers and immediately sealed. The above process is carried out under aseptic environment.

Method **III:** The drug is insoluble in water and in the base

The drug is powdered to extreme fineness and sterilised, so that the drug particles do not cause irritation to the eye. It is mixed thoroughly with a portion of the melted sterile base. Then the rest amount of melted, sterile base is mixed gradually to make a homogeneous mixture. The ointment is filled into suitable sterile containers and immediately sealed. The above process is carried out under aseptic environment.

Containers

Eye ointments are packed in small, sterilised collapsible tubes of metal or of suitable plastic material. The tube should either be fitted or provided with a suitable nozzle for easy application of the ointment without contamination and with a cap.

Generally the pack size of eye ointment is 5 g. Eye ointment can also be packed in single dose container of suitable shape to ensure easy application without contamination. Such containers should be individually wrapped.

Other requirements for the containers are described in the Pharmacopeia.

General Standards

Uniformity of weight: Should comply with the *test for content of packaged dosage forms*.

Particle size: On a microscopic slide gently spread a small quantity of the ointment as a thin layer.

- Scan under the microscope an area corresponding to 10 µg of the solid phase.
- Scan at least 50 representative fields.

Limits:

1. Not more than 20 particles have a maximum dimension greater than 25 µm,
2. Not more than 10 particles have a maximum dimension greater than 50 µm and none has a maximum dimension greater than 100 µm.

Sterility: Should comply with the *test for sterility*.

Formulations:

Product: Chloramphenicol Eye Ointment

Standard for drug: It contains not less than 98% and not more than 102% w/v of chloramphenicol, calculated as $C_{11}H_{12}Cl_2N_2O_5$ on dried basis.

Standard for product: Content of Chloramphenicol, 95-105% w/w of the stated amount.

Composition:

It contains Chloramphenicol IP 1.0% w/w in a suitable ointment basis

Use: Antibacterial

Lot size: 10 g

Manufacturing Formula:

Chloramphenicol	IP	0.10 g
Liquid Paraffin, heavy	IP	0.99 g
Wool fat	IP	0.99 g
Yellow Soft Paraffin	IP	7.22 g
Hard Paraffin	IP	0.70 g

Manufacturing Method:

- Transfer the weighed quantity of Liquid Paraffin, Wool fat, Yellow Soft Paraffin, and Hard Paraffin into a clean, dry beaker, heat the contents till they melt, stir with a clean glass rod, cover the beaker with a lid,
- Heat the basis at 150°C for one hour, remove the beaker from the oven and allow to cool in a sterile area,

- Weigh accurately the required quantity of chloramphenicol and transfer into a sterile glass mortar pestle under sterile area, powder the drug finely,

- Add the ointment basis gradually with continuous mixing, continue to mix till a uniform ointment is prepared, ensure that the sterility is maintained throughout the processing,

- Carry out the necessary tests, fill the ointment in sterile collapsible tubes, seal immediately, put a proper label.

Product: Tetracycline Hydrochloride Eye Ointment

Standard for drug: It contains not less than 950µg of $C_{22}H_{24}N_2O_8$, HCl, calculated on anhydrous basis.

Standard for product: Content of Chlortetracycline Hydrochloride, 90-115% w/w of the stated amount.

Composition:

It contains Tetracycline Hydrochloride IP 0.01% w/w in a suitable ointment basis

Use: Antibacterial

Lot size: 10 g

Manufacturing Formula:

Tetracycline Hydrochloride	IP	1.0 mg
Liquid Paraffin, heavy	IP	0.99 g
Wool fat	IP	0.99 g
Yellow Soft Paraffin	IP	7.22 g
Hard paraffin	IP	0.70 g

Manufacturing Method:

- Transfer the weighed quantity of Liquid Paraffin, Wool fat, Yellow Soft Paraffin, and Hard Paraffin into a clean, dry beaker, heat the contents till they melt, stir with a clean glass rod, cover the beaker with a lid,

- Heat the basis at 150°C for one hour, remove the beaker from the oven and allow to cool in a sterile area,

- Weigh accurately the required quantity of tetracycline hydrochloride and transfer into a sterile glass mortar pestle under sterile area, powder the drug finely,

- Add the ointment basis gradually with continuous mixing, continue to mix till a uniform ointment is prepared, ensure that the sterility is maintained throughout the processing,

- Carry out the necessary tests, fill the ointment in sterile collapsible tubes, seal immediately, and put a proper label.

Product: Neomycin Eye Ointment

Standard for drug: It contains not less than 600 units per mg of Neomycin sulphate, calculated on dried basis.

Standard for product: Content of Neomycin Sulphate, 90-115%w/w of the stated amount.

Composition:

It contains Neomycin Sulphate IP 0.5% w/w in a suitable ointment basis.

Use: Antibacterial

Lot size: 10 g

Manufacturing formula:

Neomycin Sulphate	IP	0.05 g
Liquid Paraffin, heavy	IP	0.99 g
Wool fat	IP	0.99 g
Yellow soft paraffin	IP	7.22 g
Hard paraffin	IP	0.75 g

Manufacturing Method:

- Transfer the weighed quantity of Liquid Paraffin, Wool fat, Yellow Soft Paraffin, and Hard Paraffin into a clean, dry beaker, heat the contents till they melt, stir with a clean glass rod, cover the beaker with a lid,
- Heat the basis at 150°C for one hour, remove the beaker from the oven and allow to cool in a sterile area,
- Weigh accurately the required quantity of Neomycin sulphate and transfer into a sterile glass mortar pestle under sterile area, powder the drug finely,
- Add the ointment basis gradually with continuous mixing, continue to mix till a uniform ointment is prepared, ensure that the sterility is maintained throughout the processing,
- Carry out the necessary tests, fill the ointment in sterile collapsible tubes, seal immediately, put a proper label.

Product: Gentamicin Eye Ointment

Standard for drug: It contains not less than 590 µg of Gentamicin per mg, calculated on dried basis.

Standard for product: Content of Gentamicin, 90-120%w/w of the stated amount.

Composition: It contains Gentamicin sulphate IP 1.0%w/w in a suitable ointment basis.

Use: Antibacterial.

Lot size: 10 g

Manufacturing formula:

Gentamicin sulphate	IP	0.10 g
Liquid paraffin, heavy	IP	0.99 g
Wool fat	IP	0.99 g
Yellow soft paraffin	IP	7.22 g
Hard paraffin	IP	0.75 g

Manufacturing Method:

- Transfer the weighed quantity of Liquid Paraffin, Wool fat, Yellow soft paraffin, and Hard paraffin into a clean, dry beaker, heat the contents till they melt, stir with a clean glass rod, cover the beaker with a lid,

- Heat the basis at 150 °C for one hour, remove the beaker from the oven and allow to cool in a sterile area,

- Weigh accurately the required quantity of Neomycin sulphate and transfer into a sterile glass mortar pestle under sterile area, powder the drug finely,

- Add the ointment basis gradually with continuous mixing, continue to mix till a uniform ointment is prepared, ensure that the sterility is maintained throughout the processing,

- Carry out the necessary tests, fill the ointment in sterile collapsible tubes, seal immediately, and put a proper label.

Evaluation of Eye Ointment

Common tests to be carried out for evaluation are,

1. Physical Tests
    - 1.1   Description - Colour, consistency, texture, stickiness and odour.
    - 1.2   Uniformity of mixing and smoothness.
    - 1.3   Spreadability
    - 1.4   Average content.
    - 1.5   Individual weight variation (uniformity of weights)
    - 1.6   Dissolution rate, if desired or directed
    - 1.7   Viscosity.
    - 1.8   Uniformity of container content.
    - 1.9   Particle size

2   Chemical Tests
   2.1   Identification tests
   2.2   Assay
   2.3   Uniformity of contents
3   Biological Tests
   3.1   Microbiological assay, if applicable
   3.2   Sterility

Exercises

Short Questions

1. (a) What are parenteral preparations?
    (b) Which parenteral preparations do not contain any preservative?
    (c) Name sterile preparations which are not injectables.
    (d) What are large volume parenterals and small volume parenterals?
    (e) Name at least three preparations called as large volume parenterals.
    (f) Name the additives used in ophthalmic solutions.
    (g) What special information written in eye-drops regarding its use?
    (h) What are different methods of sterilisation?
    (i) Which drugs are sterilised by filtration method?
    (j) Which water is used for manufacture of parenteral solutions?
    (k) What is pyrogen?
    (l) Which filters are used for final filtration of injection solutions?
    (m) Name the non-aqueous solvents used for parenteral preparations.
    (n) Name at least four preservatives used in injectables.
    (o) What is cold sterilisation?
    (p) Name the additives used in parenteral preparations.
    (q) At which concentration sodium chloride solution is iso-osmotic to blood plasma?
    (r) Which preparations are sterilised by gas?
    (s) Name the sproducts that sterilised by radiation?

2. Write down the general method of preparation of eye-lotion.

3. Write down the steps of manufacturing of parenteral solutions.

4. Make a list of additives, with suitable examples and function, used in injectables.

5. Describe the method of preparation of eye ointment.

6. What are the tests to be carried out for evaluation of parenteral preparations?

7. Make a list of tests to be carried out during manufacture of injectables.

8. Short notes on:

    (a) Moist heat sterilisation,

    (b) Stabilisers,

    (c) Preservatives.

6 Gaseous Dosage Form

Inhalations

Inhalations are volatile liquid preparations of drug substances. These are intended to be inhaled in the form of vapours; so that the drug substance can reach directly to the lining of the respiratory tract and exert a quick relief from bronchial and nasal congestion. When the drug substances are volatile at room temperature, it can be placed on an absorbent pad and inhaled from the pad. In some cases the preparation is added to hot (65-70°C) water to volatilise the substance and then inhaled. The vapours are inhaled for 5-10 minutes. Inhalations which are added to hot water usually contain alcoholic solutions or a mixture of alcohol and water mixed with a diffusing agent like light magnesium carbonate.

Container: Inhalations should be dispensed in white fluted bottles.

Labelling: The label should clearly mention, "Not for internal use", along with all other necessary information. When the preparation contains an insoluble diffusing agent, a direction is to be given on the label, "Shake well before use".

Formulations:

Product: Benzoin Inhalation

Standard for product: Content of total Balsamic acids, not less than 3.0% w/v, calculated as cinnamic acid, $C_9H_8O_2$, Total solids, 9.0 – 12.0% w/v.

Composition:

It contains Benzoin 10% in alcohol

Use: Expectorant

Lot size: 20 ml

Manufacturing Formula:

Benzoin, crushed	2.0 g
Prepared Storax	1.0 g
Alcohol (95%)	q.s

Manufacturing Method:

- Weigh accurately required quantity of crushed benzoin and storax,
- transfer into a clean 50 ml stopper cylinder,
- Add 15 ml of alcohol, macerate for 24 hours,
- Filter the solution through a muslin cloth, wash the filter twice with 2.5 ml of alcohol at each time, make up the volume,
- Fill the solution in a clean, dry fluted bottle, seal using a pilfer proof cap and label.

Product: Menthol and Eucalyptus Inhalation

Standard product: Total oil, 10.3 – 12.7% v/v

Use: Expectorant

Lot size: 20 ml

Manufacturing Formula:

Menthol	0.4 g
Eucalyptus oil	2.0 ml
Light Magnesium Carbonate	1.4 g
Purified water	q.s

Manufacturing Method:

- Weigh and dissolve menthol in measured volume of eucalyptus oil into a 25 ml stopper measuring cylinder,
- Weigh the quantity of magnesium carbonate, passed through a mesh no. 80,
- Transfer into the cylinder and add sufficient purified water to make up the volume, shake well,
- Fill the preparation into a clean fluted bottle, seal using a pilfer proof cap and label.

Product: Menthol and Benzoin Inhalation

Standard product: Content of total Balsamic acids, not less than 2.8%w/v, calculated as cinnamic acid, $C_9H_8O_2$, Total solids, 9.0 – 12.0% w/v.

Composition:

It contains Menthol 2.0% in benzoin inhalation.

Use: Expectorant

Lot size: 20 ml

Manufacturing Formula:

Menthol	0.4 g
Benzoin, crushed	2.0 g
Prepared Storax	1.0 g
Alcohol (95%)	q.s

Manufacturing Method:

- Weigh accurately required quantity of crushed benzoin and storax, transfer into a clean 50 ml stopper cylinder,
- Add 15 ml of alcohol, macerate for 24 hours,
- Filter the solution through a muslin cloth, wash the filter twice with 2.5 ml of alcohol at each time, make up the volume with alcohol,
- Add weighed quantity of menthol and dissolve,
- Fill the solution in a clean, dry fluted bottle, seal using a pilfer proof cap and label.

Inhalants

According to the USP, *'inhalants'* belong to special type of inhalations containing a drug or combination of drugs which are due to their high vapour pressure can be carried through a current of air to nasal passage where they exert their therapeutic effects.

Examples of this class are Amyl nitrate Inhalant USP and Propyl hexedrine Inhalant USP. Both are volatile liquids. Amyl nitrate is a vasodilator. The inhalant is prepared in sealed glass vial covered with a protective gauze cloth. Before use, the vial is broken in the fingertips and the cloth soaks the drug. The soaked cloth is then inhaled. Each vial contains 0.3 ml of amyl nitrate. It is used in the treatment of angina pain. Propyl hexedrine is a vaso constrictor and slowly volatilises at room temperature. Usually 250 mg of propyl hexedrine mixed suitable aromatics is soaked in suitable size of fibrous material and packed in plastic tube. When inhaled into the nostrils it relieves nasal congestion due to cold and hay fever. It is also used to relieve ear block and pressure pain during air travel.

Aerosol

Aerosol may be defined as a *pressurized package system which is self-propelled through a valve to expel the contents in the form of spray or foam from the container.*

Aerosol dosage form is usually considered as gaseous dosage form, as the preparation is dispensed in the form a gas, spray or mist. Sometimes, it is treated as a disperse system.

Most of the preparations, a solution, emulsion or suspension of the active ingredient, are dispersed in suitable propellant system.

This type of preparations are prepared for various types of uses like perfumes, colognes, hair sprays, hand creams, body lotions, shaving creams, deodorants, etc. apart from therapeutic use. Through this type of dosage form, a drug, e.g., epinephrine, isoproterenol hydrochloride, salbutamol sulphate, etc., can be administered for quick therapeutic action. An aerosol may by a solution or suspension of a drug substance in a mixture of solvent and inert propellant which is contained under pressure in an aerosol dispenser. The dispenser consists of a suitable container fitted with a special metering valve capable of delivering an accurate dose of a drug.

The **advantages** of aerosol package are,

- The delivery of a dose can be made without contamination of remaining material,
- Stability of the drug which may be degraded by oxygen or moisture remains unaffected,
- If the product is sterile, the sterility of the product can be maintained while dispensing a dose,
- The medicament can be delivered in a desired form smoothly over the affected area or the site of application.
- Irritation caused by mechanical application of a topical preparation can be reduced or minimized,
- Convenient to apply rapidly and easily.
- Rapid response to the medicament can be achieved,
- High concentration of the medicament can be applied over a limited area.

There are **disadvantages** of this preparation also. These are,

1. It is not economic because the container, valve, propellant and filling method are expensive,
2. Aerosol packs must not be subjected to heat,
3. Disposal, toxicity of propellants, refrigerant effect of highly volatile propellants may cause problem.

Formulation considerations:

The factors to be considered for formulation of an aerosol are,

- Physical and chemical properties of the drug or active substance,
- Particle size and shape of the drug,

- The type and amount of surfactant to be used,

- Vapour pressure and metered volume of the propellant(s), selected for use, and

- Type of aerosol container to be used.

Based on these, the aerosol formulation consists of two types of components,

1. Product concentrate consisting of active ingredient(s) and other additives,

2. Propellant system which may be a single propellant or a mixture of propellants.

For preparing the solution, the drug may be dissolved in a solvent or in suitable co-solvent which is miscible with the propellant. The particle size of the drug in a suspension or the droplet size of a solution should be controlled to such a range that, when the aerosol is inhaled, the drug can reach the region of the respiratory tract where it is desired to be deposited.

Depending on the type and use, the preparation may contain dispersing agent or surface active agent, stabilising agent, buffering agent and other additives.

The most commonly used additives are given in the Table 6.1 below;

TABLE 6.1

Additives commonly used in aerosol products.

Type of additive	Example
Antioxidant	Ascorbic acid
Dispersing agent or Surfactant	Oleic acid, Oleyl alcohol, Isopropyl myristate, Glycol ethers, Polysorbates, sorbitan esters, e.g. sorbitan trioleate, etc.
Buffers	Mixture of sodium dihydrogen phosphate and disodium hydrogen phosphate, sodium chloride.

Solvents may be water, alcohol, mixture of water and alcohol, isopropyl alcohol, vegetable oil, etc.

Propellants used for aerosol products are of three types:

1. Liquefied gas, which may be (a) hydrocarbons e.g. propane (A-108), butane(A-17), etc. or (b) fluorinated hydrocarbons, e.g. Propellant no.11 (trichloro monofluoro-methane), propellant no.12 (dichlorodifluoromethane), propellant 114 (di-chloro-tetrafluoroethane), etc.

2. Compressed gas, which may be (a) soluble gas like, nitrous oxide, carbon dioxide, etc. or (b) insoluble gas like, nitrogen, argon, etc.

3. Mixture of liquefied gas and compressed gas.

The **selection of propellant** is based on,

1. The type of aerosol system, i.e., aqueous, non-aqueous, solution, suspension or emulsion.

2. The site of application, i.e. inhalation or topical application,

3. The physicochemical properties of the propellant, i.e. molecular weight, solvent property, boiling point and vapour pressure, etc. and

4. The cost of the propellant.

A simple aerosol is a two phase system - the solution of the drug along with a liquid propellant (liquid phase) and vapours of the propellant (gas phase). The gaseous phase exerts an excess pressure on the liquid phase (solution/suspension/emulsion) and on the walls of the container. When the actuator button is pressed, the valve is opened and the liquid phase is forced to come out in the form of spray, foam or stream.

To facilitate the administration of the preparation onto the body or into the body cavity the aerosol dispenser is fitted with an appropriate adapter. For transfer through the mouth, an oral adapter is used; while for transfer through the nose, a nasal adapter is used. One type of oral adapter consists of open ended (both ends open) plastic tube is used. One end of it is fitted with the valve system and the other end functions as mouthpiece. The tube is commonly angled in the centre so that the mouthpiece can be correctly placed in the mouth. The dispenser can be held vertically either in an upright position or in an inverted position according to the instruction given by the manufacturer. The metering valve is actuated by pressing the finger on the base of the container that forces the top of the valve stem against the inner wall of the adapter.

The other type of an oral adapter has the mechanism which automatically applies pressure to the valve stem when actuated by the reduced pressure created during inhalation through the mouthpiece by the patient.

Actuation of the metering valve releases a desired quantity of the preparation, a portion of which deposits on the inner surface of the adapter and the rest is delivered. Thus, the quantity of medicament delivered to the patient with each spray is less than the quantity actually released by the valve.

An aerosol preparation being a potent, the patient should be fully made aware of proper use of the inhalation. Necessary instructions for use of the preparation must be provided with every pack of

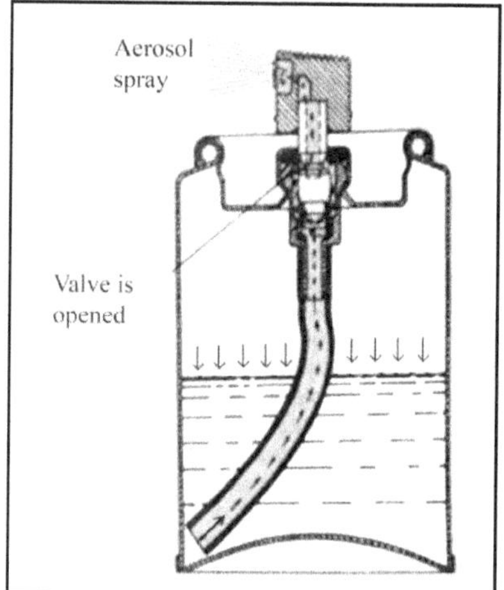

Figure 6.1 Actuation of Valve in Aerosols.

aerosol preparation in the form of a leaflet and the patient must be advised to read the instructions carefully before use.

The basic **components of aerosol** or pressure pack are; 1. Propellant, 2. Container, 3. Valve and Actuator, and 4. Product.

Containers: The containers used to pack these products are made of

1. Tinplate,
2. Aluminium,
3. Stainless steel, or tin plated stainless steel,
4. Glass either plastic coated or uncoated,
5. Plastic.

Glass laminated with a plastic coating also protects the user in case of breakage of the glass.

The type of delivery, such as foam, spray or mist of the product from an aerosol container, depends also on the valve and one of its parts, actuator attached to the container. The valve is the most basic part of any aerosol container. The amount to be discharged is also controlled by it. The valve is an assembly of,

1. Ferrule or Mounting Cup which attaches the valve perfectly to the container,
2. Valve body or Housing which contains an opening at the point of attachment of the dip tube. It may or may not have another opening known as vapour tap for escape of vaporized propellant with liquid product,
3. Stem,
4. Gasket,
5. Spring,
6. Dip tube, and
7. Actuator

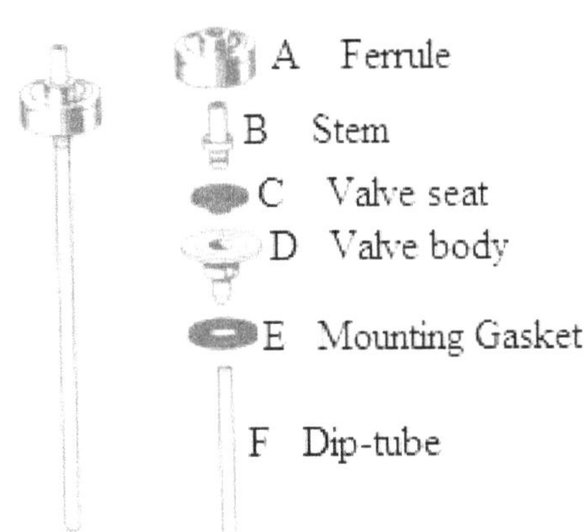

Figure 6.2 Valve Assembly of an Aerosol Pack.

General Standards

1. Contents of active ingredient delivered per spray.
2. Particle size
3. Number of deliveries per container
4. Pressure test
5. Leak test

Labelling

The label for this product should mention the following information along with other mandatory information;

1. The name of the product with the official title, if any.
2. The strength of the API (Active Pharmaceutical Ingredients) should be expressed in terms of '%w/v',
3. The quantity of drug actually delivered each time when the valve is actuated,
4. A warning that 'the container should be kept away from heat and sun, it should not be punctured, broken, or incinerated even appeared to be empty',
5. If the unit needs to be assembled before use, proper and distinctly visible marking on the container or direction on the label should be given,
6. The label should mention that 'shake the container well before use'.
7. A warning regarding the dose, that is, 'the user should not exceed the prescribed dosage and follow the instructions printed on the container or given in form leaflet or card inside the carton'.

The instruction to the user should include the following points.

1. Direction for correct use of the preparation,
2. Recommended dosage schedule and maximum number of doses in a day,
3. Direction for storage and disposal of the container.

Storage

The aerosol products should be kept in cool place, away from heat, sun and frost.

General method of manufacture

Manufacturing and packaging of aerosol preparation are done almost simultaneously. The product concentrate containing active ingredient, solvent, cosolvent, other necessary additives along with small amount of propellant(s) are mixed separately in a suitable container. The remaining portion of the propellant(s) is then mixed and filled into suitable package using either cold-fill or pressure-fill method.

The cold-fill method requires the preparation to be chilled before filling. This may be single-stage or two-stage filling process. In single-stage filling process, mixing, cooling and filling are done simultaneously in a single tank. The product is chilled to about -45 °C to -60°C before filling.

While in two-stage filling process, solution, suspension or emulsion of the active ingredient is done separately with small amount of propellant and chilled to about - 30°C, the major portion of the propellant is chilled to the same temperature separately in another tank. Before filling, the chilled propellant is mixed with the product. The tank is attached with a mixer and homogenizer. The product is passed through a filter before filling to break up the agglomerate, if formed due to chilling.

The pressure-fill method is better than the cold-fill method due to less chance pollution. The filling is done at room temperature only. In this method the filling is done under the pressure of about 300 – 600 psig when metered valve is used.

Exercises

Short Questions

1. (a) What is inhaler?

   (b) What is inhalant?

   (c) What is aerosol?

   (d) What is propellant?

   (e) Name at least three propellants.

   (f) Name the materials used for making aerosol container.

   (g) Why aerosol is called as pressurized package system?

   (h) What are the additives used in aerosol?

2. Write down the general method of manufacture of inhalations.

3. Write down the general method of manufacture of aerosol.

4. Write down the advantages and disadvantages of aerosol.

5. Name different types of propellants.

6. Define inhalant.

7. What are the storage conditions for an aerosol?

8. Classify the propellants and mention the examples of each type.

9. Explain how the propellant is selected?

10. What are advantages and disadvantages of aerosol preparation?

11. Describe briefly how an aerosol preparation is manufactured.

12. Discuss in brief the functions of different parts of valve assembly.

13. Write down the general method of manufacture of aerosol.

14. Enlist the information to be mentioned in a label of aerosol preparation.

7 Systems of Weights and Measures

The **Imperial system** is one of the many systems of English or Foot-pound-second units, first defined in the British Weights and Measures Act of (1824). Although most of the units were defined in more than one system, some subsidiary units were used to a much greater extent for different purposes. One of these systems was the US customary system derived from the British units. Units of length and area had been mostly shared between the Imperial and US customary systems. Capacity measures differed mostly due to the introduction of the imperial gallon and the unification of wet and dry measures. For example, the avoirdupois system was applied only to weights. Later in 1959 some systems were outlawed and both the US and British yard was defined identically to be 0.9144 metres, to match the International yard. The distinction among three weight systems are given below.

Weight:	Apothecary weight					Troy weight			
Pound	1					Pound	1		
Ounces	12	1				Ounces	12	1	
Drams	96	8	1			Penny weights	240	20	1
Scruples	288	24	3	1		Grains	5760	480	24
Grains	5760	480	60	20					

Avoirdupois weight							
Ton (t)	1						
Hundred weight (cwt)	20	1					
Quarter	80	4	1				
Stone (st)	160	8	2	1			
Pound (lb)	2240	112	28	14	1		
Ounce (oz)	35 840	1792	448	224	16	1	
Drachm	5 73 440	28672	7168	3584	256	16	1
Grain	15680000	784000	196000	98000	7000	437.5	27.34

Note: Troy weight, used for precious metals,

Avoirdupois weight, used for most other purposes,

Apothecaries' weight, not used because of metric system is in use.

Length: Units

League	1				
Mile	3	1			
Furlong	24	8	1		
Yard	5280	1760	220	1	
Foot	15840	5280	660	3	1
Inch	190080	63360	7920	36	12

Maritime units

Nautical mile	1		
Cable	10	1	
Fathom	600	100	1
Foot	6000	60	6 (6.08)

Gunter's survey units

Chain	1		
Pole	4	1	
Foot	66	16.5	1
Link	100	25	1.5151

Area

Units	In terms of length units	Square miles	Square rods	Square feet	Hectare
Perch	1 rod × 1 rod	$\frac{1}{10240}$	1	272.25	0.002529
Rood	1 furlong × 1 rod	$\frac{1}{2560}$	40	10 890	0.1012
Acre	1 furlong x 1 chain	$\frac{1}{640}$	160	43 560	0.4047

Volume

Units	Imperial ounce	US ounce	Imperial pint	US pint	Cubic inches
Fluid ounce (fl oz)	1	0.96076	$\frac{1}{20}$	0.060047	1.7339
Gill	5	4.8038	$\frac{1}{4}$	0.30024	8.6694
Pint (pt)	20	19.215	1	1.2009	34.677
Quart (qt)	40	38.430	2	2.4019	69.355
Gallon (gal)	160	15372	8	9.6076	277.42

After completion of legal transition the use of SI units has become mandated by law for the retail sale of food and other commodities in UK since 1995. However, some people in UK are still using the imperial units.

Metric System

This is an international decimalised system of measurement, first adopted in France in (1791). During last two centuries different variants have been considered and since 1960s it has been recognised internationally as the International System of Units (SI, Systeme International d'Unites in French). Now most of the countries in the world use this system for personal, commercial and scientific purposes.

According to the US *CIA World Factbook* in 2006, the International System of Units is the official system of measurement for all nations except for Burma, Liberia, and the Units States. In the United States, the litre is a common unit for measuring volumes, no other units of the metric system.

The metric system is decimal, all multiples and submultiples of the base units are factors of powers of ten of the unit. Fractions of a unit are not used normally. All derived units use a common set of prefixes for each multiple. For example, the prefix *kilo, meaning 1000 times of base unit, gram and metre;* which can be used for both mass and length units, kilogram and kilometre.

Weights	Length	Volume
Exagram 10^{18} gram	Exametre 10^{18} metre	Exalitre 10^{18} litre
Petagram 10^{15} gram	Petametre 10^{15} metre	Petalitre 10^{15} litre
Teragram 10^{12} gram	Terametre 10^{9} metre	Teralitre 10^{12} litre
Gigagram 10^{9} gram	Gigammetre 10^{6} metre	Megalitre 10^{6} litre
Megagram 10^{6} gram	Megametre 10^{6} metre	Megalitre 10^{6} litre
Kilogram 10^{3} gram	Kilometre 10^{3} metre	Kilolitre 10^{3} litre
Hectogram 10^{2} gram	Hectometre 10^{2} metre	Hectolitre 10^{2} litre
Decagram 10^{1} gram	Decametre 10^{1} metre	Decalitre 10^{1} litre
Gram	Metre	Litre
Decigram 10^{-1} gram	Decimetre 10–1 metre	Decilitre 10^{-1} litre
Centigram 10^{-2} gram	Centimetre 10–2 metre	Centilitre 10^{-2} litre
Milligram 10^{-3} gram	Millimetre 10^{-3} metre	Millilitre 10^{-3} litre
Nanogram 10^{-9} gram	Nanometre 10^{-9} metre	Nanolitre 10^{-9} litre
Pictogram 10^{-12} gram	Picometre 10^{-12} metre	Picolitre 10^{-12} litre
Femtogram 10^{-15} gram	Femtometre 10^{-15} metre	Femtolitre 10^{-15} litre
Attogram 10^{-18} gram	Attometre 10^{-18} metre	Attolitre 10^{-18} litre

Centimetre-Gram-Second Systems (CGS), Metre-Kilogram-Second System (MKS) and Metre-Tonne-Second System (MTS) are the three systems commonly used in metric systems.

However, millimetre-Newton-second system is used in simulation of mechanical systems.

Conversions of weights and measures

Length	Volume	Weight
1 metre = 39.4 inches	1 fluidounce = 29.6 ml	1 pound avoir = 454 g
1 metre = 3.283 ft	1 pint = 473 ml	1 pound apothecary = 373 g
1 inch = 2.54 cm	1 gallon = 3.79 lt	1 gram = 15.4 grains
	= 4 Quarts = 8 Pints	1 grain = 64.8 mg
	1 Quart = 960 cc = 2 Pints	1 kg = 2.2 lbs
	1 Pint = 480 cc = 16 OZ	1lb = 456 g
	1 OZ = 30 cc	
	1 Teaspoonful = 5 cc	
	1 tablespoonful = 15 cc	
	1 Wineglassful = 60 cc	
	1 Teacupful = 120 cc	
	1 Tumblerful = 240 cc	

8 Pharmaceutical Calculations

Weights

Minimum Weighable Quantity (MWQ)

A balance must be used within a degree of error tolerable for compounding or manufacturing purpose. USP allows a maximum error of 5% in a single operation. Each balance has range of sensitivity. The percent error depends on the amount of substance being weighed and the error increases as the amount being weighed decreases.

$$MWQ = \frac{Sensitivity \times 100\%}{Error\ in\ percent} = \frac{Sensitivity \times 100}{Error}$$

***Example* 1:** What is the MWQ of a balance with 5% error and with sensitivity of 10 mg?

Solution:
$$MWQ = \frac{Sensitivity \times 100}{Error} = \frac{10 \times 100}{5} = 200\ mg$$

***Example* 2:** What should be the sensitivity of a balance to weigh 1 mg of a substance with 2% error?

Solution: MWQ = 1 mg and Error = 2%

$$MWQ = \frac{Sensitivity \times 100}{Error} \quad \text{or} \quad 1\ mg = \frac{Sensitivity \times 100}{2}$$

Sensitivity = 50 mg

Volume

Measurement of Volume

For measuring the volume of a liquid or solution there are different types of measuring devices. Depending on the type of liquid, quantity and accuracy of the measurement a suitable measuring device should be used. For example, a cylinder is used for measuring a solvent with accuracy up to 0.5 ml, a pipette for a reagent solution with accuracy up to 0.05 ml, volumetric flask for preparing a volumetric solution.

Select the capacity of the measuring device as per the volume to be measured. For accurate measurement, view the meniscus of the liquid or solution horizontally.

For example, if the volume of a solvent to be measured is 10 ml or less, use a cylinder of 10 ml.

To measure 1 ml or less amount of a reagent or volumetric solution, use a pipette of 1 ml, but not more 5 ml.

FIGURES

Approximation of the Figures

Significant figures are the digits which have practical meaning.

For example, 2.50 and 2.5 are same. The zero is not significant and the figure 2.50 can be written as 2.5. The figure 2.5 is correct to ± 0.1.

But, if it is 2.05, the zero is a significant figure. In this case the figure is correct to ± 0.01.

Approximation

3.5473 can be approximated as follows:

   (i)   3.5 correct to first decimal, with significant figures 2 (3 and 0.5).

   (ii)   3.55 correct to second decimal with significant figures 3 (3, 0.5 and 0.05)

   (iii)   3.547 correct to the third decimal with significant figures 4 (3, 0.5, 0.04 and 0.007).

Exponent, Power and Root

$3^4 = 3 \times 3 \times 3 \times 3 = 81$ is an expression of which 81 is the *power* of the *base* 3 and 4 is the *exponent*. When 1 is the exponent it is omitted. The following laws are recalled.

A number with negative exponent: $5^{-3} = \dfrac{1}{5^3}$

Law of multiplication:

   1. *When the bases are same:* $a^x \times a^y = a^{(x+y)}$

   2. *When exponents are same:* $a^x \times b^x = (a \times b)^x$

Example: 1. $3^4 \times 3^2 = 3^{(4+2)} = 3^6$

2. $3^2 \times 5^2 \times 7^2 = (3 \times 5 \times 7)^2 = 105^2$

Law of division(:)

1. *When exponents are same:* $a^x \div b^x = \left(\dfrac{a}{b}\right)^x$

2. *When the bases are same:* $a^x \div b^y = a^{(x-y)}$

Example: 1. $3^8 \div 5^8 = \left(\dfrac{3}{5}\right)^8$

2. $3^8 \div 3^5 = 3^{(8-5)} = 3^3$

Root

The root of a power can be determined by dividing the exponent of the power by the index of the root: $\sqrt{x} = x^{1/2}$

$$\sqrt[5]{x^3} = x^{\frac{3}{5}}$$

Example: 1. $\sqrt[3]{3^5} = 3^{5/3}$

2. $\sqrt{5^8} = 5^{8/2} = 5^4$

Addition, Subtraction, Multiplication and Division

Quantities can be added or subtracted directly when these have same unit or after conversion to same unit.

Example 1: Find out total weight of the following mixture containing Paracetamol 2.5 kg, Starch 750 g, Lactose 25 g and Talcum 25 mg.

Solution:

Paracetamol	2.5 kg	= 2.5 × 1000g	= 2500 g
Starch	750 g		= 750g
Lactose	25g		= 25g
Talcum	25mg	$= \dfrac{25}{1000}$ g	= 0.025g
Total			3275.025g $= \dfrac{3275}{1000}$
			= 3.275kg

***Example* 2:** Find out the circumference of an area given the length of four sides as follows, 30 ft 4 inches, 1 yard 2 ft 8 inches, 1 yard 1 ft 11 inches and 29 ft 11 inches.

Solution:

30 ft 4 inches = 30 × 12 + 4 = 364 inches

1 yard 2 ft 8 inches = 1 × 3 × 12 + 2 × 12 + 8 = 68 inches

1 yard 1 ft 11 inches = 1 × 3 × 12 + 1 × 12 + 11 = 59 inches

29 ft 11 inches = 29 × 12 + 11 = 359 inches

Total 850 inches

Hence, the circumference of the area = 850 inches = 850/12 = 70 ft 10 inches = 23 yards 1 ft 10 inches.

***Example* 3:** What would be total weight of a mixture containing borax 27 g and glycerin 100 ml? The density of glycerin is 1.312 g /ml.

Solution:

$$Density = \frac{Mass}{Volume}$$

Weight of 100 ml of glycerin = volume × density = 100 ml × 1.312g/ml

= 131.2 g

Hence, total weight = 27g + 131.2 g = 158.2 g.

***Example* 4:** Subtract 1 litre 25 ml from 3 litres.

Solution:

3 litre = 3 × 1000 = 3000 ml

1 litre 25 ml = 1 × 1000 + 25 = 1025 ml

$$3000 - 1025 = 1975 \text{ ml} = \frac{1975 \text{ ml}}{1000} = 1 \text{ litre } 975 \text{ ml}$$

***Example* 5:** In a lot of codeine phosphate syrup 4 kg 755 g codeine phosphate has been added in place of 5 kg. How much codeine phosphate is to be added.

Solution:

Codeine phosphate to be added = 5 kg = 5 × 1000 g = 5000 g

Codeine phosphate added = 4 kg 755 g = 4 × 1000 g + 755 g = 4755 g

So, Codeine phosphate to be added = 5000 g – 4755 g = 245 g.

***Example* 6:** A syrup contains 2 mg of salbutamol sulphate per 5 ml, how much of salbutamol sulphate is present in 50 litres of syrup?

Solution: 50 litres = 50 × 1000 = 50 000 ml

5 ml of syrup contain salbutamol sulphate 2 mg

$$50000 \text{ ml of syrup contains} = \frac{2 \times 50000}{5} \text{ mg of salbutamol sulphate}$$

$$= 20000 \text{ mg} = 20 \text{ g of salbutamol sulphate}$$

***Example* 7:** The lot size of Amoxycillin capsule is 25000 and 6 kg 250 g of Amoxycillin trihydrate is used to fill the capsules. How much of Amoxycillin trihydrate is present in each capsule.

Solution: 25000 capsules contain 6 kg 250 g of Amoxycillin trihydrate

$$= 6 \times 1000 \text{ g} + 250 \text{ g} = 6250 \text{ g}$$

$$1 \text{ capsule contains } \frac{6250g}{25000} = 0.25 \text{ g} = 0.25 \times 1000 \text{ mg} = 250 \text{ mg}$$

250 mg of Amoxycillin trihydrate is present per capsule.

Reducing and Enlarging of Formulas

***Example* 8:** A formula for 7.06 kg of granules for aspirin tablet is as follows.

Aspirin	6.50 kg
Starch	0.5 kg
Talcum	0.06 kg

Enlarge the formula for 25 kg of granules.

Solution: As per the composition given

$$\text{The enlargement factor} = \frac{25 \text{ kg}}{7.06 \text{ kg}} = 3.541$$

Hence, for 25 kg granules,

Aspirin = 6.50 × 3.541 = 23.02 kg

Starch = 0.5 ×3.541 = 1.77 kg

Talcum = 0.06 × 3.541 = 0.21 kg.

***Example* 9:** As per the formula each tablet of Aspirin contains

Aspirin	335mg
Starch	25mg
Talcum	3mg

Enlarge the formula for 1000 tablets.

Solution:

$$\text{The enlargement factor} = \frac{1000 \text{ Tabs}}{1 \text{ Tab}} = 1000$$

Thus, for 1000 tablets

$$\text{Aspirin } 335\text{mg} \times 1000 = 335000 \text{ mg} = \frac{335000}{1000}\text{g} = 335\text{g}$$

$$\text{Starch } 25\text{mg} \times 1000 = 25000 \text{ mg} = \frac{25000}{1000}\text{g} = 25\text{g}$$

$$\text{Talcum } 3\text{mg} \times 1000 = 3000 \text{ mg} = \frac{3000}{1000}\text{g} = 3\text{g}$$

***Example* 10:** A 15 litres of solution contains the following ingredients.

Paracetamol 375 g

Methylparaben 30 g

Propylparaben 6 g

Sodium benzoate 15 g

Sorbitol solution 3 litres

Glycerin 2 litres

Syrup 7.5 litters

Propylene glycol 2.5 litres

Calculate quantity of each ingredient to be required for 2 lt of solution.

Solution:

$$\text{The reducing factor} = \frac{2 \text{ Lt}}{15 \text{ Lt}} = 0.133$$

Hence, the quantity to be required for 2 litres solution would be:

Paracetamol 375 g × 0.133 = 49.875 g

Methylparaben 30 g × 0.133 = 3.99 g

Propylparaben 6 g × 0.133 = 0.798 g × 1000

= 798 mg Sodium benzoate 15 g × 0.133 = 1.995 g

Sorbitol solution 3 litres × 0.133 = 0.399 litre × 1000 = 399 ml

Glycerin 2 litres × 0.133 = 0.266 litre × 1000 = 266 ml

Syrup 7.5 litres × 0.133 = 0.9975 litre × 1000 = 997.5 ml

Propylene glycol 2.5 litres × 0.133 = 0.3325 litre × 1000 = 332.5 ml

***Example* 11:** To prepare 1 litre of 1N solution 40 g of NaOH is required, for 150 ml how much of NaOH shall be required.

***Solution*:**

$$\text{The reducing factor} = \frac{150 \text{ ml}}{1000 \text{ ml}} = 0.15$$

1 litre = 1000 ml

Hence, for 150 ml NaOH shall be required = 0.15 × 40 g = 6 g.

Percentage and Ratio Strength

Percent means per hundred and expressed as %.

Percentage concentrations are expressed as follows:
- Percent weight by weight (%w/w) is the number of g per 100 g.
- Percent weight by volume (%w/v) is the number of g per 100 ml.
- Percent volume by volume (%v/v) is the number of ml per 100 ml.
- Percent volume by weight (%v/w) is the number of ml per 100 g.

***Example* 12:** In 45 g of a mixture, 9 g of talcum and 36 g of starch are present. Express the % concentration of talcum and starch in the mixture.

***Solution*:** 9g Talcum is present in 45g of the mixture

$$\text{In terms of ratio strength:} \ \frac{9g}{45g} \ \text{or 1:5}$$

$$\text{In terms of \% w/w:} \ \frac{9 \times 100}{45} = 20$$

Thus, the mixture contains 20% w/w of talcum or at a ratio of 1:5.

Similarly, 36 g of starch is present in 45 g of mixture

$$\text{In terms of ratio strength:} \ \frac{36g}{45g} \ \text{or 4:5}$$

$$\text{In terms of \% w/w:} \ \frac{36 \times 100}{45} = 80$$

Thus, the mixture contains 80% w/w of starch or at a ratio of 4:5.

***Example* 13:** How many grams of sodium hydroxide would be required to prepare 75 ml of 12.5% w/v solution.

Solution: 12.5% w/v solution means,

In 100 ml solution, sodium hydroxide is present 12.5 g

In terms of % w/v sodium required to make 75 ml $= \dfrac{75 \times 12.5}{100} = 9.375$

In terms of ratio strength: $\dfrac{9.375}{75}$ or, 1:8

***Example* 14:** A solution contains 55 g of sucrose in 80 ml. Find out the % concentration of sucrose.

Solution: 80 ml of the solution contains 55 g of sucrose

100 ml of the solution contains $\dfrac{55 \times 100}{80}$ g $= 68.75$ g of sucrose

Hence, the concentration of the sucrose solution is 68.75% w/v.

***Example* 15:** Calculate the volume of 1.5% w/v solution of A to be diluted with water to prepare 5 ml of 0.025% solution.

Solution: 0.025% solution means that

in 100 ml solution 0.025 g of solute is dissolved.

In 25 ml the solute present is $\dfrac{0.025 \times 25}{100}$ g $= 0.00625$ g

1.5% solution means that 1.5 g of solute is present in 100 ml solution.

0.00625 g of solute would be present in $\dfrac{0.00625 \times 100}{1.5}$ ml $= 0.416$ ml

Hence, 0.42 ml of solution A is to be diluted to 25 ml.

***Example* 16:** The composition of 100 ml of a tincture is given below:

Extract of crude drug	2 g
Alcohol (70%)	65 ml
Purified water	35 ml

Find out the concentration of alcohol IP (in %v/v)in the preparation.

***Solution*:**   As per IP the concentration of alcohol is 95% v/v.

As per composition, 65 ml of the alcohol (70%) is present in the tincture.

$$\text{The volume of alcohol (95\%) in 65 ml} = \frac{65 \times 70}{95} = 47.89 \text{ ml.}$$

Hence, the tincture contains 47.89ml of Alcohol IP.

Dilution

***Example* 17:** 257.5 mg of a drug is dissolved in 100 ml of 0.1 N HCl.

***Solution*:** 2 ml of this solution is diluted to 50 ml and 5 ml of this solution is further diluted to 50 ml.

Find out the concentration of the final solution.

***Solution*:** % concentration of a solution of solid means g per 100 ml.

$$257.5 \text{ mg} = \frac{257.5}{1000} \text{ g} = 0.2575 \text{ g}$$

Thus, 100 ml of the solution contains 0.2575 g of the drug and there are two dilutions:

(i)   2 ml of the solution containing $\dfrac{0.2575 \times 2}{100} = 0.00515$ g of drug is diluted to 50 ml.

So, 50 ml of the diluted solution contains 0.00515 g of the drug.

(ii)   5 ml of this solution containing $\dfrac{5 \times 0.00515}{50}$ g $= 0.000515$ g of the drug is diluted to 50 ml.

50 ml of this solution contains 0.000515 g of the drug

100 ml of this solution contains $\dfrac{0.000515 \times 100}{50} = 0.00103$ g

So, the final concentration of the solution is 0.00103%.

This can be done in a different way:

The concentration of the final diluted solution is

$$\frac{0.2575 \text{ g}}{100 \text{ ml}} \times \frac{2 \text{ ml}}{50 \text{ ml}} \times \frac{5 \text{ ml} \times 100}{50 \text{ ml}} = 0.00103\%$$

***Example* 18:** How much amount of a drug to be taken to prepare 0.002% w/v solution?

***Solution*:** The final concentration is 0.002% w/v; this means that

0.002 g of drug is present in 100 ml of solution.

Hence, 2.0 mg of the drug would be taken.

***Example* 19:** A tablet contains 3 mcg of folic acid with 50% overage and the lot size is of 100 tablets. The concentration of folic acid stock solution is 0.1%. What is the minimum quantity would be sufficient for the lot.

***Solution*:** Folic acid required per tab = 3 mcg + 50% of 3 mcg (overage)

That is, $3 + \dfrac{3 \times 50}{100} = 4.5$ mcg.

Total requirement of folic acid for 100 tabs = 100 × 4.5 mcg

$$= 450 \text{ mcg}.$$

Concentration of Stock solution is 0.1% w/v;

That is, it contains 0.1 g in 100 ml

or, 0.1g × 1000 = 100mg × 1000 = 1,00,000 mcg in 100 ml

1,00,000 mcg in 100 ml = 1000 mcg per ml.

1000 mcg of folic acid is present in 1 ml

Hence, 450 mcg of folic acid is present in $\dfrac{1 \times 450}{1000} = 0.45$ ml.

Parts Per Million (PPM)

Parts per million (ppm) means 1 part in 1 million (10^6) parts

That is, 1 g in 10,00,000 g

***Example* 20:** A powder sample contains 10 parts per million (ppm) irons; calculate the content of iron in terms of percent, w/w.

***Solution*:** 10 parts per million means 10 parts in 1000,000 parts,

i.e., 10 g in 1000 × 1000 g

In other words, 1000 × 1000 g of sample contains 10 g of iron

100 g of sample contains $\dfrac{10 \times 100}{1000000} = \dfrac{1}{1000} = 0.001\%$ w/w

So, 0.001% w/w of iron is present in the sample.

***Example* 21:** A sample of hydrochloric acid contains 0.005% w/v of lead, convert the concentration of lead in terms of ppm. Density of the acid is 1.18 g/ml at 25 °C.

***Solution*:** Concentration of lead in the HCl solution is 0.005% w/v

That is, 0.005 g of lead is present in 100 ml of the HCl solution and density of HCl solution is 1.18 g/ml.

Then, the mass of 100 ml of HCl solution = 100 × 1.18 g = 118 g

Thus, 118 g of HCl solution contains 0.005 g of lead

10,00,000 g of HCl solution contains $\dfrac{0.005 \times 1000000}{118}$ g = 42.37 g of lead.

In other words, 42.37 ppm of lead is present in HCl solution.

Mixture of Different Concentrations (Arithmetic Method)

***Example* 22:** A mixture contains 150 ml of 10% sodium chloride solution, 255 ml of 30% sodium chloride solution and 755 ml of 2.5% sodium chloride solution. Find out the concentration of sodium chloride in the mixture.

***Solution*:** Total volume of the mixture = 150 + 255 + 755 ml = 1160 ml

Content of sodium chloride in 150 ml of 10% solution = 10% of 150 ml

$$= \frac{10 \times 150}{100} = 15 \text{ g}$$

Content of sodium chloride in 255 ml of 30% solution = 30% of 255 ml

$$= \frac{30 \times 255}{100} \text{ g} = 76.5 \text{ g}$$

Content of sodium chloride in 755 ml of 2.5% solution = 2.5% of 755 ml

$$= \frac{2.5 \times 755}{100} \text{ g} = 18.875 \text{ g}$$

The total content of sodium chloride in 1160ml of mixture

$$= (15 + 76.5 + 18.875)\text{g} = 110.375 \text{ g}$$

Hence, the concentration of sodium chloride in the mixture

$$= \frac{110.375 \times 100}{1160}\% = 9.51\%.$$

***Example* 23:** Three lots A, B and C of aspirin tablets have drug content as 67.5%, 68.2% and 68.6% respectively in their granules. The rejects of three lots are 23 kg, 22.7 kg and 18.3 kg respectively. With these rejects a reprocessed lot is made. Find out the drug content in the reprocessed lot.

***Solution*:** Content of aspirin in lot A = 67.5% of 23 kg = $\dfrac{23 \times 67.5}{100}$ kg

$$= 15.52 \text{ kg}$$

Content of aspirin in lot A = 68.2% of 22.7kg = $\dfrac{222.7 \times 68.2}{100}$ kg = 15.48 kg

Content of aspirin in lot A = 68.6% of 18.3 kg = $\dfrac{18.3 \times 68.6}{100}$ kg

$$= 34.04 \text{kg}$$

Total amount of reject = 23 + 22.7 + 18.3 kg = 64.0 kg, and

Total amount of aspirin in the mixture = 15.525 + 15.481 + 12.554 kg

$$= 43.560 \text{ kg}$$

Hence, percent concentration of aspirin in the mixture = $\dfrac{43.56 \times 100}{64}$ %

$$= 68.06\%$$

Mixture of Different Concentrations (Alligation Method)

***Example* 24:** At which proportion 20% alcohol is to be mixed with 50% alcohol to make 40%.

***Solution*:**

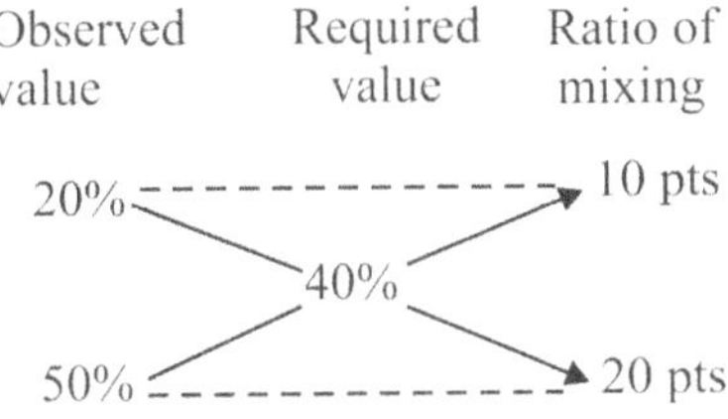

Thus, 40% of alcohol can be prepared by mixing 10 parts of 20% alcohol with 20 parts of 50% alcohol (by subtracting).

***Example* 25:** For a preparation, 10 ml of a surfactant with HLB value 9 is required. Prepare a mixture of surfactants with HLB values of 8 and 12 to get required HLB for use.

***Solution*:** Surfactant with HLB value

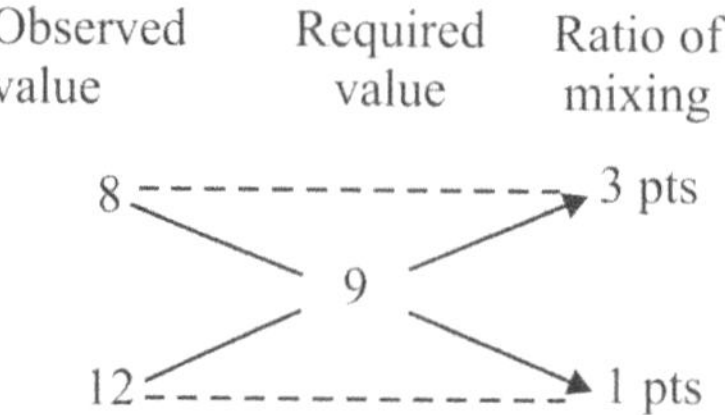

Hence, at a ratio of 3:1 the two surfactants having HLB values 8 and 12 respectively can be mixed and used.

***Example* 26:** Three paracetamol granules A, B and C having different drug contents recovered during production of three lots are 73.7%, 74.5% and 74.9% respectively. Find out at which proportion these should be mixed to get 74.6% drug content (use Alligation Method).

***Solution*:**

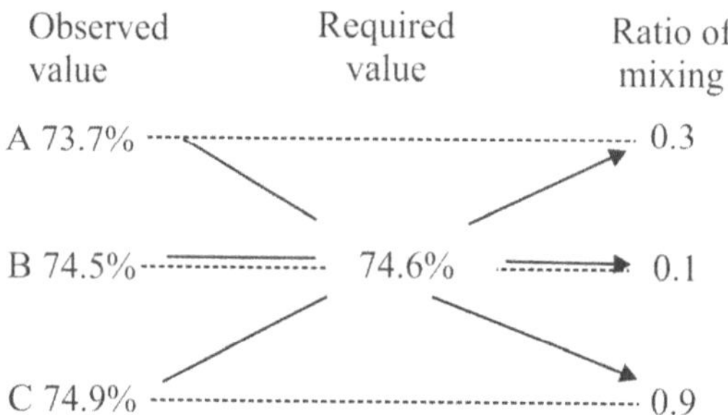

The proportion of mixing should be 0.3 parts of A, 0.1 parts of B and 0.9 parts of C.

That is 3 parts of A, 1 part of B and 9 parts of C are to be mixed.

***Example* 27:** The drug content of a solution was found 72.15%, the required content is 70.0%. How much of vehicle is to be mixed to make it 70.0%?

***Solution*:**

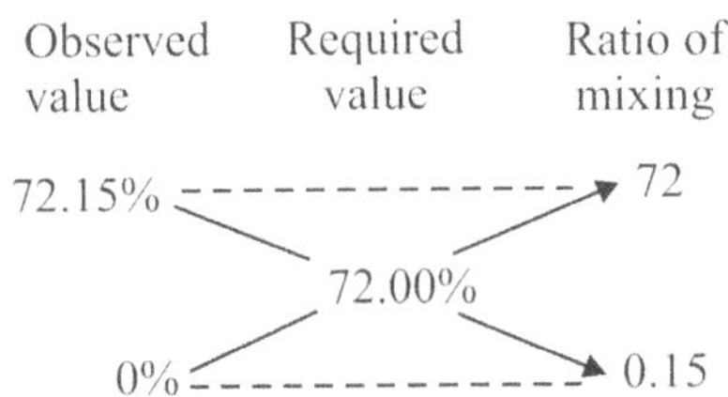

Thus, 0.15 parts of vehicle is to be mixed with 72 parts of the drug solution. In other words per 72 lts of drug solution and 150ml of the vehicle are to be mixed.

***Example* 28:** Three lots A, B and C of aspirin tablets have drug content as 67.5%, 68.2% and 68.6% respectively in their granules. The rejects of three lots are 23 kg, 22.7 kg and 18.3 kg respectively. With these rejects a reprocessed lot is made with drug content of 68.5%. Find out the ratio of mixing the three lots.

***Solution*:**

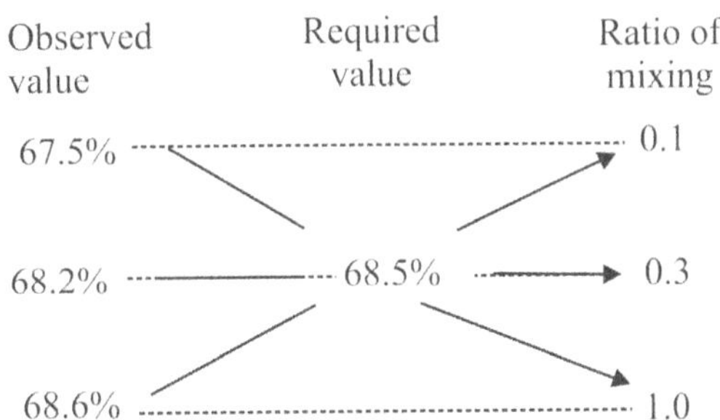

Thus, 0.1 parts of lot A, 0.3 parts of lot B and 1.0 parts of lot C are to be mixed. In other words, the proportion at which lot A, B and C are to be mixed is 1: 3: 10.

***Example* 29:** Three lots A, B and C of aspirin tablets have drug content as 67.5%, 68.2% and 68.6% respectively in their granules. The rejects of three lots are 23 kg, 22.7 kg and 18.3 kg respectively. With these rejects a reprocessed lot is made with drug content of 68.5%. Find out the ratio of mixing the three lots.

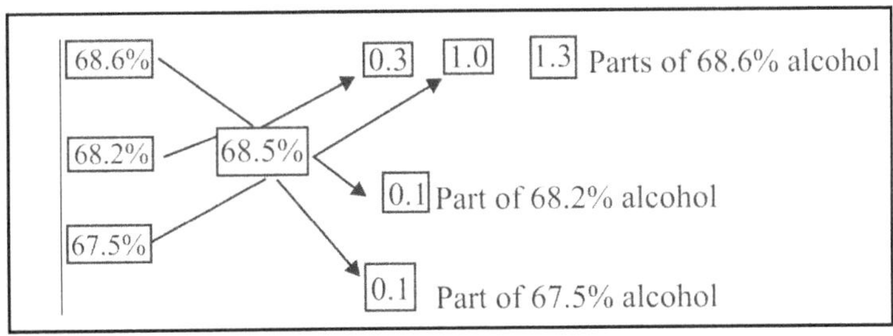

Solution: Since there are three lots to be mixed, two lots A and B, and lot A and C are grouped separately. Then the method of alligation is applied. The concentration of lot A is closer to the desired concentration, it is kept common.

Thus, 0.1 parts of lot A, 0.1 parts of lot B and 1.3 parts of lot C are to be mixed. In other words, the proportion at which lot A, B and C are to be mixed is 1: 1: 13.

Note: When the given concentrations are more than two, the calculation should be done in groups.

Proof Spirit

In Bonded laboratory (where alcoholic preparations are manufactured under the License of Excise Dept.) the alcohol is called as *spirit*.

The strength or concentration of alcohol is expressed as *Proof degrees* (°). Receipt, Issue and Duty (Tax) are calculated accordingly.

In USA,100 proof spirit is equivalent 50% v/v or 42.49% w/w of ethyl alcohol (C_2H_5OH) having specific gravity of 0.93426 at 60°F (15.56°C). Thus, 2 proof degree equals to 1% (by volume).

> In India, 57.1 volumes of C_2H_5OH (99.8%v/v) is equal to 100 volumes of proof spirit.
>
> That is, 57.1 % v/v of ethyl alcohol is equal to 100° proof.
>
> So, 1 volume of 57.1% ethyl alcohol $= \dfrac{100}{57.1} = 1.7513$ volume proof spirit.
>
> Or, 1% ethyl alcohol $= 1.7513°$ proof

The Proof strength is expressed in two ways:

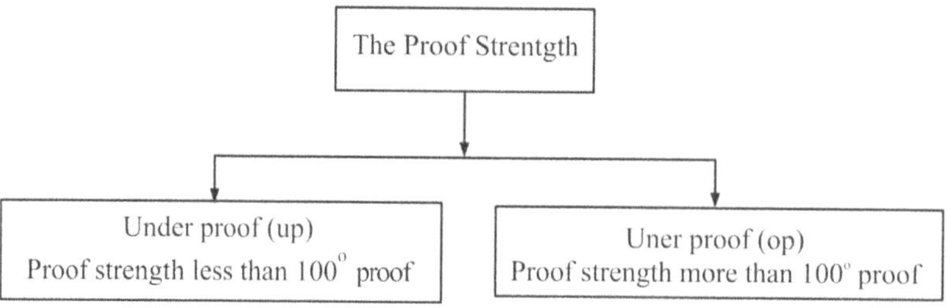

Example **30:**   What shall be the proof strength ($^\circ$proof) of 80% v/v and 20% v/v ethyl alcohol.

Solution: 1% of ethyl alcohol = 1.7513° proof

80% of alcohol = 80 × 1.7513 = 140.14° proof,

Which is more than 100 by 40.14° proof.

So, 80% alcohol is 40.14 $^\circ$ op.

Similarly, 20% v/v alcohol = 20 × 1.7513 = 35.03° proof,

which is less than 100 by 64.94° proof (100 – 35.03 = 64.97)

So, 20% alcohol is 64.97° up.

Example **31:**   Convert 25° up and 30° op into % v/v ethyl alcohol.

Solution: 1% ethyl alcohol = 1.7513° proof

Or 1.753° proof = 1% ethyl alcohol, that is 1° proof = $\dfrac{1}{1.7553}$ % v/v

25° up = 100 – 25 (as it is under proof) = 75° proof

75° proof = 75 × $\dfrac{1}{1.7553}$ % = 42.82% v/v

30° op = 100 + 30 (as it is over proof) = 130° proof

130° proof = 130 × $\dfrac{1}{1.7513}$ % = 74.23% v/v

Example **32:**   A vitamin B-complex preparation contains 10% v/v of ethyl alcohol. Express the alcohol content in terms of proof strength.

Solution: 1% ethyl alcohol is 1.7513° proof

So, 10% ethyl alcohol would be 1.7513 × 10 = 17.51 $^\circ$ proof

This is less than 100 by (100 – 17.51 = 82.49) 82.49 $^\circ$ proof.

Thus, the alcohol content of the vitamin B-complex preparation should be expressed as 82.49° up.

Equivalent Weight and Milliequivalent Weights

Type of substance	Equivalent weight (Eq.wt)
Acid	$\dfrac{\text{Molecular weight}}{\text{Basicity of the acid}}$

Contd...

Base	$\dfrac{\text{Molecular weight}}{\text{Acidity of the base}}$
Salt	$\dfrac{\text{Molecular weight}}{\text{Total valency of anion / cation}}$
Oxidizing/Reducing substance	$\dfrac{\text{Molecular weight}}{\text{Total change in oxidation No.}}$

Related Terms: The term Mole refers to 6.023×10^{23} numbers of molecules (the Avogadro's number).

gMole or mole = 1 gram molecular weight of a substance (molecular weight expressed in grams)

No. of mole = milli mole (mmole) = 1 mole expressed in mg

or, 1 gMole × 1000

Example **33:**   Molecular weight of sodium carbonate is 106. How many moles and mmoles of Na2CO3 are there in 3g of it.

Solution: Molecular weight of Na2CO3 = 106

Number of moles present in 3 g of it $= \dfrac{3}{106} = 0.0283$

mmoles in 3g = 0.0283 × 1000 = 28.3

Thus, 3g of Na_2CO_3 contain 0.0283 moles and 28.3 mmoles of it.

Example **34:**   0.7 moles of NaCl is to be added to a mixture. How many gm of it is to be taken.

Solution: Molecular weight of NaCl is 58.5

$$\text{Mole} = \dfrac{\text{weight}}{\text{molecular weight}}$$

So, $0.7 = \dfrac{\text{Weight}}{58.5}$

Or, Weight = 58.5 × 0.7 = 40.95g

Hence, 40.95g of NaCl is to be taken.

Example **35:**   Molecular weight of sulphuric acid is 98. How many moles and mmoles of the acid are there in 5ml of concentrated acid? (Density of concentrated sulphuric acid is 1.84g/ml).

Solution: 5 ml of H_2SO_4 = 5ml × 1.84g/ml = 9.2g

98g of sulphuric acid contain 1 mole

So, 9.2g of sulphuric acid contain $\dfrac{1 \times 9.2}{98} = 0.094$ moles

$$= 0.094 \times 1000 \text{ mmoles}$$

$$= 94 \text{ mmoles}$$

Equivalents (Eq) = Number of univalent counter ions required to react with one molecule of substance.

For example, there is one univalent cation (Na^+) or anion (Cl^-) in one mole of NaCl.

Thus, the total valency of NaCl = 1

gEq wt = Equivalent weight in gm

$$mEq \text{ of an i6n} = \frac{\text{ionic weigtht (mg)}}{\text{Valency}}$$

mg = mEq of atom/ion/molecule × valency

***Example* 36:** Find out the equivalent weight and gram Eq wt of $MgSO_4.7H_2O$, $CaCl_2.2H_2O$, KCl. H_2SO_4, HCl, $NaHCO_3$, NaOH, and $Na_2HPO_4.12H_2O$.

Substance	Mol. wt	Valency	Eq wt = $\dfrac{\text{Molecular / atomic / ionic wt}}{\text{Valency}}$	gEq wt
$MgSO_4$ $7H_2O$*	24 + 32 + 4 × 16 +7× 18 = 246	2	$\dfrac{246}{2} = 123$	123g
$CaCl_2,$ $2H_2O$*	40 + 2×35.5 + 2×18 = 147	2	$\dfrac{147}{2} = 73.5$	73.5g
Na_2HPO_4 $12H_2O$*	2 × 23 + 1 + 31 + 4 ×16 + 12 ×18 = 358	2	$\dfrac{358}{2} = 179$	179g
KCl	39 + 35.5 = 74.5	1	$\dfrac{74.5}{1} = 74.5$	74.5 g
H_2SO_4	2 ×1 + 32 + 4 ×16 = 98	2 (Basicity)	$\dfrac{98}{2} = 49$	49g

Table contd....

HCl	$1 + 35.5$ $= 36.5$	1 (Basicity)	$\dfrac{36.5}{1} = 36.5$	36.5g
NaHCO3	$23 + 1$ $+ 12 + 3$ $\times 16 = 84$	1 (Acidity)	$\dfrac{84}{1} = 42$	42g
NaOH	$23 + 16$ $+ 1 = 40$	1 (Acidity)	$\dfrac{40}{1} = 40$	40g

The water of crystallization must be included while calculating mol wt.

Example **37**: Calculate the mEq wt of sodium, potassium, calcium, magnesium, phosphate, chloride, citrate, sulphate, bicarbonate, carbonate ions.

Solution:

Ion	Ionic wt	Valency	Eq wt $= \dfrac{\text{atomic / Ionic wt}}{\text{valency}}$	mEq wt
Sodium, Na^+	23	1	$\dfrac{23}{1} = 23$	23 mg
Potassium, K^+	39.1	1	$\dfrac{39.1}{1} = 39.1$	39.1 mg
Calcium, Ca^{2+}	40	2	$\dfrac{40}{2} = 20$	20 mg
Magnesium, Mg^{2+}	24.3	2	$\dfrac{24.3}{2} = 12.15$	12.15 mg
Phosphate, $PO4^{2-}$	96	2	$\dfrac{96}{2} = 48$	48 mg
Bicarbonate, HCO_3^-	61	1	$\dfrac{61}{1}$	61 mg
Carbonate, CO_3^{2-}	60	2	$\dfrac{60}{2} = 30$	30 mg

Example 38: A solution contains 5 mEq/L of NaCl. What would be its concentration in mg/L?

Solution: Molecular weight of NaCl $= 23 + 35.5 = 58.5$ and its valency $= 1$

$$\text{Eq wt of NaCl} = \frac{\text{Molecular. wt}}{\text{Valency}} = 58.5$$

mEq of NaCl $= 58.5$mg

$$\text{mg/L} = \frac{\dfrac{\text{mEq wt}}{L} \times \text{mol. wt}}{\text{Valency}} = \frac{5 \times 58.5}{1} = 292.5$$

Example **39:** A powder contains 1.2 g of KCl. Calculate how many mEqs of KCl are present.

Solution: Molecular weight of KCl = 39 + 35.5 = 74.5

$$\text{Equivalent weight of KCl} = \frac{\text{Mol. wt}}{\text{Valency}} = \frac{74.5}{1} = 74.5$$

So, 74.5 mg = 1 mEq of KCl

$$1.2 \text{ g} = 1200 \text{ mg} = \frac{1200}{74.5} = 16.11$$

Example **40:** Sodium chloride and dextrose injection IP contains 5.0 g of dextrose and 0.9 g of sodium chloride per 100 ml. Convert the concentrations in terms of mEq/100 ml.

Solution:

Mol wt of dextrose, $C_6H_{12}O_6$ = 180

$$\text{Equivalent weight} = \frac{\text{Mol wt}}{\text{Valency}} = \frac{180}{1} = 180$$

mEq wt of dextrose = 180 mg

The solution contains 5 g of dextrose per 100 ml

$$\text{So, 5 g} = 5000 \text{ mg} = \frac{5000}{180} \text{ mEq} = 27.8 \text{ mEq of dextrose is present in 100}$$

ml of solution.

Similarly, mol wt of NaCl = 23 + 35.5 = 58.5 and its valence = 1

$$\text{Equivalent wt of NaCl} = \frac{58.5}{1} = 58.5 \text{ g and 1mEq of NaCl is 58.5 mg}$$

In other words, 58.5 mg = 1 mEq

$$\text{So, 0.9 g of NaCl} = 900 \text{ mg} = \frac{1 \times 900}{58.5} = 15.385 \text{ mEq}$$

Hence, in 100ml of the solution 15.4 mEq of sodium chloride is present.

Thus, Sodium Chloride and Dextrose Injection IP contains 27.8 mEq of Dextrose and 15.4 mEq of Sodium chloride per 100 ml.

Example **41:** Calculate the weight of the following salts containing 1 mEq wt of their ions: sodium phosphate, calcium chloride, magnesium sulphate.

Solution: Sodium phosphate, $Na_2HPO_4.12H_2O = 2Na^+ + HPO_4^{2-}$

Mol wt = 358,

Number of cations, $Na^+ = 2$, valency of Na+ =1,

So, the amount of sodium phosphate containing 1 mEq of $Na^+ = \dfrac{358}{2 \times 1} = 179$ mg

Similarly, No of anions, $HPO_4^{2-} = 1$, valency of $HPO_4^{2-} = 2$,

So, the amount of sodium phosphate containing 1 mEq of $HPO_4^{2-} = \dfrac{358}{1 \times 2} = 179$ mg

Calcium chloride, $CaCl_2.2H_2O = Ca^{2+} + 2Cl^-$

Mol wt = 147, No of cations = 1, valency of $Ca^{2+} = 2$

Amount of calcium chloride containing 1 mEq of $Ca^{2+} = \dfrac{147}{1 \times 2} = 73.5$ mg

No of anions = 2, valency of $Cl^- = 1$,

Amount of calcium chloride containing 1 mEq of $Cl^- = \dfrac{147}{1 \times 2} = 147$ mg

Magnesium sulphate, $MgSO_4.7H_2O = Mg^{2+} + SO_4^{2-}$

Mol wt = 246.3, No of cations = 1, valency of $Mg^{2+} = 2$

Amount of magnesium sulphate containing 1 mEq of $Mg^{2+} = \dfrac{246.3}{1 \times 2} = 123.15$ mg

No of anions = 1, valency of $SO_4^{2-} = 2$,

Amount of magnesium sulphate containing 1 mEq of $SO_4^{2-} = \dfrac{246.3}{2 \times 1} = 123.15$ mg

***Example* 42:** According to the IP there are two formulations for ORS. The composition of these is given below. Calculate the electrolyte composition of each formula in terms of mEq wt.

Each sachet contains

	ORS-A	ORS-Citrate
Sodium chloride	1.25 g	3.5 g
Potassium chloride	1.5 g	1.5 g
Sodium citrate	2.9 g	2.9 g
Dextrose, anhydrous	27.0 g	20.0 g

Solution:

Component	ORS-A	ORS-Citrate
Sodium Chloride, $NaCl = Na^+ + Cl^-$ Mol wt.= 23 + 35.5 = 58.5 Valency = 1	Eq wt = $\dfrac{58.5}{1}$; mEq = 58.5 mg mEq in 1.25 g or 1250 mg of NaCl $= \dfrac{1250}{58.5} = 21.38$ or 21.4 So, 21.4 mEqs of Na^+ ion and 21.4 mEqs of Cl^- ions are present.	Eq wt = $\dfrac{58.5}{1}$; mEq = 58.5mg mEq in 3.5 g or 3500 mg of NaCl $= \dfrac{3500}{58.5} = 59.83$ So, 59.83 mEqs of Na^+ ion and 59.83 mEqs of Cl^- ions are present.
Potassium Chloride, $KCl = K^+ + Cl^-$ Mol wt = 39 + 35.5 = 74.5 Valency = 1	Eq wt = $\dfrac{74.5}{1}$; mEq = 74.5 mg mEq in 1.5 g or 1500 mg of KCl $= \dfrac{1500}{74.5} = 20.13$ or 20.13 So, 20.13 mEqs of K^+ ion and 20.13 mEqs of Cl^- ions are present.	Eq wt = $\dfrac{74.5}{1}$; mEq = 74.5 mg mEq in 1.5g or 1500 mg of KCl $= \dfrac{1500}{74.5} = 20.13$ or 20.13 So, 20.13 mEqs of K^+ ion and 20.13 mEqs of Cl^- ions are present.
Sodium Citrate, $Na_3C_6H_5O_7$ $= 3Na^+ + C_6H_5O_7^{3-}$ Mol wt = 69 + 189 = 258 Valency = 3	Eq wt = $\dfrac{258}{3}$; mEq = 86 mg mEq in 2.9 g or 2900 mg of Na-citrate = $\dfrac{2900}{86} = 33.72$ So, 33.72 mEqs of Na^+ ion and 33.72 mEqs of $C_6H_5O_7^{3-}$ ions are present.	Eq wt = $\dfrac{258}{3}$; mEq = 86 mg mEq in 2.9 g or 2900 mg of Na-citrate = $\dfrac{2900}{86} = 33.72$ So, 33.72 mEqs of Na^+ ion and 33.72 mEqs of $C_6H_5O_7^{3-}$ ions are present.
Dextrose, Anhydrous $C_6H_{12}O_6$ Non-ionizing solute Mol wt = 180 Valency = 1	mEq wt = 180 mg mEq in 27g or 27000 mg of dextrose $= \dfrac{27000}{180} = 150$ So, 150 mEqs of $C_6H_{12}O_6$ are present.	mEq wt = 180 mg mEq in 20 g or 20000 mg of dextrose $= \dfrac{27000}{180} = 111.1$ or, 111 So, 111 mEqs of $C_6H_{12}O_6$ are present.
Total electrolyte composition is: Na^+ K^+ Cl^- $C_6H_5O_7^{3-}$ $C_6H_{12}O_6$	21.4 + 33.72 = 55.12 mEq 20.13 mEq 21.4 + 33.72 = 55.12 mEq 33.72 mEq 150 mEq	59.83 + 33.72 = 93.55 mEq 20.13 mEq 59.83 + 33.72 = 93.55 mEq 33.72 mEq 111 mEqs

Example **43:** Calculate the Eq wt of $KMnO_4$ at different mediums.

Solution: Molecular weight of KMnO4 = 158

1. **In acidic medium:** $2\ KMnO_4 + 3H_2SO_4 \rightarrow K_2SO_4 + 2MnSO4 + 3H_2O + 5O$

    Net reaction is MnO4–

    Change in Oxidation No $+7 \rightarrow +2 = 5$

    $$Eq\ wt = Eq\ wt = \frac{Molecular\ weight}{Changes\ in\ Oxidation\ No} = \frac{158}{5} = 31.6$$

2. **In neutral medium:** $2\ KMnO4 + H2O \rightarrow 2KOH + 2MnO2 + 3O$

    Net reaction is, $MnO^{4-} \rightarrow MnO2$

    Change in oxidation No $+7 \rightarrow +4 = 3$

    $$Eq\ wt = Eq\ wt = \frac{Molecular\ weight}{Changes\ in\ Oxidation\ No} = \frac{158}{3} = 52.67$$

3. **In alkaline medium:**

    Net reaction is, $MnO^{4-} \rightarrow MnO^{2-}$

    Change in Oxidation No. $+7 \rightarrow +6 = 1$

    $$Eq\ wt = \frac{Molecular\ weight}{Change\ in\ Oxidation\ No} = \frac{158}{1} = 158$$

$$\boxed{Equivalent\ wt\ of\ Oxidizing/Reducing\ substance = \frac{Molecular\ weight}{Change\ in\ Oxidation\ No}}$$

Osmolarity and Osmolality

Osmolarity: Millimoles of solute per liter (L) of solution, it is a measures of osmotic concentration.

Osmolality: Millimoles of solute per kilogram (kg) of solvent,

$$mOsmol/L = \frac{Concentation\ of\ Substance\ (g/L)}{Mol.\ wt\ (g)} \times Nos.\ of\ species \times 1000$$

Note: During such calculation the factors like solvation and interionic forces are not taken into consideration.

Example 44: The composition of a Ringer's lactate solution is as follows:

Each 1000 ml contains:

Dextrose monohydrate IP 50 g

Sodium chloride IP 6 g

Potassium chloride IP 0.3 g

Calcium chloride IP 0.2 g

Sodium lactate IP 3.1 g

Express the ionic concentration in terms of mOsmol/L.

Solution:

Dextrose, Monohydrate

Mol wt of dextrose monohydrate $= 180 + 18 = 198$

Its concentration $= 50$ g/L

Number of species it produces $= 1$

So, mOsmol of dextrose/L $= \times 1 \times 1000 = 252.52$

Sodium chloride

Mol wt of sodium chloride $= 58.5$

Its concentration $= 6$ g/L

Number of species it produces $= 2$ $(Na^+$ and $Cl^-)$

So, mOsmol of sodium chloride/L $= \dfrac{6}{58.5} \times 2 \times 1000 = 205.12$ or 205

Since, NaCl produces two species, its ionic concentration $= \dfrac{205}{2} = 102.5$

So, concentration of Na^+ ion is 102.5 mOsmol/L and concentration of Cl^- ion is 102.5 mOsmol/L.

Potassium chloride

Mol wt of potassium chloride $= 74.5$

Its concentration $= 0.3$ g/L

Number of species it produces $= 2$ $(K^+$ and Cl^- ion)

So, mOsmol of potassium chloride/L $= \dfrac{0.3}{74.5} \times 2 \times 1000 = 8.05$

Since, KCl produces two species, its ionic concentration $= \dfrac{8.05}{2} = 4.025$

So, concentration of K^+ ion is 4.025 mOsmol/L and concentration of Cl^- ion is 4.025 mOsmol/L.

Calcium chloride, $CaCl_2.2H_2O$

Mol wt of calcium chloride $= 147$

Its concentration $= 0.2$ g/L

Number of species it produces = 3 (Ca^{2+} and $2Cl^{-}$ ions)

So, mOsmol of Calcium chloride/L = $\dfrac{0.2}{147} \times 3 \times 1000 = 4.08$

Since, $CaCl_2$ produces three species, its ionic concentration = $\dfrac{4.08}{3} = 1.36$

So, concentration of Ca^{+} ion is 1.36 mOsmol/L and concentration of Cl^{-} ion is $1.36 \times 2 = 2.72$ mOsmol/L.

Sodium lactate, $NaC_6H_9O_5$

Mol wt of sodium lactate = 112

Its concentration = 3.1 g/L

Number of species it produces = 2 ($Na+$ and $C_6H_9O_5^{-}$ ion)

So, mOsmol of Sodium lactate/L = $\dfrac{3.1}{112} \times 2 \times 1000 = 55.357$ or, 55.36

Since, $NaC_6H_9O_5$ produces two species, its ionic concentration = $\dfrac{55.36}{2} = 27.68$

So, concentration of Na^{+} ion is 27.68 mOsmol/L and concentration of $C_6H_9O_5^{-}$ ion is 27.68 mOsmol/L.

Thus, the total ionic concentrations of the given Ringer's lactate solution are:

Ion /solute	Concentration (mOsmol/L)	Total concentration (mOsmol/L)
Dextrose	252.5	252.5
Sodium	102.5 + 27.68 = 130.18	130.2
Potassium	4.025	4.025
Calcium	1.36	1.36
Chloride	102.5 + 4.025 + 2.72 = 109.285	109.245
Lactate	27.68	27.68

***Example* 45:** The concentration of Ca^{2+} in a sample is 15 mg%. Calculate its concentration in terms of millimoles per L?

***Solution*:**

Atomic wt of Ca^{2+} = 40

15 mg% = 15 mg in 100 ml = 150 mg in 1000 ml = 0.15 g/L

mOsmol/L = $\dfrac{0.15\,g\,/\,L}{40g} \times 1 \times 1000 = 3.75$

Thus, per liter of solution there are 3.75 mOsmol of Ca^{2+}

Adjustment of Tonicity

There are four methods:

1. Freezing point depression method

2. Sodium chloride equivalence method, and

3. Molecular concentration method

4. Graphical method utilizing vapor pressure and freezing point data.

Freezing Point Depression Method

The blood plasma and tears freeze at -0.52°C. In other words, the dissolved substances of these fluids can depress the freezing point of pure water by 0.52°C. So, any solution that can depress the freezing point of pure water by 0.52°C will have the same osmotic pressure as blood plasma or tears, and thus, will be isotonic to blood plasma or tear fluids and it is considered that an iso-osmotic solution will be isotonic also. All hypotonic solutions will have higher freezing points. So, to adjust the tonicity of the preparation an adjusting substance is to be added to the solution

---

The working formulas:
A. When there is no other substance to adjust tonicity, the amount of the substance to be calculated as;

$$\text{The amount required} = \frac{0.52}{x}$$

Where, x is the freezing point depression of 1% solution of the substance.
B. When another substance is required to adjust the tonicity of a solution containing one ingredient,

$$\text{The amount of adjusting substance required} = \frac{0.52 - a}{b}$$

Where, a = Freezing point depression of 1% solution of the ingredient, b = Freezing point depression of 1% solution of the adjusting substance.
C. When another substance is required to adjust the tonicity of a solution containing more than one ingredient,

$$\text{The amount of adjusting substance required} = \frac{0.52 - ac}{b}$$

Where, a = Sum of freezing point depression of 1% solution of all the ingredients,
c = Sum of concentration of all the ingredients, and
b = Freezing point depression of 1% solution of the adjusting substance

---

Example **46:** What concentration of morphine hydrochloride would be iso-osmotic with blood plasma.

Solution: The freezing point depression produced by 1% solution of morphine hydrochloride is 0.086°C.

So, the percentage concentration (% w/v) of morphine hydrochloride

$$= \frac{0.52}{0.086} = 6.046.$$

Thus, 6.05% w/v solution of morphine hydrochloride will be iso-osmotic to blood plasma.

Example **47:** What concentration of sodium chloride would be iso-osmotic with blood plasma.

Solution:

The freezing point depression by 1% solution of sodium chloride is 0.576°C.

So, the percentage concentration (% w/v) of sodium chloride to be required

$$= \frac{0.52}{0.576} = 0.902$$

Thus, 0.9% w/v solution of sodium chloride will be iso-osmotic to blood plasma.

Example **48:** How much quantity of sodium chloride would be required to make 1% solution of morphine hydrochloride iso-osmotic to blood plasma?

Solution: The freezing point depression by 1% solution of morphine hydrochloride is 0.086°C and the freezing point depression by 1% solution of sodium chloride is 0.576°C.

So, % w/v of sodium chloride to be required $= \dfrac{0.52 - 0.086}{0.576} = 0.753$

Thus, 0.753% w/v solution of sodium chloride is to be added to 1% solution of morphine hydrochloride.

In other words, 1.0 g of morphine hydrochloride and 0.753 g of sodium chloride are to be present per 100 ml of solution.

Example **49:** Calculate the concentration of sodium chloride to be added to make 2% solution of quinine hydrochloride solution to make the solution iso-osmotic with blood plasma.

Solution: The freezing point depression by 1% solution of quinine hydrochloride is 0.077°C and the freezing point depression by 1% solution of sodium chloride is 0.576°C.

The amount of adjusting substance required $= \dfrac{0.52 - ac}{b}$

$$\text{So, \% w/v of sodium chloride to be required} = \frac{0.52 - 0.077 \times 2}{0.576} = 0.635$$

Thus, 0.635% w/v solution of sodium chloride is to be added to 2% solution of quinine hydrochloride to make the solution iso-osmotic with blood plasma.

Example **50:** A 50 ml solution contains 0.75 g of Pethidine hydrochloride and 0.01 g of sodium metabisulphite. Calculate the quantity of sodium chloride to be required to make the solution iso-osmotic (use freezing point depression method).

Solution: The concentration of Pethidine hydrochloride in % w/v $= \dfrac{0.75 \times 100}{50} = 1.5$

$$\text{Concentration of sodium Metabisulphite} = \frac{0.01 \times 100}{50} = 0.02$$

The freezing point depression by 1% solution of sodium chloride is 0.576°C,

Freezing point depression by 1% solution of sodium metabisulphite is 0.386°C.

Freezing point depression by 1% solution of Pethidine hydrochloride is 0.125°C.

$$\text{The amount of adjusting substance required} = \frac{0.52 - ac}{b}$$

$$ac = 1.5 \times 0.125 + 0.02 \times 0.386 = 0.1952$$

$$\text{So, \% w/v of sodium chloride to be required} = \frac{0.52 - 0.195}{0.576} = 0.564$$

Thus, 0.564 g of sodium chloride is to be added to 100 ml of the solution.

Sodium Chloride Equivalence Method

This method uses a factor, called sodium chloride equivalence, for conversion of a particular concentration of substance equivalent to the concentration of sodium chloride iso-osmotic to the blood plasma. The sodium chloride equivalent can be defined as *the weight of sodium chloride that will effect the same osmotic pressure as 1 g of a drug or substance.*

$$\text{This is calculated as: } \frac{\text{Freezing point depression by 1\% solution of the substance}}{\text{Freezing point depression by 1\% solution of sodium chloride}}$$

For example, sodium chloride equivalents of 1% potassium chloride solution

$$= \frac{\text{Freezing point depression by 1\% solution of potassium chloride}}{\text{Freezing point depression by 1\% solution of sodium chloride}} = \frac{0.439}{0.576} = 0.762$$

Hence, percentage (% w/v) of sodium chloride to be required to make 1% potassium chloride solution iso-osmotic to blood plasma = 0.9 – (sodium chloride equivalents of 1% potassium chloride solution × concentration)

$$= 0.9 - (0.76 \times 1.0)$$

$$= 0.9 - 0.76$$

$$= 0.14$$

Note:

1. 0.9% solution of sodium chloride is isotonic.

2. A list of sodium chloride equivalents (E), freezing point depression values (D) of 1% solution of some common substances has been given in **Annexure-V.**

Example **51**: How much sodium chloride would be necessary to make 50 ml solution of 1% Gentamycin sulphate isotonic? (Use *sodium chloride equivalence method*).

Solution:

0.9% solution of sodium chloride is isotonic.

50 ml solution containing $50 \times \dfrac{0.9}{100}$ g = 0.45g of sodium chloride would alone be required to make the solution isotonic.

50 ml solution contains 1% Gentamycin sulphate, means $50 \times \dfrac{1.0}{100}$ g = 0.5g Sodium chloride equivalent of 1% of Gentamycin sulphate solution is 0.05.

Now, sodium chloride would be required to make the solution isotonic

$$= 0.45g - \left[\frac{0.05}{1} \times \frac{0.5}{100} \times 50\right] g$$

$$= 0.45g - 0.0125g$$

$$= 0.4375g \text{ or, } 0.44g$$

Hence, 0.44 g of sodium chloride is to be added.

Example 52: Calculate the quantity of sodium chloride needed to make 20ml of a solution isotonic containing 0.2 g of morphine sulphate, 0.008 g of Hyoscine hydrochloride and 0.02 g of sodium metabisulphite? *(use sodium chloride equivalence method)*.

Solution:

Concentrations of the ingredients are calculated as follows:

Morphine sulphate: $\dfrac{0.2 \times 100}{20} = 1.0\%$ w/v

$$\text{Hyoscine hydrochloride} = \frac{0.008 \times 100}{20} = 0.04\% \text{w/v}$$

$$\text{Sodium metabisulphite} = \frac{0.02 \times 100}{20} = 0.1\% \text{ w/v}$$

Sodium chloride equivalents of 1% solution of morphine sulphate = 0.14

1% solution of Hyoscine hydrochloride = 0.12

1% solution of sodium metabisulphite = 0.67

So, percent of sodium chloride to be required to make 100 ml of the solution Iso-osmotic

$$= 0.9 - [(1 \times 0.14) + (0.04 \times 0.12) + (0.1 \times 0.67)]$$
$$= 0.9 - (0.14 + 0.0048 + 0.067)$$
$$= 0.9 - 0.2118$$
$$= 0.6882 \text{ or } 0.69$$

For 20 ml of the solution, $\dfrac{0.69 \times 20}{100} = 0.138$ g of sodium chloride would be required

Molecular Concentration Method

According to the colligative properties, one gram molecule of a nonionizing solute dissolved in 22.4 liters of water will have osmotic pressure of 1 atm at normal pressure and temperature. In other words, one molar solution of a non-ionizing solute will have osmotic pressure of 22.4 atm.

The osmotic pressure of blood plasma and tear fluids is approximately 6.7 atm.

Or, the concentration of these fluids will be $\dfrac{6.7}{22.4} = 0.299$ or, 0.3M (approx).

So, 0.3 M solution of any non-ionizing solute will be iso-osmotic with body fluids.

For non-ionizing solute the amount required per Lt = 0.3 × Mol wt.

While for ionizing solute, the amount to be required per litre

$$= \frac{0.3 \times \text{Mol wt}}{\text{Nos. of ions produced per molecule}} = \frac{0.3\text{M}}{\text{N}}$$

Example 53: At which concentrations (%w/v) solutions of dextrose anhydrous would be isotonic with blood plasma? (*Use molar concentration method*).

Solution:

The molecular weight of dextrose anhydrous = 180

Since, this is a non-ionizing solutes, the required amount of dextrose anhydrous per liter = 180 × 0.3 = 54 g, or, 5.4 g per 100 ml (5.4% w/v or 5% approx.)

***Example* 54:** At which concentrations (% w/v) the solutions of sodium chloride and calcium chloride would be isotonic with blood plasma? (*use molar concentration method*).

***Solution*:**

Mol wt of sodium chloride is 58.5 and that of calcium chloride (dehydrate) is 147.

Both of them ionize in water as follows:

$NaCl = Na^+ + Cl^-$, the no. of ions are 2

$CaCl_2 = Ca^{2+} + 2Cl^-$, the no. of ions are 3

Hence, the amount of sodium chloride required per liter to make the solution iso-osmotic

$$= \frac{58.5 \times 0.3}{2} \, g/L \, g/L$$
$$= 8.775 \, g/L \text{ or } 9 \, g/L,$$

That is, 0.9g per 100ml, or 0.9 % w/v.

Similarly, the amount of calcium chloride required per Lt to make the solution iso-osmotic $= \frac{147 \times 0.3}{3} \, g/L$

$$= 14.7g/L \text{ or, } 15g/L$$

That is, 1.5g per 100ml, or 1.5 % w/v.

Dose Calculation

There are various rules for conversion of adult dose to child dose. The rules are given below:

Young's Rule: Child dose $= \dfrac{\text{Age in year}}{\text{Age} + 12} \times \text{Adult dose}$

Fried's Rule: Child dose $= \dfrac{\text{Age in month} \times \text{Adult dose}}{150}$

Drilling's Rule: Child dose $= \dfrac{\text{Age in year} \times \text{Adult dose}}{12}$

Clark's Rule: Child dose $= \dfrac{\text{Weight in lbs} \times \text{Adult dose}}{150}$

$$\text{Child dose} = \dfrac{\text{Body surface area of child} \times \text{Adult dose}}{\text{Body surface area of adult}}$$

$$\text{Child dose} = \dfrac{\text{Body surface area of child} \times \text{Adult dose}}{173\text{M}^2}$$

Example 55: The adult dose of a drug is 500 mg. Calculate the dose of a child whose age is 8 yrs using different formulas.

Solution:

According to Drilling's Rule, Child dose $= \dfrac{\text{Age in year} \times \text{Adult dose}}{12} = \dfrac{8 \times 500\text{mg}}{12}$

$$= 333.33\text{mg}$$

According to Young's Rule, Child dose $= \dfrac{\text{Age in year}}{\text{Age} + 12} \times \text{Adult dose} = \dfrac{8}{8+12} \times$

500 mg $= 200$ mg

According to Fried's Rule, Child dose $= \dfrac{\text{Age in month} \times \text{Adult dose}}{150} = \dfrac{8 \times 12 \times 500 \text{ mg}}{150}$

$= 320$ mg

Example 56: The adult dose of a drug is 500 mg. Calculate the dose of a child whose body wt is 12 kg.

Solution: According to Clark's Rule, Child dose $= \dfrac{\text{Weight in lbs} \times \text{Adult dose}}{150}$

$= \dfrac{26.4 \times 500 \text{ mg}}{150} = 88\text{mg}$ [1 kg = 2.2 lbs, 12 kg = 12×2.2 lbs = 26.4 lbs]

Temperature

In Centigrade degrees, the scale operates from 0° to 100°C

In Fahrenheit degrees, the scale operates from 32° to 212°F

Hence, the relation between these two scales is $\dfrac{^\circ\text{C} - 0}{100} = \dfrac{^\circ\text{F} - 32}{180}$

Example **57:** Convert 30°C into °F.

Solution: Say, 30°C = B°F

Then,
$$\frac{B-32}{180} = \frac{30-0}{100}$$

Or,
$$\frac{B-32}{9} = \frac{30}{5}$$

Or,
$$B - 32 = \frac{30 \times 9}{5} = 54$$

$$B = 54 + 32 = 86 \ °F$$

So,
$$30°C = 86°F$$

Example **58:** Convert 84°F into °C.

Solution:

Say,
$$B°C = 84°F$$

Then,
$$\frac{B-32}{180} = \frac{30-0}{100}$$

Or,
$$\frac{B}{5} = \frac{84-32}{9} = \frac{52}{9}$$

Or,
$$B = \frac{52 \times 5}{9} = 28.88 \quad \text{or, } 28.9°C$$

Thus, 84 °F = 28.9°C

Example **59:** The temperature scale in Doctor's thermometer was in °F (degree Fahrenheit) ranging from 92.3°F to 110°F. To convert it into °C (degree Centigrade) Find out the range. The body temperature is 37°C. What would be in °F.

Solution: In Fahrenheit scale, the initial temperature of the thermometer = 92.3°F,

Say, 92.3°F = A°C

$$\frac{A-0}{100} = \frac{92.3-32}{180}$$

or,
$$\frac{A}{5} = \frac{60.3}{9}$$

or,
$$A = \frac{60.3 \times 5}{9} = 33.5°C$$

Thus, the initial temperature in Doctor's thermometer in centigrade scale is 33.5°C.

In Fahrenheit scale, the highest temperature of the thermometer = 110°F,

Say, 110°F = B°C

$$\frac{B-0}{100} = \frac{110-32}{180}$$

or,
$$\frac{B}{5} = \frac{78}{9}$$

or,
$$B = \frac{78 \times 5}{9} = 43.3°C$$

Thus, the highest temperature in Doctor's thermometer in centigrade scale is 43.3°C.

The normal body temperature is 37 °C

Say, 37 °C = X°F

$$\frac{X-32}{180} = \frac{37-0}{100}$$

Or,
$$\frac{X-32}{9} = \frac{37}{5}$$

Or,
$$X - 32 = \frac{37 \times 9}{5} = 66.6$$

Or, $$X = 66.6 + 32 = 98.6°F$$

Thus, 37°C = 98.6°F

Exercises

1. Calculate the sensitivity of a chemical balance which can weigh a minimum quantity of 1 mg with an error of 1%.

    Ans. 0.01

2. What would be the error, if a balance can weigh 0.1 mg with a sensitivity of 0.001?

    Ans. 1%

3. 1,00,000 tablets of Aspirin need to be compressed with a potency of 100% and each tablet shall contain 325 mg of Aspirin. The supplied Aspirin has the potency of 98.87%. Calculate the quantity of Aspirin required for the lot.

    Ans. 32.857 kg

4. The granules of paracetamol tablet contain 78.95% of paracetamol. Each tablet shall contain 500 mg of the drug. Calculate the average weight of the tablets.

Ans. 633.31 mg

5. Total weight of granules prepared for a tablet formulation is 68.5 kg. The drug content is 68.75%. Calculate the lot size.

Ans. 47.094 kg

6. To adjust the viscosity of a liquid preparation 25 kg of liquid glucose is to be added. The density of liquid glucose is 1.44 g/ml. How many litre of liquid glucose are to be added?

Ans. 17.36 L

7. The bulk density of tetracycline HCl supplied is 0.689 g/ml. Select the size of capsule for filling 250 mg of the drug. The average fill volume of size 0, size 1 and size 2 capsules are 0.68, 0.50 and 0.37ml respectively.

Ans. Size 2

8. Salbutamol sulphate syrup contains 2 mg of salbutamol per 5 ml. 1 mg of salbutamol sulphate is equivalent to 830 µg of salbutamol. Calculate the amount of salbutamol sulphate required to prepare 50 liters of its syrup.

Ans. 24.1 g

9. A drug has the potency of 590 µg per mg on dried basis and its loss on drying is 4.92%. If an eye drop containing 0.3% of the drug is to be prepared. Calculate the amount of drug required for preparing a lot of 25 liters.

Ans. 0.134 kg

10. Calciferol Injection should contain 7.5 mg of cholecalciferol per ml. The supplied drug has a potency of 98.25%. The bulk solution contains 7.75 mg/ml. It is required to add 5% of overage also. Calculate the quantity of the drug to be further added to a lot of 50 liters.

Ans. 6.36 g

11. According to the manufacturing formula 100 capsules contain:

    (a) Thiamine mononitrate IP 450 mg

    (b) Riboflavin IP 500 mg

    (c) Pyridoxine hydrochloride IP 150 mg

    (d) Cyanocobalamine IP 500 mcg

(e)   Niacinamide IP 4.50 g

(f)   Calcium D-pantothenate USP 500 mg

(g)   Enlarge the formula for 250 capsules.

(h)   Reduce the formula for 24 capsules.

Ans. (a) 1.125 g, 1.25 g, 375 mg, 1.25 mg, 11.25 g, 1.25 g

(b) 108 mg, 120 mg, 36 mg, 120 mcg, 1.08 g, 120 mg

12.   According to the manufacturing formula each tablet contains 2 mg of Magnesium stearate. The average weight of tablet is 465 mg. Calculate the content of Magnesium stearate in % w/w per tablet.

Ans. 0.43% w/w

13.   13.4 liters of syrup contains 380 ml of alcohol. Calculate the concentration of alcohol in terms of % v/v.

Ans. 9.5%

14.   2.5 liters of a solution contains 360 ml of glycerin. Calculate the concentration of glycerin in terms of % w/v. Density of glycerin is 1.28 g/ml.

Ans. 18.43% w/v

15.   15. A sample of water is found to contain 2 ppm of lead, 5 ppm of iron and 25 ppm of chloride. The volume of water is 25 L. Express the concentration of these in terms of % w/v.

Ans. 0.005% of lead, 0.0125% of iron and 0.0625% of chloride.

16.   The weight of vitamins mixture is 6.0kg. It contains 138 mcg of vitamin B12. Find out the concentration of vitamin B_{12} in terms of % w/w.

Ans. 0.0023%

17.   The drug content of two lots of granules, A and B, are 41% and 49% respectively. At which proportion the two lots should be mixed to prepare 2.5 kg of the granules containing 47% of the drug?

Ans. 0.625 kg of lot A and 1.875 kg of lot B (Ratio 1:3)

18.   18. The drug content of three lots of metronidazole granules - A, B and C are 32%, 36% and 41% respectively. How much quantity of each shall be mixed to prepare 5.0 kg of metronidazole granules containing 35% of the drug?

Ans. 2.69 kg of lot A, 1.15 kg of lot B and 1.15 kg of lot C (ratio 7:3:3)

19. Three lots of diluted alcohol, A, B and C containing 15%, 16% and 20% of alcohol respectively. Calculate the quantity of each lot to be mixed to prepare 3.0 liters of diluted alcohol containing 18.75% of alcohol.

Ans. 484 ml of lot A, 1064 ml of lot B and 1452 ml of lot C

20. Two lots of iodine solutions A and B having concentrations 9.75% and 10.65% are mixed at a ratio of 3:1to prepare 15 lts. Calculate the concentration of the final iodine solution.

Ans. 10%

21. A 45.5 L of 35% of alcohol has been prepared by mixing 22.4 L of 32% alcohol (A), 10.8 L of 36% alcohol (B) and 12.3 L of 41% alcohol (C). Find out the proportion of mixing using method of Aligation.

Ans. A : B : C :: 7 : 3 : 3

22. The adult dose of Ciprofloxacin is 500 mg. Calculate the Child's dose when the child is 6 years old using different formula.

Ans. 250 mg or 240 mg or 167 mg.

23. An elixir contains 10.5% v/v of ethyl alcohol. Express the concentration of ethyl alcohol in terms of proof strength.

Ans. 81.6 °up

24. One liquid preparation contains 85% of ethyl alcohol. Express the concentration of ethyl alcohol in terms of proof.

Ans. 48.9 °up

25. The alcohol content of a liquid preparation is 25° op. Express the concentration of alcohol in terms of % v/v.

Ans. 71.3%

26. The composition of sodium chloride and dextrose injection IP is as follows:

27. Each 100 ml contains:

Dextrose monohydrate IP 5 g

Sodium chloride IP 0.9 g

28. Express the ionic concentration in terms of mOsmol/L.

Ans. 252.5 mOsmol of Dextrose per liter, 205.1 mOsmol of Na+ ion and 205.1 mOsmol of Cl- ion per liter

29. Sodium chloride and dextrose injection IP contains 5.0 g of dextrose anhydrous and 0.9 g of sodium chloride per 100 ml. Calculate the concentrations in terms of mEq/100 ml.

Ans. 27.8 mEq of Dextrose /100ml and 15.4 mEq of NaCl /100 ml

30. The concentration of Ca^{2+} in a sample is 35 mg%. Calculate its concentration in terms of milliosmoles per L?

Ans. 8.75 mOsmol of Ca^{2+} per liter

31. At which concentration (% w/v) solution of metronidazole would be isotonic with blood plasma? (Use *molar concentration method,* mol wt of metronidazole 171.15 g/mole)

Ans. 5% w/v solution

32. At which concentrations (% w/v) the solutions of potassium chloride and calcium chloride would be isotonic with blood plasma? (use *molar concentration method,* mol wt of KCl is 74.55 g/mole & of $CaCl_2$ is 147.01 g/mole)

Ans. 1.1% solution of potassium chloride and 1.5% solution of calcium chloride

9 Incompatibilities

Many drugs in their official or proprietary preparations are given alone, but frequently many are given in combination. There are few which should never be given in combination with other drugs. The selection of drugs and preparations to be used in combination with each other requires a great care to avoid unwanted changes or action brought about by their admixture.

When two or more antagonistic substances are mixed, an undesirable product may be formed which can affect safety, purpose and appearance of the product. Such mixing may be done as per the prescription or manufacturing formula. Incompatibility of one substance with another is an intrinsic property of the particular substance. Incompatibility may occur between two drugs, two excipients, or between a drug with an excipient and it may be observed in two situations – prescription and formulation.

Incompatibility may be of three types:

- Physical
- Chemical, and
- Therapeutic

Incompatibility in Formulation

Physical Incompatibility

During formulation development, preformulation is the first step. The physical and chemical properties of the drug substance alone and in combination with excipients are assessed. This test is called compatibility test. The drug substance is commonly mixed with different excipients for the following purposes:

- To improve manufacturing of the formulation,
- To maximize the product's ability to administer correct dose of the drug.
- To facilitate administration
- To release the active component at desired site at desired rate, and sometimes,
- To stabilize the formulation against degradation from the environment.

Most of the excipients do not have direct pharmacological action but, they can modify useful properties of the formulation. However, they can be responsible for degradation of the drug also. Such problem occurs unintentionally.

Physical and chemical interactions between drugs and excipients can affect the chemical nature, the stability and bio-availability of drug products, and consequently, their therapeutic efficacy and safety. There are several approaches for screening drug-excipient chemical compatibility. The most useful and time saving approach is computational, which can predict drug-excipient chemical compatibility. This requires a complete database of reactive functional groups of drug and excipients, their potential impurities, and in-depth knowledge about the excipients. However, the use of this computational approach only as the sole source of information is not sufficient.

Binary mixture compatibility testing is another approach which is commonly used. In this approach, binary (1:1 or customized) mixtures of the drug and excipient are prepared with or without water. Sometimes the mixture is compacted or prepared in the form of slurry. These are then stored under stressed conditions (also known as isothermal stress testing, IST) and analyzed using a stability-indicating method, e.g. high performance liquid chromatography (HPLC). When the slurry is prepared the pH of the drug-excipient blend and the role of moisture are also investigated. Alternatively, the binary mixtures can be screened using other thermal methods, such as differential scanning calorimetry (DSC). DSC is currently the leading technique for this purpose.

There are several examples of formulation instability due to solid–solid interactions. Certain classes of compounds are known to be incompatible with particular excipients. Therefore, knowledge of the chemistry of the drug substance and excipients can often minimize formulation incompatibilities.

- Heat and water are primarily responsible (catalysts) for drug excipient interactions. They play a critical role in the degradation of a drug substance. The majority of instability reactions of 'small molecule' API (Active Pharmaceutical Ingredient) occur through hydrolysis, oxidation and Maillard reaction.

- The moisture content of the drug and excipients alone can play a critical role in their incompatibility. Heat and moisture accelerate most reactions; moisture brings molecules closer together, and heat increases the reaction rate. Excipients such as starch and povidone may possess a high water content (the equilibrium moisture content of povidone is about 28% at 75% relative humidity), which can increase drug degradation. The moisture level will affect the stability depending on how strongly it is bound and whether it can come into contact with the drug. It is generally recognized that aspirin is incompatible with magnesium salts. Higher moisture contents and humidity accelerate the degradation even further.

- Many excipients are hygroscopic, and absorb water during manufacturing; for example during wet granulation. Depending on the degree of hydrolytic susceptibility, different approaches to tablet granulation can be used to minimize hydrolysis. For example, acetylsalicylic acid readily hydrolyzes; hence, direct compression or dry granulation is recommended.

Chemical Incompatibility

Chemical interaction between the drug and excipients may lead to increased decomposition. The degradation may be due to hydrolysis, oxidation, aldehyde amine addition etc. For example,

- **Hydrolysis:** Salts of stearic acid (e.g. magnesium stearate, sodium stearate) are avoided as tablet lubricants if the drug is hydrolysable via ion-catalyzed degradation. Excipients generally contain more free moisture than the drug substance. Therefore, formulation can potentially expose the drug substance to higher levels of moisture than normal and the possibility of degradation of even stable compounds increases. In selecting excipients, it is probably best to avoid hygroscopic excipients when formulating hydrolysable compounds. However, the drug can be formulated with over-dried hygroscopic excipients (e.g. Starch 1500) to prevent the drug from coming into contact with water.

- **Humidity** is another major factor that can affect stability in solid dosage forms. Increase of relative humidity usually decreases the stability, particularly for drugs that are highly sensitive to hydrolysis. For example, nitrazepam in the solid state can degrade by interaction with excipients. Molecular mobility is also responsible for solid-solid reactions. Systems with enhanced mobility have more reactivity. Mechanical stress is also expected to accelerate such reactions by creating a larger surface area, increasing the number of defects, and increasing the amount of amorphous material.

- **Oxidation** reactions are complex and it can be difficult to understand the reaction mechanism. The best approach is to avoid excipients containing oxidative reactants such as peroxides and fumed metal oxides like fumed silica and fumed titanium dioxide. Excipients such as povidone and polyethylene glycols (PEGs) may contain organic peroxides as synthetic by-products which are typically more reactive than hydrogen peroxide. Although most compendial excipients have limits on metals, free ethylene oxide or other oxidizing agents via the peroxide or iodine value there are still some instances of oxidative degradation of drug due to presence of reactive peroxides in excipients such as povidone. For example, oxidative degradation of Raloxifene HCl occurs via peroxide impurities in povidone. Thus, it is important to understand the purity and composition of the excipient prior to formulation.

- **Aldehyde-amine addition** is another important type of reaction, which is responsible for incompatibility between excipients comprising reducing sugars (e.g. lactose, dextrose) and amine-containing drugs. Aldehyde-amine addition leads to the formation of a Schiff base, which further cyclizes to form a glucosamine followed by an Amadori rearrangement. This sequence of reactions is called the Maillard reaction, and is responsible for a large number of incompatibilities between APIs and excipients.

Common solid-state incompatibilities are shown in Table 9.1.

TABLE 9.1

List of common solid-state incompatibilities

Functional Group of the Drug	Incompatible With	Type of Reaction
Primary amine (e.g. Acyclovir)	Mono and disaccharides (e.g. lactose)	Mail lard reaction
Esters (e.g. Moexipril)	Basic components (e.g. magnesium hydroxide)	Ester hydrolysis
Lactone (e.g. Irinotecan HCl)	Basic components (e.g. magnesium hydroxide)	Ring opening (hydrolysis)
Carboxyl	Bases	Salt formation
Alcohol (e.g. Morphine)	Oxygen	Oxidation to aldehydes and ketones
Sulfhydryl (e.g. Captopril)	Oxygen	Dimerization
Phenol	Metals, Polyplasdone	Complexation
Gelatin	Cationic surfactants	Denaturation

Some of the common excipients or groups of excipients which have been found to be incompatible with drugs are given below.

- **Poly-saccharides:** Lactose is a reducing disaccharide and reactions between it and drugs containing amino groups have been reported. Lactose is one of the most common excipients in pharmaceutical oral dosage forms (tablets) and, is available in crystalline and amorphous forms. Spray dried lactose has been found to interact with dextroamphetamine sulfate.

  In fact, there are a number of reports of the incompatibility between lactose and amine-containing drugs such as aminophylline, ranitidine HCl, thiamine HCl, and acceclofenac, etc.

- **Stearates:** Magnesium stearate is widely used as a lubricant in the manufacture of pharmaceutical solid dosage forms. There are numerous reports of the incompatibility between stearates and drugs; such as aspirin, captopril, metformin, amlodipine, etc. Binary mixtures of metformin with starch and lactose showed interaction upon heating, changing the melting point of metformin. Captopril is a pyrrolidine carboxylic acid derivative used in the treatment of hypertension. It shows surface interactions with metallic stearates during grinding.

- **Povidone (Polyvinyl pyrrolidone, PVP):** In tablet formulation PVP is commonly used as a binder, as a film forming agent, and also for forming amorphous dispersions of drugs. It has been found to be incompatible with a wide range of drugs, such as sulphathiazole, oxprenolol, atenolol, haloperidol, indomethacin, ketoprofen, clenbuterol and temazepam, etc.

- **Dicalcium phosphate dihydrate (DCP):** It is commonly used as filler in tablet formulation and as a dental polishing agent in toothpaste. It has been found to be incompatible with various acidic drugs and sodium salt of poorly water soluble drugs due to its alkaline nature. For example, temazepam is acidic in nature with pKa of 1.61 interacts with DCP. Other drugs which are incompatible with DCP are oxprenolol hydrochloride, ceronapril, β-lapachone, Famotidine, nalidixic acid, quinapril and metronidazole.

- **Eudragit polymers:** These are copolymers obtained from esters of acrylic and methacrylic acid. These are available in different physical forms and widely used for making targeted and controlled release drug delivery systems. Certain drugs have been found incompatible with some Eudragit polymers. For example, ibuprofen, diflunisal, flurbiprofen, piroxicam are incompatible with Eudragit RS100 and RL100. A mild interaction between ranitidine and Eudragit E100, omeprazole and Eudragit L100 has been reported.

- **Celluloses:** In various oral and topical formulations methylcellulose is used. It is extensively used in cosmetics and food products also. MCC is used as filler in tablets and as thickener and stabilizer in processed foods. Based on the grade, HPMC is used in tablets, capsules, and in controlled release products for different purposes. MCC and several other cellulosic products such as starch, sodium starch glycolate, crospovidone, and croscarmillose sodium have been found to accelerate degradation of enalapril maleate. Isosorbide mononitrate interacts with cellulose acetate and MCC. Trichlormethiazide is stable in a solid state under humid conditions, but its tablet containing HPMC is not stable under the same conditions. Trichlormethiazide degrades faster in presence of hydroxypropyl cellulose (HPC).

- **Polyethylene glycol (PEG):** As a lubricant, cosolvent, dispersing agent PEG has been widely used in different pharmaceutical formulations. But, it also been found to cause degradation some drugs. In degradation of drugs its purity plays an important role. PEG of high purity hardly causes degradation. Ibuprofen degrades in tablets made with PEG. Similarly, aspirin undergoes pseudo-first order decomposition in presence of various grades of PEG.

  When suppository of indomethacin is prepared using PEG, indomethacin decomposes. Other drugs such as ketoprofen, calcium phosphomycin, etc. have been reported to interact with PEG and decompose.

- **Polysorbate 80:** It is commercially known as Tween 80. It is a nonionic surfactant and widely used as emulsifier in pharmaceutical and food preparations. At higher temperature in the presence of air it can affect the stability of oxidation prone drugs such as ibuprofen.

- **Sodium Lauryl Sulphate (SLS):** In tablet it is used to enhance the solubility of poorly soluble drugs. It acts as a surfactant or wetting agent. It is incompatible with certain drugs such as chlopropamide, chlordiazepoxide, clopidogrel besylate, etc.
- **Chitosan:** In a study of developing controlled release tablet of diclofenac sodium chitosan has been found to inhibit the release of diclofenac sodium from the matrix at low pH, may be due to formation of an ionic complex.
- **Magnesium oxide:** It is used as an active ingredient in antacid and sometimes, used to modify pH. For example, in Levothyroxine sodium pentahydrate tablets it is used as pH modifier. But, it interacts with ibuprofen at higher temperature ($\approx 55^{\circ}$C).
- **Silicon dioxide (Silica):** It has various applications in pharmaceutical industry. In tablets it is used as glidant, in suspensions sometimes colloidal silica is used to facilitate dispersion, etc. However, it causes the thermal decomposition of enalapril maleate.
- **Carbonates:** Many drugs are incompatible with carbonate. For example, stability of adefovir dipivoxil in solid state is affected in presence of sodium carbonate. However, insoluble carbonates, such as calcium carbonate and magnesium carbonate, enhance the stability of adefovir dipivoxil.

The incompatibilities of various drugs with excipients are summarized in Table 9.2.

TABLE 9.2

Incompalibilities of various drugs and excipients

Excipient	Drug	Therapeutic category
Saccharides		
Lactose	Acyclovir	Antiviral
	Aceclofenac , Ketoprofen	Anti-inflammatory
	Metformin, Glipizide	Antidiabetic
	Amlodipine, Ceronapril, Lisinopril, Oxprenolol	Antihypertensive
	Fluconazole	Antifungal
	Primaquine	Antimalarial
	Promethazine	Antiemetic
	Fluoxetine and Seproxetine Maleate	Antidepressant
	Picotamide	Anticoagulant
	Etamsylate	Antihemorrhagic
	Aminophylline and Clenbuterol	Bronchodilator
	Baclofen	CNS Drug;
	Ranitidine	GI Agent
	Doxylamine	Antihistaminic
	Thiamine HCL	Vitamin
	Pefloxacin	Antibiotic
Mannitol, Pearlitol (80%	Quinapril	Antihypertensive
Mannitol +20	Primaquine	Antimalarial
% Maize Starch)	Omeprazole	GI Agent
	Promethazine	Antiemetic

Table 9.2 Contd...

Starch	Seproxetine Maleate	Antidepressant
	Clenbuterol	Bronchodilator
Sodium Starch Glycolate	Clenbuterol	Bronchodilator
Dextrose	Pefloxacin	Antibiotic
Stearates	Acyclovir	Antiviral
Magnesium Stearate	Aspirin, Ibuproxam, Indomethacin, Ketoprofen	Anti-inflammatory
	Glipizide, Chlorpropamide, Glimepiride and Glibenclamide	Antidiabetic
	Captopril, Fosinopril, Moexipril, Oxprenolol and Quinapril	Antihypertensive
	Cephalexin, Erythromycin, Nalidixic Acid, Oxacillin, Penicillin G	Antibiotic
	Primaquine	Antimalarial Antiemetic
	Promethazine	Antiamoebic Anticancer
	Albendazole	Anticoagulant
	β-lapachone	Antihistaminic Hypnotic
	Clopidogrel	
	Doxylamine	
	Temazepam	
Stearic Acid	Doxylamine	Antihistaminic
Polyvinyl pyrrolidone (PVP)	Indomethacin, Ketoprofen	Anti-inflammatory
	Atenolol and Oxprenolol	Antihypertensive
	Sulfathiazole	Antibiotic Antipsychotic
	Haloperidol	GI Agent
	Ranitidine	Antihistaminic Hypnotic
	Doxylamine	Bronchodilator
	Temazepam	
	Clenbuterol	
Dicalcium Phosphate Dihydrate (DCPD)	Ceronapril, Oxprenolol and Quinapril	Antihypertensive
	Metronidazole	Antiamoebic
	β-lapachone, Parthenolide	Anticancer
	Famotidine	GI Agent
	Temazepam	Hypnotic
Eudragit Polymers		
Eudragit RS I00	Diflunisal, Flurbiprofen, Piroxicam	Anti-inflammatory
Eudragit RL100	Ibuprofen	Anti-inflammatory
Eudragit E100	Ranitidine	GI Agent
Celluloses		
Microcrystalline Cellulose (MCC), Avicel PH 101	Enalapril	Antihypertensive
	Isosorbide Mononitrate	Antiangina
	Clenbuterol	Bronchodilator
Cellulose Acetate	Isosorbide Mononitrate	Antiangina

Table 9.2 Contd...

Hydroxypropyl Cellulose	Trichlormethiazide	Diuretic
PEG	Ibuprofen, Ketoprofen	Anti-inflammatory
	Phosphomycin	Antibiotic
	Clopidogrel	Anticoagulant
Polysorbate 80	Ibuprofen	Anti-inflammatory
Sodium Lauryl Sulfate	Chlopropamide	Antidiabetic
	Clopidogrel	Anticoagulant Hypnotic
	Chlordiazepoxide	
Chitosan	Diclofenac, Piroxicam	Anti-inflammatory
Magnesium Oxide	Ibuprofen	Anti-inflammatory
Silicon Dioxide	Enalapril	Antihypertensive
Carbonates	Adefovir Dipivoxil	Antiviral
Sodium Carbonate		
Sodium Bicarbonate	Ibuprofen	Anti-inflammatory
Miscellaneous		
Plasdone	Glimepiride	Antidiabetic
Ascorbic acid	Atenolol	Antihypertensive
Citric acid	Atenolol	Antihypertensive
Butylated hydroxyanisole	Atenolol	Antihypertensive
Succinic acid	Phosphomycin	Antibiotic
Na dioctylsulfocuccinate		
Ca and Mg salts	Phosphomycin	Antibiotic
Talc	Tetracycline	Antibiotic
	Seproxetine maleate	Antidepressant

Therapeutic Incompatibility

Usually this type of incompatibility occurs when one or more drugs produces response or intensity different from that intended in the patients. This may happen due to the following reasons:

- Over doses
- Under doses
- Improper consumption by the patient
- Contraindicated drugs

Over doses: This may be divided into two groups.

Excessive single dose: Sometimes a single dose may become overdose depending on the health of the patient. The dose of a drug is based on the body weight of a normal adult person which is considered as 70 kg. The dose may become overdose if the weight of the patient is very less than the normal. However, the number of doses should not be more 2 to 3.

***Example* 1:**

> Rx
>
> | Atropine sulphate | 6 mg |
> | Phenobarbital | 360 mg |

Make capsules.

***Label*:** One capsule to be taken thrice a day.

Comments: The doses of both atropine and phenobarbital are for 12 doses and it was intended for 12 capsules. Hence, the prescription is either mistakenly prepared or incomplete one. The Pharmacist must consult the Physician before dispensing.

The correct prescription would be –

> Rx
>
> | Atropine sulphate | 6 mg |
> | Phenobarbital | 360 mg |

Make 12 capsules.

***Label*:** One capsule to be taken thrice a day.

***Example* 2:**

> Rx
>
> | Strychnine sulphate | 20 mg |
> | Iron and Ammonium citrate | 500 mg |
> | Prepare and supply 12 capsules | |

***Label*:** One capsule to be taken three times a day after meals.

Comment: Dose of strychnine hydrochloride is 10 times of the normal dose. In this case the daily dose of drug is exceeded. The pharmacist should consult the physician and obtain the permission to change the dose.

The corrected prescription would be -

> Rx
>
> | Strychnine sulphate | 2 mg |
> | Iron and ammonium citrate | 500 mg |
> | Prepare and supply 12 capsules. | |

***Label*:** One capsule to be taken thrice a day after meals.

Example 3:

> Rx
>
> | Codeine phosphate | 15 mg |
> | Ammonium chloride | 500 mg |
>
> Prepare capsules and supply 24 capsules.

Label: Two capsules to be taken every hour for cough.

Comment: The U.S.P. recommends that the prescribed dose should be taken after every four hours and not every hour. Hence the physician should be consulted.

Additive and synergistic combinations: There are certain drugs possessing similar pharmacological activity. If these drugs are combined together, they may produce additive or synergistic action. In such case advice of the physician is necessary.

Example 1:

> Rx
>
> | Amphetamine sulphate | | 20 mg |
> | Ephedrine sulphate | | 50 mg |
> | Syrup | q.s. | 100 ml |

A mixture to be made

Label: Take 25 ml every four hourly.

Comment: Both of the drugs are sympathetic and stimulants; they are prescribed in their full dose. The formulation will produce additive overdose effect. Hence, the dose of individual drug should be reduced.

Under dose: In this type of incompatibility, the effect of one drug is lesser than another one or is antagonized by the presence of another drug. This can be exemplified by combination of following types of drugs:

- Stimulants like nuxvomica, strychnine sulphate, caffeine etc. with sedatives like barbiturates, paraldehyde etc.
- Sympathomimetic or adrenergic like ephedrine, nor-adrenaline with sympatholytic drugs like ergotamine.
- Sympathetic stimulants like methamphetamine with parasympathetic stimulants like pilocarpine.
- Purgatives like castor oil, liquid paraffin etc with antidiarrheal agents like bismuth carbonates.
- Acidifiers like dilute hydrochloric acid and alkalisers like sodium bicarbonate, magnesium carbonate.

Example 2:

Rx

Aspirin	300 mg
Probenecid	500 mg

Prepare capsules.

Label: One capsule a day for gout.

Comment: Aspirin is an NSAID given to reduce the pain and swelling in case of gout attack. Probenecid blocks the active re-absorption of uric acid from the lumen of nephron, but salicylates (aspirin) blocks this action of probenecid. Hence, both of the drugs are antagonistic to each other, so its combination is therapeutically useless.

Improper consumption by the patient: In certain prescription some special directions should be written. If the patients are nor advised the drugs may not produce the desired action due to low bio-availability.

Example:

Rx

Tetracycline hydrochloride   250 mg

Prepare capsules. Supply 10 capsules.

Label: Take one capsule every six hourly.

Comments: Calcium present in milk inactivates the tetracycline, hence a patient may not get any therapeutic effect if he/she takes the capsule with milk.

Remedy: The pharmacist should advise the patient to take the capsule with water and not with milk. The patient should not take antacid containing calcium salts.

Contra-indicated drugs

Certain drugs should not be given in particular disease condition. Some examples are given below;

(i)   Corticosteroids are contraindicated in patients with peptic ulcer.

(ii)   Vasoconstrictors are contraindicated in hypertensive patients

(iii)   Some drugs should not be given in asthmatic patients e.g. barbiturates, morphine etc.

(iv)   If a person is allergic to a drug (e.g. penicillin injection) then it should not be given to the patient.

(v)   Certain combination of drugs contraindicates.

Example:

    Rx

Sulphadiazine	0.25 g
Sulphamerazine	0.25 g
Ammonium chloride	0.50 g

Prepare capsules

Label: Take two capsules six hourly for cough.

Comment: In this prescription ammonium chloride is a urinary acidifier and it could cause deposition of sulphonamide crystals in the kidney.

Incompatibility in Prescriptions

Now-a-days, official or proprietary formulations of drug are being prescribed. Hardly the physicians write the names and quantities of ingredients in the prescription and indicate the form in which these are to be mixed and dispensed. However, incompatibilities may occur due to dilution or mixing of these products. This may be due to physicochemical with or without therapeutic interactions.

Physical incompatibility includes:

Usually, physical incompatibility occurs due to immiscibility or insolubility. It can cause invisible, non-uniform products from which removal of an accurate dose is very difficult.

Classification:

- Immiscibility
- Insolubility
- Liquefaction

- *Immiscibility*
  - o Oils are immiscible with water and hence, combination of oily drugs with water produces a product possessing two separate layers.
    Remedy: This problem can be overcome by emulsification or solubilization.
  - o Care must be taken when concentrated hydroalcoholic solutions of volatile oils such as spirits and concentrated waters, are used as adjuncts (e.g. as flavoring agents) in aqueous preparations. Large globules of oils may be separated.

Remedy: To prevent the formation of large globules, the hydroalcoholic solution should either be gradually diluted with the vehicle before admixture with the remaining ingredients or poured into the vehicle with constant stirring.

o Addition of high concentrations of electrolytes to a saturated aqueous solution of a volatile oil causes separation of the oil which deposits as a surface layer.

Example: This happens in Potassium Citrate Mixture B.P.C. in which large quantity of soluble solids salts out the lemon oil.

Remedy: To disperse the droplets evenly, quillaia tincture is to be added as wetting agent.

- *Insolubility*

o Liquid preparations containing indiffusible solids such as chalk, aromatic chalk powder, succinyl sulfathiazole and sulphadimidine (in mixtures); calamine and zinc oxide (in lotions).

Remedy: A thickening agent is necessary to obtain uniform product from which uniform doses can be removed.

o Some insoluble powders such as sulphur and certain corticosteroids (hydrocortisone acetate) and antibiotics are difficult to wet with water.

Remedy: Wetting agents such as saponins for lotions containing sulphur; polysorbates in parenteral suspensions of corticosteroids and antibiotics are used to distribute the powder and to prevent formation of slow dispersing, solid stabilized foam on shaking.

o When a resinous tincture is added to water, the water insoluble resin agglomerates and forms indiffusible clots.

Remedy: This is prevented by adding the undiluted dispersion of protective colloid (Tragacanth mucilage) slowly.

Example: Lobelia & Stramonium tincture which should be mixed with tragacanth mucilage and stirred constantly. This will produce a stable preparation.

o High concentrations of electrolytes cause cracking of soap emulsions (ionic) by salting out the emulsifiers.

- *Liquefaction*

When certain low melting solids are powdered togetherly, a liquid or soft mass is produced due to lowering of the melting point of the mixture to below room temperature. A eutectic mixture is formed.

Any two of the following exhibits this type of behaviour, camphor, menthol, phenol, thymol and chloral hydrate, and sodium salicylate with phenazone.

Example:

    Rx

Thymol	250 mg
Camphor	2 mg
Menthol	2 mg

  Make powder.

Comments: If these ingredients are triturated together, they form a eutectic mixture.

Method **I:**

All the ingredients are triturated. A eutectic mixture (liquid) is formed. Then the liquid is triturated with enough absorbent powder e.g. light kaolin or light magnesium carbonate. This produces a free flowing powder.

Method **II:**

Each ingredient is triturated separately with small amount of adsorbent or diluent and then these powders are lightly mixed (by tumbling action) and packed.

The diluent largely prevents contact between the ingredients and adsorbs any liquid that may be produced.

Example:

    Rx

Chloral hydrate	250 mg

    Prepare capsules. Supply 10 capsules.

Label: Take the capsules at night time.

Comment: Chloral hydrate is hygroscopic in nature. It will absorb moisture and soften the hard gelatin capsule shells and the shape of the capsule may change physically.

Remedy: An equal quantity of light magnesium oxide should be mixed with chloral hydrate. Other adsorbents such as kaolin, talc, starch etc. may be used.

Example:

    Rx

Aminopyrine	0.3 g
Acetyl salicylic acid	0.2 g
Codeine sulphate	0.015 g
Belladonna extracts	0.010 g

  Prepare capsules.

Comment: In this prescription aminopyrine and acetyl salicylic acid form eutectic mixture and wetting of belladonna extract give green colour.

Remedy: Light magnesium oxide (approximately 65 mg) may be added. The half quantity of magnesium oxide is mixed with aminopyrine and the other half is mixed with acetyl salicylic acid separately. The two are then mixed gently and thereafter other ingredients are added and mixed gently.

Chemical Incompatibility includes

The incompatibility due to chemical changes occurred between preparations dispensed together is known as Chemical Incompatibility. The changes may be of several types and may be classified as follows:

1. Chemical change without any visible change; such as

   - The neutralization of acids by bases.

   - The glucosides break down into acids.

   - The action of acids on the activity of pancreatic ferments and of alkali on gastric ferments.

2. Precipitation of newly formed chemical substances as a result of the interaction between two chemical substances in solution.

   - Salts of the alkaline earths react with alkali hydroxides and carbonates, phosphates, borates, oxalates. The corresponding insoluble salts of the alkaline earths formed are precipitated. The corresponding free acids formed are also incompatible.

   - Salts of the metals in solution are incompatible with hydrates, carbonates, phosphates, oxalates and the corresponding acids; in many cases these are incompatible with proteins, tannins, acacia, and sometimes with alkaloids and phenozone. Salts of silver, mercurous, lead, and bismuth are also incompatible with bromides and iodides. Similarly the metals such as calcium, barium and strontium are incompatible with sulphates and sulphuric acid.

   - Hydrates or carbonates of the alkalies such as sodium, potassium, and ammonia are incompatible with salts of metals and alkaline earths, and with alkaloids and with some glucosides.

   - Alkaloids form insoluble salts with other organic acids than acetic and citric acid; the free alkaloid is very much less soluble than the salts, and it is precipitated by alkali hydrates and carbonates and by borax. Ammonium carbonate and bicarbonates do not cause precipitation so readily. Iodides, bromides, salicylates, benzoates, usually cause a precipitation of tannic acid, and iodine in a solution of mercuric iodide; precipitation may be prevented in many of these cases using

15-50% alcohol. Alkaloids may cause precipitation with many metallic salts especially of mercury.

- Proteins are precipitated by alkaloids, many metal salts, tannin and alcohol.

3. Change of colour due to the formation of some soluble but undesired substance.

   - An objectionable appearance of preparations containing tannic acid, gallic acids and iron salts; ammonia and carbolic acid; gallic acid and thymol; ferric chloride and salicylates, carbolic acid, creosote, guaiacol, salol, acetanilide, phenazone, phenacetin, oils of wintergreen, cloves, pimenta, and thyme, podophyllin, aloin, gamboges, asafoetida, storax, myrrh, balsam of Peru, balsam of Tolu, morphine and apomorphine.

   - The change in colour is the indication of a chemical change. Such changes occur in mixture of salicylates, phenozone, and acetanilide with the free nitrous acid in Spirits of Nitrous Ether (isonitroso-compounds are formed).

4. Chemical splitting of one of the substances and the formation of an undesired substance. This may result the following;

   - Release of a volatile component, in part or entirely, depending upon the amount formed in the solution. For example, hydrochloric acid react with nitric acid and releases nitrous oxides; strong acids when reacts with alcohol releases ethers; chloral and butyl chloral react with alkalies and chloroform is released.

   - Dextrose or other sugar is formed when glucosides react with acids and alkalies.

   - Sudden liberation of gas which may be sufficient to cause an explosion. For example, reaction between chromic acid, concentrated nitric acid, nitrates, permanganates, chlorates, with substances like sulphur and sulphides, sulphites, iodides, phosphorus, hypophosphite, reduced iron, and many organic substances such as sugar, tannin, etc. These reactions occur only when the dry substances are triturated together or in some cases when mixed in very concentrated solutions.

5. In some cases when two solids are triturated together a soft sticky or a damp mass, or a liquid is formed; probably the chemical reaction takes place. Such substances are camphor, carbolic acid, thymol, phenozone, phenacetin, chloral, sodium phosphate, lead acetate.

Exercises

   1. Define the term incompatibility.
   2. What are different types of incompatibility?
   3. What is physical incompatibility?
   4. What is chemical incompatibility?

5. What is therapeutic incompatibility?

6. What is antagonism?

7. What are the factors that accelerate degradation of drug?

8. What is over dose?

9. What is under dose?

10. What is additive combination?

11. Classify incompatibilities and explain with relevant example.

12. Explain with example drug-drug incompatibility.

13. Explain with suitable example drug-excipient incompatibility.

14. Explain with suitable example how heat and moisture can accelerate degradation of a drug.

15. Briefly exemplify 'food-drug interaction'.

16. Discuss in brief the physical incompatibility with relevant examples.

17. Discuss in brief the chemical incompatibility with relevant examples.

18. Explain the reasons for therapeutic incompatibility.

19. Explain how incompatibility can take place in prescription.

20. Explain with relevant examples the incompatibility between two excipients.

Index

C

W

Y

Z